Sustainable Development Goals Series

The **Sustainable Development Goals Series** is Springer Nature's inaugural cross-imprint book series that addresses and supports the United Nations' seventeen Sustainable Development Goals. The series fosters comprehensive research focused on these global targets and endeavours to address some of society's greatest grand challenges. The SDGs are inherently multidisciplinary, and they bring people working across different fields together and working towards a common goal. In this spirit, the Sustainable Development Goals series is the first at Springer Nature to publish books under both the Springer and Palgrave Macmillan imprints, bringing the strengths of our imprints together.

The Sustainable Development Goals Series is organized into eighteen subseries: one subseries based around each of the seventeen respective Sustainable Development Goals, and an eighteenth subseries, "Connecting the Goals", which serves as a home for volumes addressing multiple goals or studying the SDGs as a whole. Each subseries is guided by an expert Subseries Advisor with years or decades of experience studying and addressing core components of their respective Goal.

The SDG Series has a remit as broad as the SDGs themselves, and contributions are welcome from scientists, academics, policymakers, and researchers working in fields related to any of the seventeen goals. If you are interested in contributing a monograph or curated volume to the series, please contact the Publishers: Zachary Romano [Springer; zachary.romano@springer.com] and Rachael Ballard [Palgrave Macmillan; rachael.ballard@palgrave.com].

Dom Conroy • Fiona Measham
Editors

# Young Adult Drinking Styles

## Current Perspectives on Research, Policy and Practice

Second Edition 2025

palgrave
macmillan

*Editors*
Dom Conroy
Faculty of Arts and Social Science
The Open University
London, UK

Fiona Measham
Department of Sociology
Social Policy and Criminology
University of Liverpool
Liverpool, UK

ISSN 2523-3084 ISSN 2523-3092 (electronic)
Sustainable Development Goals Series
ISBN 978-3-031-98527-0 ISBN 978-3-031-98528-7 (eBook)
https://doi.org/10.1007/978-3-031-98528-7



This Palgrave Macmillan imprint is published by the registered company Springer Nature Switzerland AG.
The registered company address is: Gewerbestrasse 11, 6330 Cham, Switzerland

If disposing of this product, please recycle the paper.

# Preface

The phrase 'young adult drinking' conjures up evocative images, at least until recently, of excess, anti-social behaviour and harm. More recently the images of young adults on our screens have been of a more restrained, and indeed often strained, ilk, associated with a prioritisation of health and wellness in image and deed, plant-based diets (evident in the growing popularity of vegan products marketed at young adults) and concerns about their own future and the future of the planet, with movements like Extinction Rebellion reflecting a shift from a culture of consumption to a culture of restraint and sustainability.

At the close of the second decade of the twenty-first century, research and scholarly discussion concerning young adult alcohol use increasingly recognises the myriad ways in which alcohol can be understood and researched. Evidence now consistently points to broad demographic shifts in drinking behaviour among young adults. This is reflected in changes in expectations and stereotypes around drinking styles and behaviours among women and men and in the significant increase in the number of non-drinkers found among young adults in many developed countries. The rapid rise of social media use and mobile/smartphone technology also hold significant implications for future trends in alcohol, not just for drinkers but also for health promotion, and for alcohol industry manufacturing, marketing and retail practices.

Views on drinking behaviour and approaches to alcohol among young adults continue to evolve. Accordingly, new research agendas and some evidence of movement away from a purely 'pathological' model for thinking about drinking behaviour among young adults have occurred. This new research climate is partly reflected in the great increase in qualitative and mixed methods research and a growth in multi-disciplinary collaborations involving anthropologists, epidemiologists, psychologists, criminologists and sociologists, to name but a few. This diversification of topic focus and method application in the field of alcohol research is critically important from both clinical and policy perspectives. Progressive, successful modes of promoting more moderate drinking over the life course among young adults seem likely to benefit from the 'real world' emphasis of some contemporary alcohol research.

Why should the drinking practices among individuals whom we are terming 'young adults' (those aged approximately 18–30 years) warrant particular attention? Some authors consider that there are typical characteristics and decisions involved in this life stage—for example, relating to living arrangements; acquiring secure/meaningful employment; initiation and experimentation with illicit drugs and altered states of intoxication; engaging with choices and meanings associated with identity and sexuality—that qualitatively distinguish young adulthood from earlier or later life stages. While early phases of experimentation may be behind them, many young adults are leaving the protective influences of family and local community for university, work and cohabiting with friends and partners, and beginning to lay down particular understandings about alcohol's role in their life, which may form the basis for how alcohol is used (or not) for the remainder of that individual's life. Therefore, from their late teens onwards, young adults are presented (in most cases) with a relatively unfamiliar but considerable range of settings and occasions which demand decisions and action relating to alcohol use (and non-use).

How might 'drinking styles' provide a useful shift of focus? The lexicon for describing and understanding drinking behaviours and practices, and for identifying particular 'types' of drinkers is vast but is also culturally and historically situated. For example, we can think of drinking behaviour in terms of 'social drinking', 'moderate drinking', 'problem drinking', 'anti-social drinking', 'binge drinking', 'light drinking' and the list continues. Given the constructive power of the terminology surrounding alcohol consumption in the context of young adult drinking practices, questions are raised about possible alternatives that manage to navigate a route through these hard definitions to produce a more coherent appreciation of young adult drinking practices, cultural and policy change surrounding alcohol consumption, and new trends in research. The term 'drinking styles', which has appeared previously on occasions in the alcohol literature, helps guide the development of theory that accounts for fluidity and inconsistency in drinking practices over time. In terms of 'real world' advantages, the term 'drinking styles' provides a term that recognises that drinking behaviour is chosen and re-chosen between and within events involving the potential for alcohol consumption. Put another way, to discuss an individual's (or group's) drinking styles provides a way of acknowledging the multiple factors (and therefore multiple sites) for pursuing a health promotion agenda to promote safe, sustainable drinking practices among young adults.

Whilst there is persistent coverage of alcohol-related issues in the media, academic, policy and broader cultural settings, what is much less clearly available is a space dedicated to a consideration of the trends, nuances and contexts for young adult drinking linked with life stage transitions and identity/identities in the post-Internet world. In exploring the complexities of drinking behaviour among young adults the contributors to this collection avoid traditional understandings of young adult drinking that pathologise and generalise. We advocate instead for an inclusive approach evident in the wide range of disciplinary backgrounds, cultural perspectives and international settings represented in this book, in order to better understand the economic, cultural and pharmacological crossroads at which we now stand.

Never before has there been such a wide range of methods and approaches to considering drinking behaviour and practices among young adults. Our collection reflects this diversity with a range of methodological traditions which help expose nuance and difference in young adult drinking behaviour. Much of this is comprised of interview-based data, but this book also contains research based on focus groups, on studies of policy documents and on analyses of large-scale survey data. We think this variety has helped to produce a more engaging and stimulating text but has also offered a collection that acknowledges the range of methodological lenses that can be applied to alcohol research focused on young adults and, as such, offers a more representative reflection of current field research.

We have structured the book into five short but distinct sections. Part I is organised around the theme of 'Changing Trends in Young Adult Drinking' reflecting both growing interest in what appears to be a decline in alcohol consumption among young people in recent years but also how drinking practices in young adulthood may transition to different drinking practices later in life. Part II is titled 'Diversity in Young Adult Drinking' and presents a series of examples of the diversity of young adult drinking behaviour with focus in the new edition on under-represented groups.

Part III turns attention to non-drinkers and non-drinking in newly titled section, 'Young Adults Who Drink Little or No Alcohol' which is designed to highlight and explore contemporary aspects of drinking practices among young adults (or, indeed, anyone) including focus on, illustratively, participation in abstinence challenges, and experiences of sober dating among young adults.

Part IV presents chapters under the section heading 'Young Adult Drinking Spaces: Staying Inside; Going Outside; Digital Spaces' and suggests how young adult drinking styles might be usefully framed in a contextualised sense involving specific places, time periods, online spaces or particular groups of people. Part V titled 'Young Adult Drinking Styles Since COVID-19: Policy and Practice' shifts attention to consider topic areas with perhaps particular relevance to alcohol policy, with two final book chapters which explore, respectively, violence associated with alcohol consumption and connections between alcohol consumption and mental health and policy implications relevant to young adults.

London, UK — Dom Conroy
Liverpool, UK — Fiona Measham

# Acknowledgments

Thank you to all our contributors and collaborators for their willingness to engage with this project initially and for revising chapters for the second edition of this book. Without the generosity of spirit of our academic colleagues in the alcohol field in engaging with the process of feedback and discussion involved in developing chapter content, this collection would not have been possible.

We would also like to thank Palgrave Macmillan for their consistent support and patience throughout the production of this book.

We have made every effort to trace all copyright holders in the production of this book. If, however, any have been overlooked, the publishers will be willing to make the required arrangements to address this at the earliest opportunity.

**Competing Interests Statement** The editors do not have any competing financial and/or non-financial interests in relation to the content of the book to declare. Similarly, no competing financial and/or non-financial interests in relation to the content of the book are declared by the editors on behalf of the contributors.

**Ethics Approval** Where original research is described in book content this research was ethically approved and required individuals to sign informed consent before participating in research.

# Contents

## Part II Diversity in Young Adult Drinking



## Part III Young Adults Who Drink Little or No Alcohol

# Notes on Contributors

**Marie Fjellerup Bærndt** is a postdoctoral researcher at VIVE, the Danish Center for Social Science Research, Denmark and did her PhD studies on young Muslim women and the Danish (youth) alcohol culture. She has focused on young Muslim women's subjective experiences with an interest in how youth drinking can advance as well as complicate issues of community, belonging and inclusion. Currently she is doing research on STX (upper secondary school) students' different ways to find and develop communities of cohesion within their school, with a particular interest in relations that cut across differences such as ethnicity and gender. Her theoretical interests are broad and cover, for example, intersectionality, belonging, sociologyof emotions, phenomenology and storytelling.

**Emma Banister** is a Professor of Consumption and Society at the University of Manchester. Her research expertise is in Transformative Consumer Research, informing policy outcomes and addressing inequalities and vulnerabilities in the marketplace and the workplace. Her research mainly focuses on issues connected with identity, consumer culture, and policy in relation to alcohol, parenting, and parental leave. She is co-chair of the Academy of Marketing's 'Consumer Research with Social Impact' Special Interest Group. Her work has been published in a range of sociology and business journals.

**Ashlea Bartram** is a senior research fellow at the National Centre for Education and Training on Addiction at Flinders University, Australia. She is a mixed-methods researcher with over seven years of experience in research and evaluation related to alcohol, tobacco, and other drugs, with work that spans the spectrum from prevention and policy to treatment and workforce development. She has a particular interest in the ways people do 'non-drinking' and the implications of these for health promotion.

**Alexandra Bogren** is Associate Professor of Sociology at Södertörn University, Sweden. She is currently doing research on young people's experiences of sexual encounters and sexual violence in drinking settings. She is also the Principal Investigator (PI) on a Swedish Research Council funded project on the uses of body-worn cameras within the Swedish Police. Her previous work has examined how the mass media (re)produce, communicate, and challenge gendered discourses of alcohol and drug use.

**Gabriel Caluzzi** is a postdoctoral research fellow at the Centre for Alcohol Policy Research, La Trobe University. His work aims to understand how drug and alcohol practices among young people are informed by sociocultural context. He is particularly interested in the cultural meanings young people associate with alcohol, and how recent declines in young people's drinking might be understood within the context of broader generational changes.

**Dom Conroy** is an associate lecturer at The Open University. Dom has expertise in qualitative and mixed methods research and has conducted health-related research focusing on alcohol consumption among young people, non-drinking, sobriety and temporary abstinence challenges. Over the last 15 years, Dom has produced over 30 peer-reviewed articles in addition to the first volume of Young Adult Drinking Styles which, in 2021, won a British Medical Association category award.

**Claire Davey** is a researcher of contemporary sobriety culture, particularly women's use of online sobriety communities. Claire holds a PhD from Canterbury Christ Church University obtained in 2024 and was a recipient of their University Research Scholarship. Her research has been published in numerous peer-reviewed journals, including *Frontiers in Global Women's Health*, *Drug and Alcohol Review* and *Journal of International Women's Studies*. In 2023, Claire won the Feminist Studies Association's Student Essay Prize. She is currently writing a book titled *Sober Sisterhood: Women's Recovery Culture within Online Sobriety Communities*, based on her PhD research.

**Vibeke Asmussen Frank** is Head of Research Center for Social Marginalisation, VIA University College, Denmark and has done social science alcohol and drug research for over 20 years. A main interest has been substance users' own perspectives and experiences, and how these are embedded within cultural, societal, and political contexts. She has focused on young peoples' alcohol intoxication and use of nitrous oxide, substance use by prison inmates, and marginalized citizens in drug use treatment. Frank has engaged with theories related to the subjective experiences of substance use, including theories of intoxication, addiction, recovery, intersectionality, gender, welfare institutional sociology and policy-in-practice.

**Millie Gooch** is the founder of the Sober Girl Society and is one of the voices leading the sobriety movement in the UK. As a journalist, she has written for a range of publications and has been featured everywhere from Elle and Stylist to the BBC and British Vogue. Her debut book, *The Sober Girl Society Handbook*, was released in 2021, and in 2022 she received the Media Award from the Research Society on Alcoholism for her contributions in helping disseminate empirical research on alcohol and creating a safe space for people to explore alcohol-free living. Millie is a proud ambassador for Alcohol Change UK and has just completed her master's degree in Addiction and Mental Health. Her second book *Booze Less* was released in November 2024.

**Ian Goodwin** is Associate Professor of Communication at Waipapa Taumata Rau/University of Auckland. With a background in cultural studies Ian's research has been wide-ranging and inter-disciplinary yet centres on understanding the societal changes associated with the rise of digital media technologies. In the last few years, he has focused particularly on social media. He is currently interested in exploring intersections between algorithmic culture, health and well-being, alcohol consumption, unhealthy product marketing, consumer activism, citizenship, and media policy.

**Laura Goodwin** is a senior lecturer in Mental Health and theme lead for Public Mental Health at Lancaster University. She conducts research on the comorbidity of mental health and alcohol problems, with specific expertise in understanding the complexity of these issues in trauma exposed population, such as in military veterans. She has been funded by the MRC, ESRC, NIHR and third sector organisations and is currently leading NIHR funded work on how we can improve treatment pathways for people with co-occurring problems. Her work has informed policy and practice, for example in the recent "UK clinical guidelines for alcohol treatment".

**Geoffrey Hunt** a social anthropologist, is Professor at the Centre for Alcohol and Drugs Research at Aarhus University, Denmark and Director at the Institute for Scientific Analysis, in San Francisco. Hunt is the Principal Investigator (PI) on a US NIH funded project on Intoxication and Sexual Encounters and also PI on a Danish Research Council funded project establishing a Network of gender researchers among the five Nordic countries. His book publications include: *Youth Drugs and Nightlife* (Routledge, 2010), *Drugs and Culture* (Ashgate, 2011), *Sage Handbook of Drug and Alcohol Studies* (2017) and *The Routledge Handbook of Intoxicants and Intoxication* (2022).

**Patricia Irizar** is a research fellow in the Department of Sociology at the University of Manchester. Her research focuses on understanding co-occurring alcohol and mental health problems, particularly in trauma-exposed occupations, using both quantitative and qualitative methods. Irizar's wider research involves examining the levels and drivers of ethnic inequalities in physical and mental health, including ethnic inequalities in adolescent well-being. As an interdisciplinary researcher, Irizar collaborates with academics across a range of disciplines, as well as third sector organisations and people with lived experience, to address health inequalities.

**Susan Kiene** is Professor of Global Health at San Diego State University School of Public Health and Honorary Professor at Makerere University School of Public Health. Kiene is a social and behavioral epidemiologist who studies the multilevel (e.g., social environment, behavioral, structural) factors that affect health and inequities in access to health services among underserved and historically marginalized populations. Kiene's research is primarily in infectious diseases, sexual and reproductive health, alcohol and substance use, and implementation science, with a focus on developing, testing, and preparing for multilevel interventions to improve health and health equity.

**Emmanuel Kyasanku** is the Program Director and a researcher at the Africa Medical and Behavioral Sciences Organization (AMBSO) and a PhD candidate at Karolinska Institutet. Emmanuel has an extensive training in Public Health, clinical medicine and community health, and leads AMBSO's initiatives in research and community-based service delivery. He is a key investigator on the AMBSO Population Health Surveillance program (APHS) that nests alcohol and substance use studies and he is also expanding AMBSO's research scope into clinical trials. His role at AMBSO and his academic pursuits at Karolinska Institutet underscore his dedication to advancing public health both locally and internationally.

**Carly Lightowlers** is a Reader in Criminology at the University of Liverpool with experience as an academic as well as conducting research in local and central government settings. Her research primarily makes use of secondary data sources and quantitative methods with which to study alcohol-related violence, the processing of such cases through the courts, as well as the unequal distribution of associated harm.

**Michael Livingston** is an associate professor at the National Drug Research Institute in Australia. He worked at the Centre for Alcohol Policy Research and the National Drug and Alcohol Research Centre and has a long history of research on alcohol policy and epidemiology. His work focuses on the impact of alcohol policy changes and general trends in alcohol consumption and harm, with a particular emphasis on youth drinking patterns.

**Antonia Lyons** is Director of the Centre for Addiction Research at the University of Auckland, Aotearoa New Zealand. She brings a critical health psychology perspective to her work in multidisciplinary teams. Her research has focused on the social and embodied contexts of behaviours related to well-being and developing pathways towards improving outcomes. Her work has explored digital media, identity, drinking practices and cultures and alcohol consumption at different life stages.

**Sarah MacLean** is a professor in Social Work and Social Policy and is affiliated with the Centre for Alcohol Policy Research at La Trobe University. She has published extensively on alcohol and inhalant use and, in recent years, also on gambling. During 2019–2022 she was joint Editor-in-Chief of *Health Sociology Review*. Sarah works collaboratively to identify responses that can be implemented by alcohol and drug services, local communities and governments.

**Marjana Martinic** is an independent consultant with an interest in cross-cultural dimensions of drinking patterns, lifestyle, and health. She has an extensive background in alcohol policy and its supporting evidence base. Marjana led the Science and Policy workstream at the International Alliance for Responsible Drinking (IARD) and its predecessor, the International Center for Alcohol Policies (ICAP). Her past work and publications have explored youth drinking, risk, the evolution of drinking patterns, and opportunities for engagement among public and private sector entities in helping to reduce alcohol-related harm.

**Fiona Measham** has been Chair in Criminology at the University of Liverpool since 2019. She has spent over three decades researching trends in drug use, their relationship with drug policy and the wider socio-cultural contexts to use. Fiona has authored and co-authored over 100 publications, most recently exploring aspects of drug cultures, harm reduction and the interface of drugs and sexuality, as well as engagement in nightlife, underpinned by critical understandings of power, pleasure and deviance in society. Fiona is founder and trustee of The Loop (2012–) and The Loop Australia (2018–), award-winning charities best known for introducing drug checking in the UK and three Australian states.

**Amanda Miller** is a Research Assistant Professor at San Diego State University. She earned her PhD in Public Health through a joint doctoral program between San Diego State University and the University of California, San Diego. Miller also holds a Master of Science in Global Health Sciences from the University of California, San Francisco, and a Bachelor of Arts in Anthropology from the University of California, Santa Barbara. With over a decade of experience in alcohol research, her work focuses on understanding and addressing substance use and its impact on public health.

**Stephen Mugamba** is a Ugandan researcher and public health expert with experience in epidemiology, clinical trials, and public health program management. He is currently the Deputy Program Director at Africa Medical and Behavioral Sciences Organization (AMBSO) in Uganda. Mugamba's background training is in Health Communication and Public health and for the last 20 years, he has made significant contributions to the field of HIV prevention science. His research work focuses on improving HIV prevention outcomes, particularly in resource-limited settings and has been published in several peer-reviewed journals.

**Emily Nicholls** is a Senior Lecturer in Sociology at the University of York, UK. Her work focuses on contemporary lived experiences of drinking and non-drinking, including the role of alcohol in 'doing' femininity on a 'girls' night out', drinking during the COVID-19 pandemic, women's experiences of early sobriety and the consumption and marketing of No- and Low-Alcohol drinks.

**Amy Pennay** is a Senior Research Fellow and the Deputy Director of the Centre for Alcohol Policy Research at La Trobe University. Amy's research investigates how social and cultural factors influence drinking practices and health outcomes. Her recent work has focused on youth drinking practices, (sub)cultures of drinking, and intersections of drinking and policy with social determinants such as gender, class, race, place and sexuality.

**Margit Anne Petersen** is an associate professor at the Centre for Alcohol and Drug Research, Aarhus University, Denmark. She has a background in social and medical anthropology. Her work primarily focuses on young people's uses and perceptions of legal and illegal substances (alcohol, illicit drugs and pharmaceuticals) and how these in different contexts contribute to developing or changing a gendered self. She is Principal Investigator of several large research projects that cover different aspects of intoxicated youth.

**Maria Piacentini** is Professor of Consumer Research at Lancaster University Management School and Director of the Centre for Consumption Insights. Her research focuses on consumer vulnerability, and she has explored this theme in a number of contexts of public policy concern. Her work has been published in *Sociology*, *Sociology of Health & Illness*, *European Journal of Marketing*, *Journal of Business Research*, *Journal of Marketing Management and Marketing Theory*. Maria was co-editor of 'Consumer Vulnerability: Conditions, contexts and characteristics', published as part of the Routledge Studies in Critical Marketing series. Maria was a co-chair of the ESRC seminar series on Vulnerable Consumers (2012–2014). Along with Emma Banister and Kathy Hamilton, she is co-chair of the Academy of Marketing's 'Consumer Research with Social Impact' Special Interest Group.

**Jo-Anne Puddephatt** is a senior lecturer at Edge Hill University with a background in better understanding co-occurring alcohol and mental health problems. Jo-Anne's research is interested in the mechanisms between alcohol and mental health problems and identifying groups at risk of experiencing these problems through a range of epidemiological and qualitative methodologies. Her research also focuses on how people with co-occurring problems can be identified earlier and better supported in their treatment journey. Jo-Anne is a member of the Health Research Institute at Edge Hill University and has supported the delivery of NIHR and charity funded projects.

**Tim Turner** is Senior Lecturer in Criminology at Coventry University. He worked as a forensic mental health nurse, and is the joint editor of Critical Issues in Mental Health (Palgrave). As a Registered Intermediary, Tim has worked extensively with vulnerable witnesses in the criminal justice system. His doctorate research, an ethnography of British youth in Ibiza, was conducted over three summers and examined the situated social meaning of poly-drug use in the context of tourism. His research interests are focused on the relationship between drug use, pleasure and space.

**Rakhi Vashishtha** is a seasoned implementation scientist and mixed-method researcher specializing in quantitative methodologies, including clinical and economic evaluations. Her research focuses on innovative digital interventions for alcohol misuse management, leveraging technology to tackle public health challenges. With expertise in designing and analyzing complex interventions, she aims to improve health outcomes by embedding research findings into real-world healthcare settings. Passionate about health equity, she is committed to ensuring that digital health solutions, such as mHealth and AI-driven tools, are accessible to diverse populations, bridging the gap between research and practice.

**Emma Vieira** is an early career researcher and PhD Student with the National Drug Research Institute at Curtin University. Emma has a background in psychology, graduating from the University of Western Australia. Her PhD uses a mixed-methods approach to explore how gender impacts alcohol consumption and related harms for young adults in Australia.

# List of Tables

# 1

# Book Introduction: Young Adult Drinking Styles

Dom Conroy and Fiona Measham

**Abstract** Alcohol consumption among young adults conjures up images of unrestrained, excessive consumption. However, alcohol use among young adults is increasingly understood using different lenses and with different emphases. This chapter introduces book aims and outlines contributions that reflect this range of lenses and emphases. Contributions cover alcohol's role in initiating and maintaining friendship groups; changes in alcohol use over time among young adults; links between identity and alcohol use including online identities; and how alcohol policy has responded to (and may be shaped by) young adults' alcohol consumption. The chapter emphases the inter-disciplinary, international

D. Conroy (✉)
Faculty of Arts and Social Science, The Open University, London, UK
e-mail: d.conroy@open.ac.uk

F. Measham
Department of Sociology, Social Policy and Criminology, University of Liverpool, Liverpool, UK
e-mail: f.measham@liverpool.ac.uk



D. Conroy, F. Measham (eds.), *Young Adult Drinking Styles*, Sustainable Development Goals Series, https://doi.org/10.1007/978-3-031-98528-7_1

focus of the book and also the importance of a focus on young adults, as a group of individuals at a distinctive life stage.

The phrase 'young adult drinking' has, historically at least, conjured up evocative images of excess, anti-social behaviour and harm. These images linking alcohol consumption by young adults with personal and social harms remain readily available in mass media depictions of archetypal leisure time activities involving drinking and drunkenness. The dangers posed to young adults by alcohol as a substance that too readily leads to over-indulgence, dependence and an array of other risks such as personal injury and potentially higher risk sexual encounters are often closely woven into the assumptions of empirical research in the social sciences. More recently the images of young adults on our screens have been of a more restrained, and indeed often strained, ilk, associated with a prioritisation of health and wellness in image and deed, plant-based diets (evident in the growing popularity of vegan products marketed at young adults), and concerns about their own future and the future of the planet, with movements like Extinction Rebellion reflecting an apparent shift from a culture of consumption to a culture of restraint and sustainability.

At the close of the first quarter of the twenty-first century, research and scholarly discussion concerning young adult alcohol use increasingly recognises the myriad ways in which alcohol can be understood and researched. This more nuanced attitude towards alcohol research acknowledges alcohol's varied role within social rituals (such as pre-loading and drinking games) and permits scope for increased recognition of alcohol's valued role in initiating and maintaining friendships among young adults.

Since the first edition of this collection was published six years ago, the evidence base has increasingly consolidated around broad shifts in young adult drinking behaviours previously, and more tentatively, explored here. This is reflected in changes in expectations and stereotypes around the gendering of drinking-related attitudes and behaviours and in the significant increase in the number of non-drinkers found among young adults, as well as the growth in the popularity of 'sobriety' or 'mindful drinking' communities in many developed countries. The central role of mobile/smartphone technologies and associated social media engagement also hold significant implications for future trends in alcohol, not just for drinkers but also for wider health promotion, and for alcohol industry manufacturing, marketing and retail decisions.

Traditionally, the peer-reviewed empirical research on young adult alcohol consumption has primarily focused on drinking in higher income countries and the global north, despite a growing body of work providing insights into young adult drinking in middle- or lower income countries (e.g. Huckle et al., 2020; Xu et al., 2022). There is increasing recognition of the tendency in social science research to extrapolate findings from research conducted in higher income countries and of the limits of these 'universalist' theories designed to explain drinking in particular demographics (including young adults). Relatedly, there have been important drives to address these tendencies towards 'grand theories' of drinking behaviour in work exploring the role of context, of how social identifiers like class, gender and sexuality interact with alcohol-related decisions and actions, and of varied drinking styles.

Views on drinking behaviour and approaches to alcohol among young adults continue to evolve. Accordingly, social scientists have recognised the importance of efforts to shift the emphasis of research agendas towards less traditional models of young adult drinking. One notable characteristic of this shift is a conscious movement away from a purely 'pathological' model for thinking about drinking behaviour in which 'problem cognitions' (e.g. alcohol beliefs) or 'problem dispositions' (e.g. personality) are identified as key 'drivers' of higher risk drinking among young adults. This new research climate is partly reflected in the great increase in qualitative and mixed methods research used to explore alcohol-related attitudes, behaviours, experiences and practices. In addition, exploring alcohol use among young adults has been recognized as an ongoing multi-disciplinary project with continued important contributions from anthropologists, epidemiologists, psychologists, criminologists and sociologists, to name but a few. This diversification of topic focus and method application in the field of alcohol research is critically important from both clinical and policy perspectives. For example, health promotion approaches for successfully raising awareness about alcohol harms or modes of promoting more moderate drinking over the life course among young adults seem likely to benefit from the 'real world' emphasis of some contemporary alcohol research.

This empirical work and theoretical debate that we allude to above has helped generate greater awareness of young adult drinking as something nuanced, complex, both pleasurable and problematic, and, critically, tightly bound within broader social contexts, relationships and the life course. Our aim for the first edition of this book was to present a sample of the breadth of this research and to explore where the emphases of progressive alcohol research concerning young adults may usefully go from here. For the second edition of this collection, we have been fortunate to secure an even wider range of contributions from authors whose work can help us to deepen and enrich understanding of the diverse and sometimes contradictory nature of young adult drinking styles.

## Who Are 'Young Adults'?

There is great variety in terms of how young adults are defined, both in the academic literature and in wider public discourse. We choose the term 'young adults' to refer to individuals aged approximately 18–30 years. We prefer this term to 'adolescents' which would span younger demographic groups, and 'youths' and 'young people', which are less clearly defined terms, usually include early and mid-teenage groups and may be associated with different connotations and theoretical emphases. This is a group who, for most countries (with the notable exception of the USA), is legally allowed to purchase alcohol and therefore operate in a distinctly different legal context to those who are in their early and mid-teens. In approaching this book we are mindful, however, that different terms will have particular currency for our readership in different international settings and within different disciplines.

We turn now to the term 'young adults' and consider how this was reached and how this works in relation to terminology used to describe the focal group of interest for our contributors. Accounting for consumption in the life stage(s) which follows adolescence but precedes the years of established adulthood has attracted theoretical interest. Most prominent here is Arnett's (2000) theory of 'emerging adulthood' designed to articulate an understanding of the experiences of young adults aged roughly 18–25 years, which was conceptualised in part in appreciation of the changes in the life stages of younger adults which have taken place in industrialised societies in recent decades, which replace the more traditional theories of life stage transition (e.g. Erikson, 1950). The advantages of this theoretical approach is that it draws attention to important and distinctive features which may be experienced during this period of the lifespan characterised by identity exploration, formation and uncertainty. However, we take the position that any rigid categorisation of lifespan stages risks impinging on our understanding of the heterogenous, diffuse and changing nature of the experience of young adulthood which is inevitably situated in terms of their distinct history, culture and socio-economic context.

When we wrote the first edition of this book, 'young adults' were crudely identified in media, social media and marketing terms as 'Millennials/Generation Y' (i.e. born between 1981 and 1996) and to a lesser extent, 'Zoomers/Generation Z' (i.e. born between 1997 and 2012). Another six years on and these categories have changed, with a greater proportion of current young adults identifiable as Zoomers/Generation Z. While we do not seek to frame discussion of young adults within social generations derived from culturally restricted (Western) and theoretically driven starting points in this edition, we draw attention to this in our introductory chapter simply to illustrate the rapid change and state of flux that the category 'young adulthood' has experienced, even within the relatively brief period between the two editions of this book.

Research involving young adults, as the preparation for this book has borne out time and again, is frequently conflated with research involving significantly younger individuals in a life stage more like middle adolescence (e.g. 15–17-year-olds) or even early adolescence (e.g. 11–14-year-olds). In focusing on 'young adults' we have a particular editorial view and definition which we believe helps narrow focus to a group of individuals who warrant particular attention and dedicated focus in the alcohol literature. The term 'young adults' targets individuals aged over eighteen and therefore adults for at least some purposes, in a legal sense, in the UK and many other jurisdictions.

Imposing an upper limit is more problematic of course, and this is acknowledged in longstanding theoretical discussion on emerging and established adulthood (Green, 2016; Levinson, 1986). In this edited collection our starting point was a desire to focus on 'young adults' aged approximately 18–30 years. Given that different terms mean different things to different people anyway (who may, quite reasonably, have little interest or investment in particular terms to describe the age range of the sample on whom their own research focuses), but also to promote the principle of academic freedom, we have adopted an inclusive approach and you will see variations in terminology and age ranges in this book including, predominantly, the terms 'young people' and 'young adults'.

## What Is 'Drinking'?

As with the other elements of our title, pinning down what is meant by drinking presents not dissimilar challenges. The alcohol literature is, once again, surrounded by different meanings and associations attached to the wide-ranging (and ever-increasing) vernacular for defining the focal activities of interest and relevance to this book and to this field. To illustrate, we could refer to these activities using the following expressions: 'drinking', 'drinking behaviour', 'drinking practices', 'alcohol intake', 'alcohol consumption'. A parallel and growing range of terms exist to define and encapsulate the behaviour (and individuals) who do not drink alcohol (sometimes a health decision, a lifestyle choice, situated within a particular community or a particular time/place): 'non-drinking', 'abstinence', 'alcohol abstinence', 'sobriety', 'sober curiosity', 'mindful drinking', 'temporary sobriety' or 'social non-drinking'. Further terms refer to types of drinking practices, with emphasis on the characteristics and often the intensity of these practices, with illustrations including: 'harmful drinking', 'excessive drinking', 'binge drinking' and 'high intensity drinking'. This final list of words presents particular difficulties, partly because there is often no agreed clear and operational definition of these terms and partly because definitions and meanings themselves can be seen to carry moral values and judgements, especially when used in particular contexts or in relation to particular groups in society (e.g. 'binge drinking' in the context of young adults who are also women).

Each descriptive term brings its own point of emphasis, its advantages and caveats. The expression 'drinking behaviour' would be broadly acceptable from a post-positivist psychology research perspective, where an understanding of alcohol use would typically prioritise activity located at the level of the individual, which can be understood in discrete and objectively definable 'behavioural' terms. Other social science research perspectives would more likely problematise this starting point, noting that 'drinking behaviour' artificially disaggregates an understanding of alcohol use (including, e.g., an understanding of motivations to initiate and to drink in large quantities) from the social and environmental context to which it is intimately tied. By contrast, there are advantages to referring to 'drinking practices' over more individually orientated terms such as 'drinking behaviour', because it blurs the individual and the social and does not imply clearly defined time frames for alcohol consumption, and therefore it is favoured in this book. No arrangement of terminology can attract or appease all audiences, however. We are aware here that, as an editorial team, as with the first edition, we approach this book collection from our own disciplinary and sub-disciplinary perspectives. Like other decisions relating to terminology in this book, we have taken a loose, non-prescriptive approach both to our contributors' choice of vocabulary and to our own terms for defining alcohol use among young adults.

A final complexity with the question 'what is drinking?'—relating to changes in the availability, settings, costs and types of alcoholic drinks—is considered here. We will explore the post-pandemic context in which drinking takes place in more detail below, but note here that drinking practices have been impacted significantly by the COVID-19 pandemic and associated lockdowns, whose rise, fall, ebbs and flows have changed the world in which we live in the years between these first and second editions. Research has identified increased home drinking, reduced visits to traditional 'on license' drinking premises, alongside an international, post-pandemic 'cost of living crisis' involving rapid inflation of goods including alcoholic drinks. Another factor relates to the greatly increased diversification of 'NoLo' beverages containing no or low alcoholic content including, particularly, the growing market in 'low alcohol' products which contain between 0.5% and 1.2% alcohol by volume (ABV) and 'alcohol free' products which are below 0.5% ABV (Okaru & Lachenmeier, 2022). From a research perspective, this diversification is challenging and one priority of research concerning young adult drinking is to understand the implications of the increased availability of these 'NoLo' alcoholic products, as well as the variations in how and where they are consumed (Piatkowski et al., 2024).

## Why an Interest in Young Adult Drinking?

To this point we have drawn attention to the changed and changing landscape of alcohol-related research concerning young adults and note the exciting opportunities and challenges ahead for research in this field. We have considered some of the terminology that can or should be used to define the group of individuals who are the focus of our attention for this collection, and similarly, the activities relating to alcohol that will be focused on. Putting this together, we now turn to the question in the title of this sub-section: why should the drinking practices among individuals whom we are terming 'young adults' warrant particular attention? Different perspectives are helpful in addressing this question.

One might draw on Arnett's (2000) account of emerging adulthood again here to consider what have been presented as typical characteristics of this life stage and how they might have a bearing on drinking practices during this period. Indeed, this has been the focus of specific discussion and research in the emerging adulthood literature (e.g. Arnett, 2005; Maynard et al., 2015). These might include pivotal decisions relating to living arrangements and lifestyle choices; embarking on higher education; acquiring secure/meaningful employment; accessing licensed leisure and underground parties in adult nightlife; initiation and experimentation with illicit drugs and altered states of intoxication; identifying whether and what relationship circumstances suit an individual; and similar issues relating to choices and meanings associated with identity and sexuality. These important considerations mark 'young adults' as a group for whom alcohol use is one in a constellation of factors to consider from a research and policy perspective.

Another perspective might draw greater attention to the particular pressures faced by young adults in the closing quarter of the twenty-first century to work with (whether to adhere to or resist) cultural understandings of what becoming and 'being' a young adult could or should entail. The visibility and importance of alcohol use as a feature of 'being young' is something which is recognised and capitalised on by the alcohol, hospitality, events and festival industries when considering their own marketing strategies (Hastings et al., 2010). Alcohol branding and sponsorship have a near omniscient presence in much young adult leisure from the naming of entertainment arenas and live music stadia to festival bars, not unrelated to the growing restrictions on sponsorship of sporting events and of alcohol marketing more generally in many developed countries (Rowley & Williams, 2008).

A pragmatic approach to health promotion offers a further perspective to help explain why focusing on alcohol use among young adults might attract research attention. While secondary school has traditionally provided an important opportunity for formal educational input on health education and life skills, the expansion of higher education to cover nearly half of young adults in many developed countries results in young adults representing an additional and under-recognised demographic group to target with age and life stage-appropriate health promotion, education and prevention campaigns. While reviews have identified the most effective prevention programmes for secondary school youth being those that focus on normative education and enhancing social and social resistance skills, more consideration is needed regarding their efficacy with young adults (Botvin & Griffin, 2007) in both healthcare and community settings (Derges et al., 2017). For while the earliest phase of experimentation may be behind them, many young adults are leaving the protective influences of family and local community to engage with the pleasures and possibilities but also the demands and pressures of an increasingly independent life involving university, work, and cohabiting with friends, partners or classmates. Indeed, these demands create a unique period in some respects which may be an important factor in shaping decisions around consumption of legal and also illegal drugs and their role in their lives. Young adulthood may well involve the beginning, the extension or the consolidation and even entrenchment of particular understandings about alcohol's role in their lives which may form the basis for how alcohol is used (or not) for the remainder of that individual's life. Therefore, from their late teens onwards, young adults are presented (in most cases) with a relatively unfamiliar but considerable range of settings, occasions and opportunities which demand decisions relating to alcohol use (and non-use).

## Why Drinking 'Styles'?

Clarity of terminology, as discussed in the sections above, is central to clarity of understanding. The lexicon for describing and understanding drinking behaviours and practices, and for identifying particular 'types' of drinkers, is vast but is also culturally and historically situated. For example, we can think of drinking behaviour in terms of 'social drinking', 'moderate drinking', 'problem drinking', 'anti-social drinking', 'binge drinking', 'light drinking' and the list continues. We might also think about 'risky drinking', 'harmful drinking', 'immoderate drinking' and, increasingly visibly, the terminology of 'responsible drinking' in the USA and other international settings (e.g. International Alliance of Responsible Drinking, 2019). These terms help to influence the polarising parameters within which we might think about drinking behaviour, and drinking behaviour among young adults particularly, as morally acceptable/unacceptable, as harmful/beneficial to the self and as harmful/beneficial to others in our immediate and wider vicinity. Moreover, these terms set down yardsticks by which research questions are framed, by which research projects are designed and implemented, by which research evidence informs and governs the development and delivery of alcohol policy, and by which evidence also informs the justification, choice and delivery of interventions and clinical practice relevant to alcohol consumption.

Discussion here is intended partly to draw attention to the constructive power of the terminology surrounding alcohol consumption in the context of young adult drinking practices, and the theoretical and practical difficulties that rigid definitions can produce for understanding behaviour that is inherently complex and multi-faceted. For example, contemporary use of the term 'binge drinker' would serve to produce an understanding of an individual's approach to alcohol consumption as excessive and harmful regardless of the company and environment in which the individual finds themselves in; the cultural and sub-cultural norms pertinent to that individual; wider circumstances and demands; and how drinking practices can be understood from the perspective of life narrative including transition between particular life stages. Historically, the term 'binge' was often associated with a prolonged and intense drinking session or 'bender' (Herring et al., 2008). Therefore, drinker categories like 'binge drinker', useful as they may be in academic and everyday language, can create a persistently decontextualised understanding of young adult drinking practices, where the focus again returns to the individual and ignores the political, socio-cultural, corporate and economic contexts within which that individual's drinking occurs and is understood.

This raises questions about possible alternatives which manage to navigate a route through these rigid definitions to produce a more coherent appreciation of young adult drinking practices; cultural and policy change surrounding alcohol consumption; and new trends in research. The term 'drinking styles' has both conceptual and real world advantages. In conceptual terms, 'drinking styles' shifts the emphasis of young adult drinking behaviour to account for the fluidity and inconsistency in drinking practices over the course of a social event, a week, a month, a life stage or a lifespan. This shifts the research agenda towards an emphasis on contradictory and counter-intuitive features of drinking practices which may fluctuate in association with contextual considerations. Additionally, it links young adult drinking practices with wider sociological discussions around leisure lifestyles, friendship networks, subcultures, neo-tribes and the associated indicators around music, clothing, nightlife, consumption and stylistic 'scenes' (Bennett, 2004).

In practical terms, 'drinking styles' is a term which recognises that drinking behaviour is chosen and re-chosen between and within events involving the potential for alcohol consumption. As a term, drinking styles also provide a rhetorical way of acknowledging that a given young adult has possibilities open to them in terms of how they understand the role of alcohol, its subjective effects, its social role, and its community and cultural understandings. Moreover, to discuss an individual's (or group's) drinking styles provides a way of acknowledging the multiple factors (and therefore multiple sites) for pursuing a health promotion agenda to promote safe, sustainable drinking practices among young adults.

The notion of 'styles' in the context of health behaviour or health practices is rare. This is perhaps surprising given the appearance of this term among, for example, educationalists, where theories of differing 'learning styles' have proven influential (e.g. Messick, 1984; Peterson et al., 2009) and, from the perspective of some educational commentators, controversial (Kirschner, 2017; Willingham et al., 2015). Researchers with an interest in health behaviours do not conventionally refer to 'eating styles', 'styles of sexual practice', 'physical activity styles' or 'drinking styles'.

Drinking styles is not a new term, however. It has appeared in discussion of patterns of drinking behaviour among individuals with a diagnosis of alcoholism and the children of alcoholics (e.g. Johnson et al., 1989; Olenick & Chalmers, 1991). However, deployment of the term in a way that aligns with our suggested use—to recognise variations in drinking behaviour and the context-dependent nature of drinking practices—is present in the work of Betsy Thom and colleagues who, for example, have documented the nuances in young men's motivations to drink and their drinking practices (Harnett et al., 2000). These nuances are also evident in work on 'peer attachment styles' (Bartholomew & Horowitz, 1991) and 'romantic attachment styles' (Hazan & Shaver, 1987) in young adulthood. The expression 'drinking styles' rarely appears in its present intended meaning. For example, although Bai (2021) used the term 'drinking styles' in their research article, their operational measure—'weekly average drinking amount'—is traditional and typical within the alcohol field. In developing the second edition of this collection, the term 'drinking styles' remains a rarely used term and, where used, typically acts as a synonym for a traditional, post positivist and individually located meaning around individual alcohol consumption patterns, or acts as a rhetorical flourish, perhaps for the title of a research article.

## What Is the Purpose of This Book?

While there is persistent coverage of alcohol-related issues in the media, academic, policy and broader cultural settings, what is much less clearly available is a space dedicated to a consideration of the trends, nuances and contexts for young adult drinking linked with life stage transitions and identity/identities in the rapidly evolving and globally connected world. Studies are now turning their attention to considering the socio-cultural context to drinking in a world shifting from cultures of consumption to cultures of austerity, alongside the growing impact of online, digital and virtual worlds. We have seen the ebbs and flows of both alcohol consumption and of licensed leisure more broadly, with a rise in binge drinking and recreational drug use across developed countries in the late 1990s and early 2000s, associated with growing disposable income and notions of extended adolescence delaying life stage milestones like marriage, mortgage and parenthood (Measham et al., 2011). Then in the post millennial decade there has been an apparent downturn in alcohol and in consumption more generally, associated with economic recession and associated austerity measures leading to growing economic restrictions on licensed leisure and a turn against conspicuous consumption.

In exploring the complexities of drinking behaviours among young adults, the contributors to this collection take a deliberate discursive turn away from traditional understandings of young adult drinking that seek to pathologise and generalise. We advocate instead for an inclusive approach evident in the wide range of disciplinary backgrounds, cultural perspectives and international settings represented in this book, in order to better understand the economic, cultural and pharmacological crossroads at which we now stand.

Never before has there been such a wide range of methods and approaches to considering drinking behaviour and practices among young adults, particularly in relation to digital methods associated with new communication technologies. Online surveys, photo ethnography and participatory methods are just some of the methods increasingly utilised in the field to gain a broader and deeper understanding of drinking practices than enabled by previous traditional qualitative and quantitative data collection. One of the increasingly prominent strands of alcohol research involves discursive methods which explore how individual rhetoric and interactions are involved in shoring up credentials with a particular kind of drinker identity (e.g. non-drinkers, Nairn et al., 2006; Conroy & de Visser, 2014; Conroy et al., 2022) or in positioning particular drinking styles in pejorative terms (e.g. Conroy & de Visser, 2013). The book also reflects different methodological traditions in exposing nuance and difference in young adult drinking behaviour. Much of this is comprised of interview-based data, but this book also contains research based on focus groups, on studies of policy documents and on analyses of large-scale survey data. Several methods are described across the book including in situ face-to-face data collection in licensed leisure space (Turner and Measham, Chap. 14), discourse analysis (Banister, Conroy & Piacentini, Chap. 8) and online social media analysis (Goodwin and Lyons, Chap. 12). We think this variety has helped to produce a more engaging and stimulating text but has also offered a collection which acknowledges the range of methodological lenses that can be applied to alcohol research focused on young adults and, as such, offers a more representative reflection of current field research.

For the second edition of this collection, published almost a decade after the first edition's original conception, we have revisited its purpose, particularly to account for the complex effects on drinking resulting from living through the COVID-19 pandemic and lockdowns, alongside the new challenges and opportunities presented to young adult drinkers and non-drinkers in a post-pandemic world.

A cumulative body of evidence has started to illuminate changes in alcohol use and alcohol-related problems before, during and after the COVID-19 pandemic. For example, a systematic review of 27 studies has pointed to changes which include decreased total alcohol consumption (in Australia), more frequent drinking (in the USA) and increases in the proportion of individuals identified as having problem alcohol use in the UK (Sohi et al., 2022). A longitudinal research project involving 234 heavy drinking young adults assessed at pre- and two-year post-pandemic timepoints revealed significant reductions in both the quantity and frequency of alcohol consumption, fewer alcohol problems and an indication that these reductions were partly due to decreased weekend drinking (Creswell et al., 2024).

The impact of home-based drinking, increasingly familiar for many young adults in a post-pandemic world, has been the focus of discussion for some of our own research (Conroy & Nicholls, 2022; Nicholls & Conroy, 2021, 2023), alongside the pandemic-linked rise in preferences for and the incidence of home deliveries (see Grossman et al., 2022; Noel & Rosenthal, 2023) which are also likely to have a distinctive bearing on young adult drinking styles.

## Overview of the Book

One of our starting points with this book is that one way in which drinking practices can be meaningfully and productively understood is with reference to culture, to context, and to historical period and change. Accordingly, the second edition of this book has involved some structural changes, particularly in terms of considering alcohol consumption practices in a post-pandemic world where changing trends in license drinking/drinking in public spaces/new familiarity with home-based drinking all have implications for how, when, where and with whom young adults consume alcohol.

In this second edition, we present eight chapters fully updated from the original book, alongside eight brand new chapters written specifically for this revised edition. As such, this second edition remains fully in the spirit of the original edition but includes new perspectives and topic areas to ensure a contemporary, refreshed approach to understanding young adult drinking styles. We are very fortunate to be able to present original empirical findings in several chapters in this revised edition, evident in Chap. 9 (Bartram and Conroy's interviews with temporary abstinence challenge participants), in Chap. 10 (Davey and Gooch's autoethnographic reflections on sober dating) and in Chap. 11 (Nicholls' analysis of 'no and low' alcohol consumption practices).

Similarly, we have made some changes to the structure of this second edition, evident in the structuring into five parts. Some parts have revised titles and others are entirely new, better suited to the contributions to the revised edition. These book parts (or sections) are summarised below.

Part I is organized around the theme of 'Changing trends in young adult drinking' reflecting the increasingly well-established phenomenon of declining alcohol consumption among young adults in the first quarter of the twenty-first century relative to earlier decades and how drinking practices in young adulthood may transition to different drinking practices in later adult life.

Changing trends in alcohol consumption have been well documented over the last two decades but perhaps have been more challenging to decipher. In Chap. 2, Michael Livingston and Rakhi Vashishtha provide an updated authoritative overview of this international phenomenon contrasting different European and English-speaking countries in turn and illustrating the progression from adolescent to adult trends in each case drawing on new available data. Within this, the authors discuss the complexity and nuance involved in presenting a standardized picture of drinking behaviour trends across different countries. Given these trends, the clear question arises: 'why have drinking trends changed?' and more specifically to the purposes of this book 'why are young adults all around the world, living in different countries, socio-cultural and policy contexts, drinking less than previously?' There are no easy answers to this question and Chap. 3 written and updated by Gabriel Caluzzi and Amy Pennay is a nuanced critical consideration of a range of theoretical perspectives which link these changes in alcohol consumption to the changing nature of family, leisure, identities, digital technologies and both physical and mental health considerations. In their updated chapter, Caluzzi and Pennay contextualise decreased young adult drinking in a wider decline in 'risky' practices traditionally associated with young adulthood and a shift from associating alcohol with sociability and social wellbeing, to negative mental health outcomes, and warn that this in itself might have negative consequences for wellbeing. Then, in Chap. 4, Marjana Martinic discusses in her revised chapter how drinking patterns can be understood as being in a state of flux and how drinking trajectories involve multiple, interweaving factors including socio-economic and cultural factors alongside family dynamics and the changing experience of employment, parenthood and gender in contemporary adult lives.

Martinic draws on the epidemiological literature to unpack the evolving relationship that young adults have with alcohol and the wider changing social visibility and meanings of alcohol consumption for young adults.

Part II is titled 'Diversity in Young Adult Drinking' and presents a series of illustrations of young adult drinking in the context of under-researched contexts involving under-represented social groups.

Chapter 5 begins this section with Alexandra Bogren and colleagues' chapter titled 'Gender, Drinking, and Drunkenness: From Discourses of Gender Difference to Youthful Femininities and Masculinities'. This revised chapter examines four strands of gendered discourse relating to young adult drinking practices as evident from studies of everyday talk and media presentations of alcohol consumption among young adults. Young adult drinking in Swedish popular and policy discourse is represented as risky, as pleasurable or as problematic, in relation to female respectability and male aggressiveness.

The section continues with Chap. 6 which presents Marie Bærndt and Vibeke Frank's chapter 'Understanding Experiences/Perceptions of Young Muslim Women in the Danish Youth Alcohol Culture'. This chapter presents key patterns from relevant field literature leading to the presentation of three themes derived from interviews with young Muslim women concerning, in part, the intersection between alcohol cultures and national identities.

Chapter 7 concludes this section with Amanda Miller, Stephen Mugamba and Susan Kiene's chapter which draws on a Ugandan national context to explore mental health and alcohol use in low- and middle-income countries during the country's period of stringent COVID-19 lockdowns. Miller and colleagues unpack the constellation of factors involved in diverse patterns of alcohol use among young adults during this period.

Part III is titled 'Young Adults Who Drink Little or No Alcohol' and focuses on key illustrations from the large and growing body of work concerning non-drinking, sobriety and abstinence-related topic areas in relation to young adult drinking styles.

This section starts with an updated version of Chap. 8 by Banister and colleagues which presents a review on research and scholarly debate concerning non-drinkers and non-drinking. These authors review relevant empirical research on social experiences and perceptions of non-drinkers, before problematising relevant terminology and outlining considerations for future research, policy and practice. They highlight a concern that many previous studies on this subject have framed non-drinkers as a culturally homogeneous and problematised 'outgroup', having as their starting point that drinking is a normalised leisure activity among young adults.

Chapter 9 continues this section with Ashlea Bartram and Dom Conroy's chapter which focuses on temporary alcohol abstinence initiatives (TAIs, i.e., challenges to abstain from alcohol consumption for typically one month) from the perspective of young adults. Bartram and Conroy begin with a review of recent international literature on TAIs before presenting illustrative qualitative interview study findings concerning young adults' immediate plans relating to alcohol consumption post participation in a temporary alcohol challenge (e.g., 'Dry January' in the UK).

Chapter 10 continues this section with Claire Davey and Millie Gooch's contribution which examines UK-based young women's lived experiences of sober dating. Davey and Gooch examine the rise of sobriety including the growth of 'sober curious' online communities and draw on interview data and autoethnographic reflections to understand women's lived experiences of sober dating and explore areas for future research in this emerging field.

The section concludes with Chap. 11, written by Em Nicholls, which explores the rapidly expanding market of No and Low (NoLo) alcohol drinks in high-income countries where drinking rates among young adults are declining. Nicholls draws on original primary research to highlight how NoLos are used and young adults' motivations for consuming them.

Part IV is titled 'Young Adult Drinking Spaces: Staying Inside; Going Outside; Digital Spaces' and presents a series of examples of how young adult drinking behaviour might be usefully framed in a contextualized sense involving specific places, time periods, online spaces or particular groups of people.

This section starts with Chap. 12 by Ian Goodwin and Antonia Lyons, updated from the original edition, which explores the relationship between social media, online drinking cultures and young adult identities and the wider implications of this for a health promotion agenda. Goodwin and Lyons highlight how ripe this field is for future research exploring the holistic ecology of young adults' social media engagement and the social dynamics and synchronization of these new forms of communication and representation within young adult drinking cultures.

Chapter 13 continues this section with Dom Conroy and Sarah MacLean's updated chapter now titled 'Friendship and Alcohol Use Among Young Adults: What Do We Know and Where Could Things Go?' which considers reciprocal pathways between young adult friendships and social networks and young adult drinking styles. The updated chapter concludes by focusing on recent work concerning friendship in the context of mental health interventions. Conroy and MacLean present the case that young adult friendships, in their many forms and dynamics, appear to be underutilized within alcohol harm reduction interventions.

Chapter 14 continues this section with Tim Turner and Fiona Measham's consideration of licensed leisure locations which appear to buck the general trend in falling rates of young adult alcohol consumption. Utilising qualitative and quantitative data from a number of their studies, it contextualises young adult drinking in the polydrug repertoires which occur in the unusual, occasional or spectacular settings of music festivals and nightlife tourist resorts. Turner and Measham argue that some young adult drinking patterns—characterised here as 'atypical intoxication'—are a central feature of the literal and symbolic journeys many take through woodland festivals and nightlife tourist resorts. Using the three-phase monomyth of separation, immersion and return, Turner and Measham explore the tensions of transgressive leisure and intoxication within these commodified play spaces. It is this increasingly atypical intoxication—of both alcohol and other drugs—which results in additional risk, but also additional opportunity, in terms of potential engagement by young adults in health and harm reduction services.

The section concludes with Chap. 15, newly written by Dom Conroy and Em Nicholls, which takes a post-pandemic perspective to focus on home drinking and solitary home-based drinking practices among young adults. Conroy and Nicholls review the extant literature on home-based drinking to set the scene for an exploration of interview data from the UK-based Drinking in Lockdown project to illustrate what may be a renewed interest in home-based drinking, and perhaps new understandings and norms relating to solitary drinking, among younger adults.

Our fifth and final book section shifts attention to consider young adult drinking styles since COVID-19: policy and practice across two final book chapters.

Chapter 16 is authored by Carly Lightowlers and is titled 'What the COVID-19 Pandemic Has Taught Us About Alcohol Drinking and Associated Violence'. In this chapter, Lightowlers explores evidence about the alcohol-violence relationship, including insights gleaned before, during and after the pandemic. Lightowlers presents readers with a challenge to assumed associations between alcohol-related violence problem and young adults in the night-time economy.

The second and final section chapter, Chap. 17, is authored by Laura Goodwin and colleagues and articulates relevant key theories regarding co-occurring alcohol and mental health problems among young adults, before considering evidence and current treatments relating to these issues.

Together we hope that these chapters contribute to a growing understanding of the diversity of post-pandemic young adult drinking practices and suggest something of what might be learnt from building bridges across disciplines, methodologies and countries in order to shine a light on this topic.

## References

Arnett, J. J. (2000). Emerging adulthood: A theory of development from the late teens through the twenties. *American Psychologist, 55*(5), 469.

Arnett, J. J. (2005). The developmental context of substance use in emerging adulthood. *Journal of Drug Issues, 35*(2), 235–254.

Bai, Z. (2021). Does frequent prayer help reduce alcohol use? Heterogeneity in religious contexts and drinking styles. *Mental Health, Religion & Culture, 24*(2), 151–163.

Bartholomew, K., & Horowitz, L. M. (1991). Attachment styles among young adults: A test of a four-category model. *Journal of Personality and Social Psychology, 61*(2), 226.

Bennett, A. (2004). Consolidating the music scenes perspective. *Poetics, 32*(3–4), 223–234.

Botvin, G. J., & Griffin, K. W. (2007). School-based programmes to prevent alcohol, tobacco and other drug use. *International Review of Psychiatry, 19*(6), 607–615.

Conroy, D., & Nicholls, E. (2022). 'When I open it, I have to drink it all': Push and pull factors shaping domestic alcohol consumption during the COVID-19 pandemic UK Spring 2020 lockdown. *Drug and Alcohol Review, 41*(6), 1275–1283.

Conroy, D., & de Visser, R. O. (2013). 'Man up!': Discursive constructions of non-drinkers among UK undergraduates. *Journal of Health Psychology, 18*(11), 1432–1444. https://doi.org/10.1177/1359105312463586

Conroy, D., & de Visser, R. O. (2014). Being a non-drinking student: An interpretative phenomenological analysis. *Psychology & Health, 29*(5), 536–551. https://doi.org/10.1080/08870446.2013.866673

Conroy, D., Griffin, C., & Morton, C. (2022). Defending, contesting and rejecting formal drinker categories: How UK university students identify as 'light-drinkers' or 'non-drinkers'. *Drugs: Education, Prevention and Policy, 29*(5), 509–518.

Creswell, K. G., Hisler, G. C., Lyons, G., Carrillo-Álvarez, F. A., Fairbairn, C. E., & Wright, A. G. (2024). Changes in alcohol consumption and alcohol problems before and after the COVID-19 pandemic: A prospective study in heavy drinking young adults. *Nature Mental Health, 2*, 1–12.

Derges, J., Kidger, J., Fox, F., Campbell, R., Kaner, E., & Hickman, M. (2017). Alcohol screening and brief interventions for adults and young people in health and community-based settings: A qualitative systematic literature review. *BMC Public Health, 17*, 562.

Erikson, E. (1950). *Childhood and society*. Norton.

Green, L. (2016). *Understanding the life course: Sociological and psychological perspectives*. John Wiley & Sons.

Grossman, E. R., Benjamin-Neelon, S. E., & Sonnenschein, S. (2022). Alcohol consumption and alcohol home delivery laws during the COVID-19 pandemic. *Substance Abuse, 43*(1), 1141–1146.

Harnett, R., Thom, B., Herring, R., & Kelly, M. (2000). Alcohol in transition: Towards a model of young men's drinking styles. *Journal of Youth Studies, 3*(1), 61–77.

Hastings, G., Brooks, O., Stead, M., Angus, K., Anker, T., & Farrell, T. (2010). Alcohol advertising: The last chance saloon. *BMJ, 340*, 184–186.

Hazan, C., & Shaver, P. (1987). Romantic love conceptualized as an attachment process. *Journal of Personality and Social Psychology, 52*(3), 511.

Herring, R., Berridge, V., & Thom, B. (2008). Binge drinking: An exploration of a confused concept. *Journal of Epidemiology and Community Health, 62*, 476–479.

Huckle, T., Callinan, S., Pham, C., Chaiyasong, S., Parker, K., & Casswell, S. (2020). Harmful drinking occurs in private homes in some high-and middle-income alcohol markets: Data from the international alcohol control study. *Drug and Alcohol Review, 39*(6), 616–623.

International Alliance of Responsible Drinking. (2019). Mission statement. http://www.responsibledrinking.org/

Johnson, S., Leonard, K. E., & Jacob, T. (1989). Drinking, drinking styles and drug use in children of alcoholics, depressives and controls. *Journal of Studies on Alcohol, 50*(5), 427–431.

Kirschner, P. A. (2017). Stop propagating the learning styles myth. *Computers & Education, 106*, 166–171.

Levinson, D. J. (1986). A conception of adult development. *American Psychologist, 41*(1), 3.

Maynard, B. R., Salas-Wright, C. P., & Vaughn, M. G. (2015). High school dropouts in emerging adulthood: Substance use, mental health problems, and crime. *Community Mental Health Journal, 51*(3), 289–299.

Measham, F., Williams, L., & Aldridge, J. (2011). Marriage, mortgage, motherhood: What longitudinal surveys can tell us about gender, 'drug careers' and the normalisation of adult drug use. *International Journal of Drug Policy, 22*(6), 420–427.

Messick, S. (1984). The nature of cognitive styles: Problems and promise in educational practice. *Educational Psychologist, 19*, 59–74.

Nairn, K., Higgins, J., Thompson, B., Anderson, M., & Fu, N. (2006). 'It's just like the teenage stereotype, you go out and drink and stuff': Hearing from young people who don't drink. *Journal of Youth Studies, 9*(3), 287–304.

Nicholls, E., & Conroy, D. (2021). Possibilities and pitfalls? Moderate drinking and alcohol abstinence at home since the COVID-19 lockdown. *International Journal of Drug Policy, 88*, 103025.

Nicholls, E., & Conroy, D. (2023). 'I've gone from one extreme to the other': Critical junctures in relationships with alcohol during the COVID-19 pandemic. *Drugs: Education, Prevention and Policy, 30*(6), 613–622.

Noel, J. K., & Rosenthal, S. R. (2023). Impact of alcohol home delivery and other methods of obtaining alcohol in young adults. *Alcohol and Alcoholism, 58*(6), 606–611.

Okaru, A., & Lachenmeier, D. (2022). Defining no and low (NoLo) alcohol products. *Nutrients, 14*(18), 3873.

Olenick, N. L., & Chalmers, D. K. (1991). Gender-specific drinking styles in alcoholics and nonalcoholics. *Journal of Studies on Alcohol, 52*(4), 325–330.

Peterson, E. R., Rayner, S. G., & Armstrong, S. J. (2009). Researching the psychology of cognitive style and learning style: Is there really a future? *Learning and Individual Differences, 19*, 518–523.

Piatkowski, T., Patel, M., Puljević, C., Davies, E., Barratt, M., Winstock, A., & Ferris, J. (2024). Why, where, and with whom? Understanding the set and setting influencing the consumption of NoLo beverages. *Drugs: Education, Prevention and Policy*, 1–13.

Rowley, J., & Williams, C. (2008). The impact of brand sponsorship of music festivals. *Marketing Intelligence & Planning, 26*(7), 781.

Sohi, I., Chrystoja, B. R., Rehm, J., Wells, S., Monteiro, M., Ali, S., & Shield, K. D. (2022). Changes in alcohol use during the COVID-19 pandemic and previous pandemics: A systematic review. *Alcoholism: Clinical and Experimental Research, 46*(4), 498–513.

Willingham, D. T., Hughes, E. M., & Dobolyi, D. G. (2015). The scientific status of learning styles theories. *Teaching of Psychology, 42*(3), 266–271.

Xu, Y., Geldsetzer, P., Manne-Goehler, J., Theilmann, M., Marcus, M. E., Zhumadilov, Z., et al. (2022). The socioeconomic gradient of alcohol use: An analysis of nationally representative survey data from 55 low-income and middle-income countries. *The Lancet Global Health, 10*(9), e1268–e1280.

# Part I

## Changing Trends of Young Adult Alcohol Use

# 2

# Have Recent Declines in Adolescent Drinking Continued Into Young Adulthood?

Michael Livingston, Emma Vieira, and Rakhi Vashishtha

**Abstract** Livingston, Vieira and Vashishtha explore whether the widely established declines in adolescent drinking have continued as these cohorts age into young adult. They compile key trends from surveys conducted across twelve countries, providing the first systematic attempt to assess trends in drinking for people in early adulthood. The data highlight declining drinking for young adults across many countries since the early 2000s, although there remain significant inconsistencies in the global trends. Importantly, the data collated demonstrate the diversity of approaches to measurement of drinking in adult populations—we argue that the development of consistent and comparable approaches to data collection and measurement is critical to improve the reliability of estimates in future.

M. Livingston (✉) • E. Vieira
National Drug Research Institute, Curtin University, Perth, WA, Australia
e-mail: michael.livingston@curtin.edu.au; Emma.Vieira@curtin.edu.au

R. Vashishtha
Programme in Health Services and Systems Research, Duke-NUS Medical School, Outram, Singapore
e-mail: rakhi.vashishtha@nus.edu.sg


D. Conroy, F. Measham (eds.), *Young Adult Drinking Styles*, Sustainable Development Goals Series, https://doi.org/10.1007/978-3-031-98528-7_2

# Introduction

Studies from around the world highlight that alcohol consumption typically peaks in early adulthood, at least in intoxication-oriented drinking cultures. For example, in Britton et al.'s (2015) combination of nine UK cohort studies, men aged 25 were estimated to consume around 23 units of alcohol per week, while those in their 50s consumed less than 15. Similar patterns are evident in studies from the USA (Kerr et al., 2009), Sweden (Kraus et al., 2015), the UK (Meng et al., 2014) and Australia (Livingston et al., 2016). These patterns are reflected in acute alcohol-related harms: Alcohol is the number one risk factor for injury and disease globally for people aged between 15 and 44 (Institute for Health Metrics and Evaluation, 2021). It is a particularly important risk factor for adolescents and young adults, contributing to around 8% of the total disease burden in this population (and substantially more than this in high income countries) (Institute for Health Metrics, 2016).

Understanding changes in how young adults drink is therefore critical to understanding the public health implications of alcohol consumption in a society. Governments and other public health actors spend considerable resources in trying to reduce drinking in this age group, with public campaigns, health promotion interventions and policies often targeted at their drinking. Historically however, monitoring of drinking patterns in this age group has been inconsistent and often entirely lacking. Researchers and governments have long wanted to understand trends in alcohol consumption within populations, and a tradition of regular population surveys measuring alcohol consumption (and often the use of other substances) was developed through the latter part of the twentieth century. Despite this, changes to questionnaire design, survey methodologies and inconsistent funding have meant that consistent long-term trends in survey-related measures of drinking are often lacking. While there are some exceptions where long-term survey data are available (e.g. Härkönen et al., 2017, Meng et al., 2014), sub-analyses for young adults remain rare.

This is in stark contrast to adolescent drinking, where regular and comparable data collection provides detailed and consistent trend data. This is largely driven by two major cross-national studies that have been conducted since at least the 1990s. These two studies—the European School Survey Project on Alcohol and Other Drugs (ESPAD) and the Health Behaviour in School Children Study (HBSC)—both provide multi-country trends on adolescent alcohol use and have been running for more than twenty years. Furthermore, countries not included in these studies often have their own long-running (and broadly comparable) school surveys—for example, Australia's School Student Alcohol and Drug Survey (ASSAD) has been running since 1984 (White & Williams, 2016). Thus, our knowledge of trends in adolescent drinking is much more comprehensive than it is for trends in drinking among young adults.

## Adolescent Drinking Trends

A series of research studies from across Europe, North America and Australasia have identified sharp declines in alcohol consumption for adolescents since the early 2000s (de Looze et al., 2015; Kraus et al., 2018; Livingston, 2014). In a key overview paper, Vashishtha et al. (2021) summarise data from 39 high-income jurisdictions, highlighting declines in the vast majority. Importantly, the magnitude and timing of the declines vary—Anglo and Nordic countries have the steepest and longest declines, while other parts of Europe have seen less dramatic changes. Similarly, de Looze et al. (2015) examined data on teenagers between 11 and 15 years of age from the Health Behaviour in School Children (HBSC) survey between 2002 and 2010, finding sharp declines in past-week alcohol use in 20 of 28 countries examined, while Pape et al. (2018) presents data from the European School Survey Project on Alcohol and Other Drugs from 26 countries, finding significant declines in past-month drinking between 2003 and 2015 for 22 of these countries. These trends appear to have affected multiple drinking behaviours, with marked increases in abstention, delayed onset of drinking and reduced rates of heavy episodic drinking, and there is increasing evidence that a range of other risky or adult behaviours (fighting (Pickett et al., 2013), driving (Delbosc & Currie, 2013), etc., have declined alongside the reductions in drinking. There remain debates about the implications of these trends for these cohorts as they age into adulthood. Will their consumption levels remain lower than they were for previous cohorts in early adulthood or will they simply 'catch up' once they age out of adolescence, where particular factors (e.g. parenting practices, legal supply issues) may be holding them back?

There is a substantial body of evidence demonstrating strong associations between alcohol consumption in adolescence and heavy drinking in adulthood (Englund et al., 2008; Grant & Dawson, 1997; Wechsler et al., 1995). Similarly, studies have repeatedly shown that earlier age of onset of drinking is associated with higher rates of alcohol use disorders and other problems in adulthood (Dawson et al., 2008; Hingson & Zha, 2009). With this in mind, we would expect the decline in adolescent drinking described here to flow through into lower rates of heavy drinking and reduced alcohol-related harm among young adults. Given that the adolescent trends appear to have established in many countries by the early 2000s, there has been sufficient time to observe the initial impacts of the decline in youth drinking on adult consumption, but we could find no comprehensive attempt to do so. A number of Australian studies have shown falls in young adult alcohol consumption in recent years (Livingston et al., 2018; Livingston & Dietze, 2016), and a series of analyses of cohort and repeated cross-sectional surveys have highlighted that generational differences in drinking narrow as recent cohorts reach adulthood, but are still significantly lower (Callinan et al., 2020, Leggat et al., 2021, Livingston et al., 2022). In contrast, analyses from Sweden and Finland argue that declines in adolescent drinking have mostly dissipated by early adulthood, especially among heavier drinkers (Kraus et al., 2024, Lintonen et al., 2016).

A key complication of course is the impact of the COVID-19 pandemic on drinking trends. Our empirical review does not explicitly focus on this question, given the marked variations in pandemic experiences between countries, but it is worth briefly outlining the published evidence here. In an early review of the relatively low quality literature, Acuff et al. (2022) found roughly equivalent proportions of people increasing and decreasing consumption during the pandemic, but increases slightly more likely among young adults. In contrast, a later systematic review focussed specifically on young adult consumption, Hussong et al. (2023)

note that robust evidence remains relatively scarce, with most studies relying on convenience samples and retrospective assessments. Still, combining the handful of representative studies with the broader literature, they find a generally consistent picture that drinking for young adults generally declined during the initial 12 months of the pandemic, but subsequently rebounded strongly. Thus, it is likely that data from 2020 onwards in the review below reflect specific pandemic impacts, as well as broader long-running trends in young adult drinking.

## Methods

We have compiled data from 12 countries on recent trends in drinking for young adults. The lack of the systematic multi-country surveys that are run within schools (e.g. ESPAD, HBSC, Global School-based Student Health Survey (GSHS)) make this a more challenging task. For this reason, the data here are likely to be incomplete. Systematic online searches were conducted to identify either peer-reviewed publications outlining trends in young adult drinking for particular jurisdictions or, more commonly, grey literature summarising survey data within countries. We limited searches to high-income countries with a strong tradition of alcohol research likely to have conducted regular high-quality population surveys—thus our data come from predominantly Anglo countries and Western Europe. References in media reports and other publications were used to identify data sources for some countries. We also used our network of contacts in alcohol research groups around the world where published data for specific countries could not be located (e.g. for Norway). Many survey reports were written in languages other than English so, where necessary, Google Translate was used to extract key data from survey reports. Gender breakdowns are provided where they were readily available in published reports.

We have not attempted to produce comparable measures across countries. Reporting practices vary markedly—different countries use different measures of standard drinks (Kalinowski & Humphreys, 2016) and different thresholds for risky drinking (National Health and Medical Research Council, 2009), meaning standard reports in surveys are inconsistent between countries. Instead, we group the results in two sets—firstly, any measure of *risky* drinking however it is defined, and secondly any other drinking measure not specifically focussed on risk (frequency, abstinence vs past year drinking, etc). Similarly, there are no standardised age groups for reporting age-specific drinking trends, so we have relied on the specific age breakdowns provided in published reports. In some countries this includes respondents below the legal purchase age of alcohol (e.g. 15–24-year-olds in Canada), but generally data span the late teens and early twenties. The time periods for which data are available are also inconsistent—we attempted to collate data from the early 2000s onwards to provide a similar timeframe to that used in previous work on adolescent drinking declines. These variations in reporting practices across countries thus make it almost impossible to compare drinking patterns *between* countries. Fortunately, we are mainly interested here in understanding whether changes in drinking *within* countries look similar around the world.

## Results

### Australia

Data on risky drinking for Australia come from the National Drug Strategy Household Survey (NDSHS). Table 2.1 includes the trends in two measures of risky drinking for 18–24-year-olds between 2007 and 2019, extracted from the most recent survey report (Australian Institute of Health and Welfare, 2017). Rates of both measures of risky drinking have declined sharply for both men and women over the period, although there were increases in both measures between 2016 and 2019 for men. For example, male long-term risky drinking fell markedly between 2007 (39%) and 2016 (23%), but increased again slightly in 2019 (27%).

**Table 2.1** Risky drinking trends among young adults

| | | | | | | | | | | | | | | | | | | | |
|---|---|---|---|---|---|---|---|---|---|---|---|---|---|---|---|---|---|---|---|
| | Australia | | | | 2007 | | | 2010 | | | 2013 | | | 2016 | | | 2019 | | |
| 18–24 | Long-term risky drinking[a] | Men | | | 39% | | | 39% | | | 28% | | | 23% | | | 27% | | |
| | | Women | | | 20% | | | 22% | | | 23% | | | 13% | | | 10% | | |
| | Risky single occasion drinking[b] | Men | | | 61% | | | 60% | | | 55% | | | 46% | | | 47% | | |
| | | Women | | | 46% | | | 47% | | | 41% | | | 38% | | | 34% | | |
| | England | | 2005 | 2006 | 2007 | 2008 | 2009 | 2010 | 2011 | 2012 | 2013 | 2014 | 2015 | 2016 | 2017 | 2018 | 2019 | | 2021 |
| 16–24 | Long-term risky drinking[c] | Men | | | | | | | 27% | 31% | 28% | 24% | 24% | 21% | 20% | 22% | 19% | | 20% |
| | | Women | | | | | | | 20% | 17% | 14% | 17% | 14% | 14% | 13% | 12% | 11% | | 10% |
| | Risky single occasion drinking[d] | Men | 45% | 41% | 44% | 43% | 35% | 32% | 32% | 31% | 27% | 31% | 36% | 28% | 30% | | | | |
| | | Women | 41% | 40% | 40% | 38% | 37% | 31% | 30% | 29% | 29% | 31% | 32% | 27% | 31% | | | | |
| | USA | | 2005 | 2006 | 2007 | 2008 | 2009 | 2010 | 2011 | 2012 | 2013 | 2014 | 2015 | 2016 | 2017 | 2018 | 2019 | 2020 | 2021 |
| 19–20 | Heavy episodic drinking[e] | Both | 36% | 34% | 31% | 31% | 28% | 28% | 30% | 30% | 27% | 28% | 24% | 23% | 22% | 20% | 21% | 17% | 23% |
| 21–22 | | Both | 40% | 42% | 46% | 42% | 41% | 39% | 39% | 39% | 40% | 38% | 35% | 38% | 40% | 34% | 35% | 31% | 33% |
| 23–24 | | Both | 39% | 43% | 40% | 42% | 42% | 40% | 40% | 38% | 38% | 34% | 35% | 35% | 31% | 36% | 34% | 31% | 35% |
| 25–26 | | Both | 38% | 36% | 38% | 40% | 40% | 37% | 39% | 36% | 37% | 32% | 35% | 35% | 34% | 33% | 37% | 32% | 35% |
| | Sweden | | 2005 | 2006 | 2007 | 2008 | 2009 | 2010 | 2011 | 2012 | 2013 | 2014 | 2015 | 2016 | 2017 | 2018 | 2019 | 2020 | 2021 |
| 17–29 | Intensive drinking (past month)[f] | Both | 50% | 49% | 47% | 43% | 40% | 40% | 40% | 43% | 42% | 44% | 47% | 48% | 45% | 45% | 44% | 41% | 42% |
| | Germany | | 2005 | | | 2008 | | 2010 | 2011 | 2012 | | 2014 | 2015 | 2016 | | 2018 | 2019 | | 2021 |
| 18–25 | Long-term risky drinking[g] | Men | 24% | | | 24% | | 20% | 22% | 19% | | 17% | 16% | 16% | | 21% | 19% | | 17% |
| | | Women | 14% | | | 12% | | 11% | 15% | 13% | | 14% | 12% | 13% | | 15% | 14% | | 16% |
| | Heavy episodic drinking[h] | Men | 53% | | | 53% | | 49% | 54% | 53% | | 44% | 45% | 46% | | 46% | 48% | | 40% |
| | | Women | 25% | | | 28% | | 26% | 29% | n.a. | | 26% | 25% | 22% | | 26% | 25% | | 19% |

*(continued)*

**Table 2.1** (continued)

| | | | | | | | | | | | | | | | | | | |
|---|---|---|---|---|---|---|---|---|---|---|---|---|---|---|---|---|---|---|
| | Norway | | | | | | | | 2012 | 2013 | 2014 | 2015 | 2016 | 2017 | | | | |
| 16–24 | Heavy episodic drinking[i] | Both | | | | | | | 70% | 73% | 63% | 64% | 65% | 66% | 66% | 69% | 68% | 65% |
| | Denmark | | | | | | | | | | 2014 | 2015 | 2016 | 2017 | | 2019 | | |
| 15–25 | Frequent risky drinking[j] | Both | | | | | | | | | 48% | 39% | 34% | 35% | | 37% | | |
| | New Zealand | | | 2006–2007 | | | | | 2011–2012 | 2012–2013 | 2013–2014 | 2014–2015 | 2015–2016 | 2016–2017 | 2017–2018 | 2018–2019 | 2019–2020 | 2020–2021 |
| 18–24 | Hazardous drinking[k] | Both | | 43% | | | | | 30% | 32% | 33% | 34% | 33% | 33% | 32% | 36% | 33% | 35% |
| | Monthly 6+ drinking[l] | Both | | 44% | | | | | 36% | 42% | 35% | 37% | 35% | 36% | 36% | 38% | 33% | 41% |
| | Canada | | 2004 | | 2008 | 2009 | 2010 | 2011 | 2012 | 2013 | | 2015 | | 2017 | | 2019 | | |
| 15–24 | Drinking above acute guidelines[m] | Both | 14% | | 18% | 17% | 15% | 13% | 13% | 15% | | 14% | | 14% | | 14% | | |
| | Drinking above chronic guidelines[n] | Both | 19% | | 23% | 20% | 18% | 15% | 17% | 19% | | 17% | | 18% | | 18% | | |
| | Spain | | 2005 | 2007 | | 2009 | | 2011 | | 2013 | | 2015 | | | 2018 | | 2020 | |
| 15–34 | Prevalence of past year intoxication[o] | Men | 40% | 39% | | 44% | | 41% | | 43% | | 38% | | | 39% | | 42% | |
| | | Women | 21% | 23% | | 26% | | 24% | | 26% | | 23% | | | 25% | | 27% | |
| | France | | 2005 | | | | 2010 | | | 2014 | | | | | 2017 | | | |
| 20–25 | Risky drinking[p] | Both | 11% | | | | 18% | | | | | | | | | | | |

|  |  |  |  |  |  |  |
|---|---|---|---|---|---|---|
| 18–24 | Occasional heavy drinking (once per week) in the last 12 months | Men | 12% | 17% | 16% | 14% |
|  |  | Women | 2% | 6% | 6% | 6% |
| 18–24 | At least 10 drunken events (last 12 months) | Men | 10% | 19% | 21% | 19% |
|  |  | Women | 2% | 5% | 8% | 7% |

[a] Long-term risky drinking involves consuming at least 20g of pure alcohol per day (on average) over the past 12 months, National Drug Strategy Household Survey

[b] Risky single-occasion drinking involves consuming more than 40g of alcohol in a single occasion at least 12 times in the past 12 months, National Drug Strategy Household Survey

[c] Average of >2 units per day (16g of pure alcohol), Health Survey for England

[d] At least one occasion of >32g (men) or >24g (women) of pure alcohol in the past week, Opinion and Lifestyle Survey, England

[e] At least one occasion of >70g alcohol in the past fortnight, Monitoring the Future Survey

[f] >80g of pure alcohol in a session, CAN (Centralförbundet för Alkohol- och Narkotikaupplysning) Survey

[g] >24g/12g of pure alcohol per day for men/women, Federal Centre for Health Education Surveys

[h] >60g of pure alcohol in a given day, Federal Centre for Health Education Surveys

[i] >60g pure alcohol on at least one occasion in the past year, Alkoholbruk i den voksne befolkningen Survey

[j] At least 2 occasions of >60g of pure alcohol in the past month, Full of Life Survey

[k] AUDIT score of 8 or higher (34), New Zealand Health Survey

[l] 60g of pure alcohol at least once per month, New Zealand Health Survey

[m] >41 grams of pure alcohol (women)/>54 grams of pure alcohol on any one day in the past week, CAS, CADUMS, CTADS and CADS Surveys

[n] >136 grams of pure alcohol (women)/>204 grams of alcohol (men) in the past 7 days, CAS, CADUMS, CTADS and CADS Surveys

[o] Self-reported intoxication in the past year, Encuesta Sobre Alcohol y Otras Drogas en España Survey

[p] 50g of pure alcohol or more in a session at least monthly, French Health Barometer Survey

## England and the United Kingdom

England has seen marked reductions in adolescent drinking since the early 2000s (Bhattacharya, 2016). Data on long-term risky drinking and risky single-occasion drinking were available in two different surveys. The Health Survey for England collects data on the proportion of the population drinking an average of more than 2 UK units per day (16g of pure alcohol per day), while the Opinion and Lifestyle Survey collected data on past-week heavy drinking (>32g in a session for men, >24g for women) up until 2017. Trends in both measures are presented in Table 2.1 for 16–24-year-olds.

Both measures showed substantial declines for both men and women in recent years. Both data series also show signs of declines stabilising—rates of long-term risky drinking for men were stable between 2016 and 2021, while for women declines were marginal. For risky single occasion drinking the decline in drinking was concentrated around 2008–2010 for both men and women. In fact, on this measure, drinking rates were relatively stable in the last five survey waves up to 2017. An overview of UK data from a range of sources suggests that these declines have been driven by both an increase in abstention among young people and a reduction in the amount of alcohol consumed by drinkers (Oldham et al., 2018).

## United States of America

The USA has quite a different context to most other countries discussed in this chapter. The minimum legal purchase age for alcohol is 21, the highest in the world (World Health Organisation, 2018b) and in recent years regulations around cannabis have relaxed markedly, with as yet unclear effects on drinking patterns (Hall & Lynskey, 2016). The declining trend in adolescent drinking in the USA also predates most other countries with rates of drinking falling since the 1990s (Jang et al., 2017; Johnston et al., 2006a, 2006b; Patrick et al., 2017).

The USA also has some of the most comprehensive data sources on alcohol consumption in the world, with multiple sources available to assess recent trends. In Table 2.1 we present data on heavy episodic drinking from Monitoring the Future, a long-running study of youth substance use, as published in Patrick et al. (Patrick et al., 2022). These data point to declines in drinking, although the declines are much steeper for those under the legal drinking age, with prevalence dropping by more than half between 2005 and 2015 for 19–20-year-olds compared with much smaller declines in the older age groups—among 25–26-year-olds, risky drinking rates have been relatively stable across the period.

Across a broader range of sources, Grucza et al. (2018) found no significant recent trends for heavy drinking among 18–29-year-olds when they compiled data from six other national surveys. It is worth noting that US data on adolescent drinking show substantial declines between 1991 and 2013 (Patrick et al., 2022) but, while some sources of data have identified recent declines in drinking for young adults, the overall picture appears to be one of stability.

## Sweden

Sweden is another country that has seen a marked decline in adolescent drinking since the early 2000s (Hallgren et al., 2012; Larm et al., 2019; Norström & Svensson, 2014; Svensson & Andersson, 2016). In general, Sweden has a relatively restrictive approach to alcohol policy, with a government monopoly on retail sales, relatively high taxes, and restrictions on advertising and opening hours of outlets. The 'Europeanisation' of alcohol policy in Sweden to comply with European Union regulations has led to some relaxation of these policies (Cisneros Örnberg, 2009) and gradual increases in per-capita consumption since the early 2000s (even while youth drinking declined sharply) (Norström & Ramstedt, 2018).

We present here data on young adult drinking from a monthly monitoring survey conducted by CAN (Centralförbundet för Alkohol- och Narkotikaupplysning). The most recent report (Guttormsson, 2022) provides a series of different measures of alcohol consumption for 17–29-year-olds. These data are summarised in Tables 2.1 and 2.2.

On most measures, alcohol consumption for young adults in Sweden has declined, but that decline was concentrated between 2004 and

**Table 2.2** Trends in other drinking measures among young adults

| | | | | | | | | | | | | | | | | | | | |
|---|---|---|---|---|---|---|---|---|---|---|---|---|---|---|---|---|---|---|---|
| | Sweden | | 2005 | 2006 | 2007 | 2008 | 2009 | 2010 | 2011 | 2012 | 2013 | 2014 | 2015 | 2016 | 2017 | 2018 | 2019 | 2020 | 2021 |
| 17–29 | Any drinking (past month)[a] | Both | 80% | 78% | 78% | 75% | 74% | 72% | 72% | 72% | 72% | 75% | 77% | 77% | 74% | 72% | 72% | 71% | 71% |
| | Number of drinking days in the past month[a] | Both | 4.2 | 4.1 | 4.0 | 3.8 | 3.6 | 3.4 | 3.4 | 3.4 | 3.5 | 3.9 | 4.1 | 4.1 | 4.0 | 4.1 | 3.6 | 3.3 | 3.5 |
| | Volume of alcohol (past month)[a] | Both | 1.2l | 1.0l | 1.1l | 0.9l | 0.8l | 0.8l | 0.8l | 0.9l | 0.9l | 0.8l | 0.8l | 0.9l | 0.8l | 0.9l | 0.9l | 0.7l | 0.9l |
| | Germany | | 2005 | | | 2008 | | 2010 | 2011 | 2012 | | 2014 | 2015 | 2016 | 2017 | 2018 | 2019 | 2020 | 2021 |
| 18–25 | Weekly drinking[b] | Men | 55% | | | 53% | | 48% | 55% | 52% | | 47% | 46% | 41% | | 45% | 42% | | 40% |
| | | Women | 25% | | | 20% | | 20% | 24% | 24% | | 23% | 20% | 20% | | 22% | 23% | | 23% |
| | Finland | | 2000 | | | | | 2008 | | | | | 2016 | | | | | | |
| 15–19 | Median volume of pure alcohol consumed in the past year[c] | Men | 1.9 | | | | | 0.8 | | | | | 0.5 | | | | | | |
| | | Women | 1.1 | | | | | 0.8 | | | | | 0.3 | | | | | | |
| 20–29 | Median volume of pure alcohol consumed in the past year[c] | Men | 3.7 | | | | | 3.7 | | | | | 1.8 | | | | | | |
| | | Women | 1.0 | | | | | 1.0 | | | | | 0.9 | | | | | | |
| | Norway | | | | | | | | | 2012 | 2013 | 2014 | 2015 | 2016 | 2017 | 2018 | 2019 | 2020 | 2021 |
| 16–24 | Past year drinking[d] | Both | | | | | | | | 87% | 86% | 82% | 80% | 80% | 80% | 77% | 85% | 85% | 82% |
| | Denmark | | | | | | | | | | | 2014 | 2015 | 2016 | 2017 | | | | |

| 15–25 | Lifetime abstainer[e] | Both | | | | | | | | | 11% | 12% | 18% | 19% | | 15% | | |
|---|---|---|---|---|---|---|---|---|---|---|---|---|---|---|---|---|---|---|
| | New Zealand | | | 2006–2007 | | | | | 2011–2012 | 2012–2013 | 2013–2014 | 2014–2015 | 2015–2016 | 2016–2017 | 2017–2018 | 2018–2019 | 2019–2020 | 2020–2021 |
| 18–24 | Past year drinking[f] | Both | | 89% | | | | | 85% | 86% | 84% | 86% | 85% | 84% | 84% | 86% | 85% | 86% |
| | Canada | | 2004 | | 2008 | 2009 | 2010 | 2011 | 2012 | 2013 | | 2015 | | 2017 | | 2019 | | |
| 15–24 | Past 12-month use[g] | Both | 83% | | 78% | 76% | 72% | 71% | 70% | 73% | | 72% | | 71% | | 65% | | |

[a] CAN (Centralförbundet för Alkohol- och Narkotikaupplysning) Survey
[b] Federal Centre for Health Education Surveys Denmark
[c] Drinking Habits Survey, Finland
[d] Alkoholbruk i den voksne befolkningen
[e] Full of Life Survey, Norway
[f] New Zealand Health Survey
[g] CAS, CADUMS and CTADS Surveys

2010—in subsequent years, drinking has been relatively stable and, for some measures, increased. Thus, for example, the prevalence of risky drinking by 17–29-year-olds in the past month fell from 50% to 40% between 2005 and 2009, but has not dropped below 40% in the subsequent 12 years. Similar patterns are evident for other Swedish measures (e.g. any drinking fell from 80% in 2005 to 74% in 2009 and has been broadly stable ever since).

## Germany

Overall, alcohol consumption in Germany has been steadily declining from its peak of nearly 14 litres of pure alcohol per person in the late 1970s down to less than 10 litres per person in the most recent data available (Anderson & Pinilla, 2017). Data on adolescent drinking from the 2014 HBSC report (World Health Organisation, 2018a) found that weekly drinking had roughly halved for both boys and girls between 2002 and 2014, although the most recent HBSC report shows an uptick in drinking (albeit using past 30 day consumption, not a weekly drinking measure) (Inchley et al., 2020).

The most reliable data on German data on young adult drinking patterns come from a series of surveys run by the Federal Centre for Health Education. These surveys have been run irregularly between 2005 and 2021, with occasional years not available. Three different measures of drinking for 18–25-year-olds are presented in Tables 2.1 and 2.2.

These data show declines for all measures of drinking, especially for men. For example, between 2005 and 2021, the prevalence of heavy episodic drinking for men fell from 53% to 40%, while the decline for women was from 25% to 19%. In contrast to Sweden, the declines in Germany mostly occurred in more recent years (i.e. after 2012).

## Finland

Finland has seen some major alcohol policy changes in recent years, with spirits and beer taxes cut by around one-third in 2004 before increasing by 10% in 2009. Per-capita consumption moved as expected following these tax changes, increasing between 2003 and 2008 and then declining after the tax increase in 2009 (Anderson & Pinilla, 2017). In contrast, adolescent drinking fell across the period, seemingly unaffected by tax policy changes (Raitasalo et al., 2018). In 2018, a broader range of alcohol products were made widely available in grocery stores (up to 5.5% alcohol by volume), greatly expanding availability (Karlsson et al., 2020).

Finnish data for young adults comes from their long-running Drinking Habits Survey that has been collecting detailed and comparable data on Finnish drinking every eight years since the late 1960s (Härkönen et al., 2017). Because of the idiosyncratic nature of the questions used, the clearest measure of change over time is the median volume of pure alcohol reported by respondents. Trends for men and women among older teenagers (15–19) and younger adults (20–29) are presented in Table 2.2.

These data show a significant decline between 2000 and 2016, especially for men. Median drinking for older teenagers fell sharply for both men and women between 2000 and 2016 (dropping by more than half), while for 20–29-year-olds there was a sharp drop for men between 2008 and 2016, but little change for women. New data should be available in 2024, with the recent changes to availability potentially impacting consumption trends.

## Norway

Norway is another country with broadly restrictive alcohol policies. Per-capita consumption steadily increased by nearly 50% between 1993 and 2008 but has since been in decline. Drinking for 15-year-olds in the ESPAD survey has fallen by half, with 24% of respondents reporting past-month alcohol consumption in 2019, down from 48% in 2003 (ESPAD, 2023).

Consistently recorded data on Norwegian drinking is available only from 2012 onwards, via the Alkoholbruk i den voksne befolkningen (Alcohol consumption in the adult population) survey (Folke Helse Instituttet, 2022). Data on past-year drinking and past-year risky drinking are available across the period and are presented in Tables 2.1 and 2.2.

For both measures, trends were relatively stable for Norwegian young adults (aged 16–24), with some suggestion of a decline in the early years of the surveys (2012–2014), followed by broad stability over the remaining seven years of survey data available.

## Denmark

Denmark has the most liberal alcohol policy of the Nordic countries, with widespread alcohol availability and relatively relaxed drinking age laws. Per-capita consumption there has historically been high, although it has fallen by 20% since a peak of 10.1 litres of pure alcohol per person in 1996 (Anderson & Pinilla, 2017). These declines come during a period when adolescent drinking was a key policy focus, with a minimum purchase age of 16 implemented in 2004, even as taxes were cut in 2003. Danish adolescents have historically been among the heaviest drinking adolescents in Europe, but there have been steep declines there as in many other countries since 2002 (Andersen et al., 2014).

Consistently collected, long-term data on drinking by Danish young adults could not be located. Instead, we rely on recent surveys conducted as part of the 'Full of Life' campaign conducted between 2014 and 2019 (Kræftens Bekæmpelse (The Danish Cancer Society), 2021). The most consistent alcohol use measures were (1) abstinence from alcohol and (2) the frequency of binge drinking (more than 5 drinks (60g pure alcohol) on a single occasion) in the past month for 15–25-year-olds. Trends for these measures are presented in Tables 2.1 and 2.2.

Young adults are increasingly choosing not to drink at all, with the proportion reporting no alcohol consumption at all increasing from 11% in 2014 to 19% in 2017, but then dropping back to 15% in 2019. Risky drinking rates fell sharply, from 48% to 35% between 2014 and 2017, but have also increased slightly by 2019 to 37%.

## New Zealand

Per-capita consumption in New Zealand has been relatively stable since the early 2000s, while adolescent consumption has declined sharply (Clark et al., 2013).

Data for New Zealand come from the New Zealand Health Survey (NZHS). The NZHS was conducted in 2006–2007 and then annually in 2011–2012. The drinking questions were changed in 2016–2017, but trends appear relatively unaffected (New Zealand Ministry of Health, 2022). There are three measures collected over the period: hazardous drinking as measured by the AUDIT score, regular drinking occasions of 6+ standard drinks (60g or more of pure alcohol) and any past year drinking.

There were no clear trends in any measures in New Zealand, with decreases between the earliest survey in 2006–2007 and 2011–2012 largely washing out over the remaining decade of data.

## Canada

Per-capita consumption in Canada increased slightly through the early part of the 2000s and has been stable since about 2008. Adolescent alcohol consumption has also fallen substantially in Canada (de Looze et al., 2015).

Canadian alcohol consumption data for young adults come from a variety of sources: The Canadian Addiction Survey (CAS, 2004), the Canadian Alcohol Drug Use Monitoring Survey (CADUMS, 2008–2012) and the Canadian Tobacco Alcohol and Drugs Survey (CTADS, 2013–2019). These three surveys are closely related and, while the methodologies have changed across waves, key alcohol questions are consistent across time allowing for some tentative comparisons. We have relied on published estimates for 15–24-year-olds from the CAS, CADUMS and CTADS (Health Canada, 2012, 2020) but had to manually combine estimates for 15–19 and 20–24-year-olds (based on population estimates provided in the results) from the CTADS (Health Canada, 2018) due to changes in reporting practices. Risky drinking prevalence trends are presented in Table 2.1 (for both acute and chronic risks), while trends in any alcohol consumption are presented in Table 2.2.

The data presented show a decline in past 12-month use, especially between 2004 and 2010. In contrast, risky drinking rates were stable across the study period.

## Spain

Alcohol research has been a much lower priority in Southern European countries than in the Anglo and Northern European countries discussed above. Per-capita consumption in Spain has historically been markedly higher than most of the countries discussed thus far, but drinking patterns have tended to be less intoxication oriented and the risks of alcohol consumption have been less of an emphasis in research and public policy (Room & Mäkelä, 2000). Despite the substantially different context, adolescent drinking in Spain appears to show the same trends as many of the other countries discussed in this chapter, with weekly drinking declining by around half between 2010 and 2018 (Leal-López et al., 2021).

Data on alcohol consumption trends for young adults in Spain come from the Encuesta Sobre Alcohol y Otras Drogas en España (EDADES—Survey on Alcohol and Drugs in Spain), reported in a major compendium of alcohol and drug data for the period 1995–2022 (Observatorio Espanol de las Dragas y las Addiciones, 2023). Age-specific trend data were only reported for the past year prevalence of intoxication (self-reported), which is largely subjective and potentially influenced by changing norms around what 'intoxication' might mean. Trends are presented in Table 2.1 for men and women aged 15–34.

Self-reported rates of intoxication were stable for men and slightly increasing for women between 2005 and 2020.

## France

Per-capita consumption has declined in France since the 1950s, falling by more than half from nearly 20 litres of pure alcohol per person to around 9 (Anderson & Pinilla, 2017). Adolescent drinking in France has declined, but not as steeply as it has in many other European countries (World Health Organisation, 2018a).

Data from France's public health Barometer series suggests that for 18–24-year-old men and women, two measures of risky drinking—occasional heavy drinking and at least 10 drunken events in the past 12 months—rose sharply between 2010 and 2014 compared to 2005 and then dropped slightly by 2017. For example, for 18–24-year-old men, occasional drinking increased sharply from 12% to 17% between 2005 and 2010 and showed slight decline by 2014 to 14%. Similarly, for women occasional heavy drinking rose from 2% to 6% from 2005 to 2010 and plateaued thereafter, until 2017.

## Discussion

The data presented here provide relatively mixed evidence that alcohol consumption for young adults had declined across a range of high-income countries. The time periods, measures and age groups for which data are available vary markedly, which makes drawing the data together into a simple summary difficult. It is clear, however, that some countries have seen marked declines in drinking among young adults. In Australia and the UK, measures of risky drinking have fallen by at least a quarter since 2007, while Denmark has seen a similar sized drop in recent years. Young adults below the age of 23 in the USA have also seen marked decreases in drinking, while trends for those in their mid/late twenties have been more stable. In general, where sex-specific data were available, trends for men and women have been similar, with the notable exception of Finland, where the median amount of pure alcohol consumed by men aged 20–29 fell from 3.7l in 2000 to 1.8l in 2016, while for women of the same age consumption fell from 1.0l to 0.9l.

There were also countries where a significant decline in young adult drinking was not identified or where declines had been largely short-lived. Notably traditional wine cultures, France and Spain saw no evidence of declines in drinking. Quite a few countries reported some declines in drinking, but not in recent years. Thus, for example, all measures of drinking for Swedish young people (aged 17–29) fell between 2004 and 2010, but there has been stability or increases in subsequent years. Similar patterns were evident in Norway, Canada and New Zealand. Even in England, Denmark and Australia, where declines have been substantial, the trends seem to have stabilised or even begun to reverse in recent survey waves.

Thus, the overall picture does not strongly suggest that declines in drinking during adolescence is leading to long-running generational drinking declines in many countries. While in some places drinking is clearly lower than for previous generations, there remains significant variation to consider. These variations raise fascinating questions. Why, for example, do we see no decline in young adult drinking in Spain despite dramatic reductions in adolescent drinking? Why do Swedish and Australian trends for young adults look so different when adolescent drinking statistics for the two countries are markedly similar? These questions require much more in-depth research data than that which can be attained using monitoring surveys. We have not included here any analysis of key socio-demographic factors likely to influence the experience of being young adults across these countries—for instance, employment prospects for young adults are likely to vary considerably. Cultural practices around alcohol and young adulthood are similarly unlikely to be consistent around the world and research from a range of theoretical and methodological traditions is necessary to provide a more nuanced understanding of the drivers of the trends reported here.

The data presented here provide only limited opportunities to assess how the disruption of the COVID-19 pandemic in 2020 (and beyond) has influenced young adult drinking trends. There are no startling outliers among the countries where monitoring data for 2020 or 2021 have been published, suggesting potentially limited impacts, but much more in-depth and country-specific work is necessary given the wildly varying approaches to and experiences of the pandemic across the countries examined.

Of course the data presented here are limited in numerous ways—age-specific alcohol consumption data relies inherently on self-report surveys which are prone to a wide range of biases that have the potential to change over time (Gmel & Rehm, 2004). These issues are magnified by the marked changes in survey methodologies that have occurred in many of the series we report on, not to mention the diversity of measures and survey practices between countries. These limitations contrast with the general consistency of methods and approach in the two major cross-national studies of adolescent drinking (HBSC and ESPAD) and raise the question as to whether a similar standardisation of approach is necessary to ensure we better understand the changing patterns of alcohol consumption in young adulthood, a period where the risk of alcohol-related harm is substantial.

The data reported here represent fascinating differences in behaviour over time and between jurisdictions that require urgent examination. While there is an increasing body of work exploring the reasons for the decline in teenage drinking (Caluzzi et al., 2022; Vashishtha et al., 2020) and initial attempts have been made to assess how these trends play out over the life course in some countries (Kraus et al., 2024; Livingston et al., 2022), there remains little work exploring whether, how and why these declines continue into adulthood. Understanding the longer-term outcomes of declines in teenage drinking is crucial to better assess the public health implications, and ongoing qualitative and quantitative research in this space is crucial.

## References

Acuff, S. F., Strickland, J. C., Tucker, J. A., & Murphy, J. G. (2022). Changes in alcohol use during COVID-19 and associations with contextual and individual difference variables: A systematic review and meta-analysis. *Psychology of Addictive Behaviors, 36*(1), 1.

Andersen, A., Rasmussen, M., Bendtsen, P., Due, P., & Holstein, B. E. (2014). Secular trends in alcohol drinking among Danish 15-year-olds: Comparable representative samples from 1988 to 2010. *Journal of Research on Adolescence, 24*(4), 748–756.

Anderson, K., & Pinilla, V. (2017). Annual Database of Global Wine Markets, 1835 to 2016. Wine Economics Research Centre, University of Adelaide. Retrieved 18 December 2024, from https://economics.adelaide.edu.au/wine-economics/databases#annual-database-of-global-wine-markets-1835-to-2023

Australian Institute of Health and Welfare. (2017). 2016 National Drug Strategy Household Survey - Detailed Report. Canberra, AIHW. Retrieved 9 January 2025, from https://www.aihw.gov.au/reports/illicit-use-of-drugs/2016-ndshs-detailed/data

Bhattacharya, A. (2016). *Youthful abandon: Why are young people drinking less?* Institute for Alcohol Studies. Retrieved 18 December 2024, from http://www.ias.org.uk/uploads/pdf/IAS%20reports/rp22072016.pdf

Britton, A., Ben-Shlomo, Y., Benzeval, M., Kuh, D., & Bell, S. (2015). Life course trajectories of alcohol consumption in the United Kingdom using longitudinal data from nine cohort studies. *BMC Medicine, 13*(1), 47.

Callinan, S., Pennay, A., Livingston, M., & Kuntsche, E. (2020). Patterns of alcohol consumption in 16 cohorts of Australian young adults aged 15–24 between 2001 and 2016. *Addiction, 115*(8), 1452–1458.

Caluzzi, G., Livingston, M., Holmes, J., MacLean, S., Lubman, D., Dietze, P., Vashishtha, R., Herring, R., & Pennay, A. (2022). Declining drinking among adolescents: Are we seeing a denormalisation of drinking and a normalisation of non-drinking? *Addiction, 117*(5), 1204–1212.

Cisneros Örnberg, J. (2009). *The Europeanization of Swedish alcohol policy.* Statsvetenskapliga institutionen. Retrieved 9 January 2025, from https://www.diva-portal.org/smash/get/diva2:200235/FULLTEXT01.pdf

Clark, T. C., Fleming, T., Bullen, P., Denny, S., Crengle, S., Dyson, B., Fortune, S., Lucassen, M., Peiris-John, R., Robinson, E., Rossen, F., Sheridan, J., Teevale, T., & Utter, J. (2013). *Youth'12 overview: The health and wellbeing of New Zealand secondary school students in 2012.* The University of Auckland. Retrieved 9 January 2025, from https://www.fmhs.auckland.ac.nz/assets/fmhs/faculty/ahrg/docs/2012-overview.pdf

Dawson, D. A., Goldstein, R. B., Patricia Chou, S., June Ruan, W., & Grant, B. F. (2008). Age at first drink and the first incidence of adult-onset DSM-IV alcohol use disorders. *Alcoholism: Clinical and Experimental Research, 32*(12), 2149–2160.

de Looze, M., Raaijmakers, Q., ter Bogt, T., Bendtsen, P., Farhat, T., Ferreira, M., Godeau, E., Kuntsche, E., Molcho, M., & Pförtner, T.-K. (2015). Decreases in adolescent weekly alcohol use in Europe and North America: Evidence from 28 countries from 2002 to 2010. *The European Journal of Public Health, 25*(suppl 2), 69–72.

Delbosc, A., & Currie, G. (2013). Causes of youth licensing decline: A synthesis of evidence. *Transport Reviews, 33*(3), 271–290.

Englund, M. M., Egeland, B., Oliva, E. M., & Collins, W. A. (2008). Childhood and adolescent predictors of heavy drinking and alcohol use disorders in early adulthood: A longitudinal developmental analysis. *Addiction, 103*(s1), 23–35.

ESPAD. (2023). *European School Survey Project on alcohol and other drugs, data tool.* EMCDDA Joint Publications. Retrieved 9 January 2025, from https://data.espad.org/

Folke Helse Instituttet. (2022). *Alkoholbruk i den voksne befolkningen* (Alcohol Consumption in the Adult Population). Norwegian Institute of Public Health.

Retrieved 23 November 2023, from https://www.fhi.no/le/alkohol/alkoholinorge/omsetning-og-bruk/alkoholbruk-i-den-voksne-befolkningen/?h=1&term=

Gmel, G., & Rehm, J. (2004). Measuring alcohol consumption. *Contemporary Drug Problems, 31*, 467–540.

Grant, B. F., & Dawson, D. A. (1997). Age at onset of alcohol use and its association with DSM-IV alcohol abuse and dependence: Results from the national longitudinal alcohol epidemiologic survey. *Journal of Substance Abuse, 9*, 103–110.

Grucza, R. A., Sher, K. J., Kerr, W. C., Krauss, M. J., Lui, C. K., McDowell, Y. E., Hartz, S., Virdi, G., & Bierut, L. J. (2018). Trends in adult alcohol use and binge drinking in the early 21st-century United States: A meta-analysis of 6 National Survey Series. *Alcoholism: Clinical and Experimental Research, 42*(10), 1939–1950.

Guttormsson, U. (2022). *Självrapporterade alkoholvanor i Sverige 2004–2021* (Self-reported alcohol habits in Sweden 2004–2021). Centralförbundet för alkohol- och narkotikaupplysning, CAN. Retrieved 9 January 2025, from https://www.can.se/app/uploads/2022/11/can-rapport-213-sjalvrapporterade-alkoholvanor-i-sverige-2004-2021.pdf

Hall, W., & Lynskey, M. (2016). Why it is probably too soon to assess the public health effects of legalisation of recreational cannabis use in the USA. *The Lancet Psychiatry, 3*(9), 900–906.

Hallgren, M. L., Hakan, L., & Andreasson, S. (2012). Drinking less but greater harm: Could polarized drinking habits explain the divergence between alcohol consumption and harms among youth? *Alcohol and Alcoholism, 47*(5), 581–590.

Härkönen, J., Savonen, J., Virtala, E., & Mäkelä, P. (2017). *Suomalaisten alkoholinkäyttötavat 1968—2016* (Finnish Drinking Habits, 1968-2016). Terveyden Ja Hyvinvionnin Laitos. Retrieved 9 January 2025, from https://www.julkari.fi/bitstream/handle/10024/134585/URN_ISBN_978-952-302-873-9.pdf

Health Canada. (2012). *Canadian alcohol and drug use monitoring survey - survey tables*. Health Canada. Retrieved 9 January 2025, from https://www.canada.ca/en/health-canada/services/canadian-alcohol-drugs-survey/canadian-alcohol-drug-use-monitoring-survey-summary-results-2011.html

Health Canada. (2018). *Canadian tobacco, alcohol and drugs survey*. Health Canada. Retrieved 9 January 2025, from https://www.canada.ca/en/health-canada/services/canadian-alcohol-drugs-survey/2017-summary.html

Health Canada. (2020). *Canadian tobacco, alcohol and drugs survey 2019 summary*. Health Canada. Retrieved 9 January 2025, from https://www.canada.ca/en/health-canada/services/canadian-alcohol-drugs-survey/2019-summary.html

Hingson, R. W., & Zha, W. (2009). Age of drinking onset, alcohol use disorders, frequent heavy drinking, and unintentionally injuring oneself and others after drinking. *Pediatrics, 123*(6), 1477–1484.

Hussong, A. M., Haik, A. K., & Loeb, H. M. (2023). Generation COVID: Young adult substance use. *Current Opinion in Psychology, 52*, 101640.

Inchley, J., Currie, D., Budisavljevic, S., Torsheim, T., Jastad, A., Cosma, A., Kelly, C., Arnarsson, A., & Samdal, O. (2020). *Spotlight on health and wellbeing: Findings from the 2017/18 HBSC Survey in Europe and Canada*. WHO Regional Office for Europe. Retrieved 9 January 2025, from https://www.who.int/europe/publications/i/item/9789289055000

Institute for Health Metrics. (2016). GBD compare data visualization. University of Washington. Retrieved 9 January 2025, from http://vizhub.healthdata.org/gbd-compare

Institute for Health Metrics and Evaluation. (2021). *GBD results tool, global health data exchange*. University of Washington. Retrieved 9 January 2025, from https://www.healthdata.org/data-tools-practices/interactive-visuals/gbd-results

Jang, J. B., Patrick, M. E., Keyes, K. M., Hamilton, A. D., & Schulenberg, J. E. (2017). Frequent binge drinking among US adolescents, 1991 to 2015. *Pediatrics, 139*(6), e20164023.

Johnston, L., O'Malley, P., Bachman, J., & Schulenberg, J. (2006a). *Monitoring the Future national survey results on drug use, 1975–2005: Volume I: Secondary school students*. University of Michigan. Retrieved 9 January 2025, from https://monitoringthefuture.org/wp-content/uploads/2022/08/mtf-vol1_2010.pdf

Johnston, L., O'Malley, P., Bachman, J., & Schulenberg, J. (2006b). *Monitoring the Future national survey results on drug use, 1975–2005: Volume II: College students and adults*. University of Michigan. https://files.eric.ed.gov/fulltext/ED514367.pdf

Kalinowski, A., & Humphreys, K. (2016). Governmental standard drink definitions and low-risk alcohol consumption guidelines in 37 countries. *Addiction, 111*(7), 1293–1298.

Karlsson, T., Mäkelä, P., Tigerstedt, C., & Keskimäki, I. (2020). The road to the alcohol act 2018 in Finland: A conflict between public health objectives and neoliberal goals. *Health Policy, 124*(1), 1–6.

Kerr, W. C., Greenfield, T. K., Bond, J., Ye, Y., & Rehm, J. (2009). Age–period–cohort modelling of alcohol volume and heavy drinking days in the US National Alcohol Surveys: Divergence in younger and older adult trends. *Addiction, 104*(1), 27–37.

Kræftens Bekæmpelse (The Danish Cancer Society). (2021). *Danskernes alkoholvaner 2020 (Danes' alcohol habits 2020)*. Danish Cancer Society. Retrieved 9 January 2025, from https://www.cancer.dk/forebyg/drik-mindre-alkohol/rapporter-og-forskning/rapporter/

Kraus, L., Loy, J. K., Olderbak, S., Trolldal, B., Ramstedt, M., Svensson, J., & Törrönen, J. (2024). Does the decline in Swedish adolescent drinking persist into early adulthood? *Addiction, 119*(2), 259–267.

Kraus, L., Tinghög, M. E., Lindell, A., Pabst, A., Piontek, D., & Room, R. (2015). Age, period and cohort effects on time trends in alcohol consumption in the Swedish adult population 1979–2011. *Alcohol and Alcoholism, 50*(3), 319–327.

Kraus, L., et al. (2018). 'Are The Times A-Changin'? Trends in adolescent substance use in Europe. *Addiction, 113*(7), 1317–1332.

Larm, P., Raninen, J., Åslund, C., Svensson, J., & Nilsson, K. W. (2019). The increased trend of non-drinking alcohol among adolescents: What role do internet activities have? *European Journal of Public Health, 29*(1), 27–32.

Leal-López, E., Sánchez-Queija, I., Rivera, F., & Moreno, C. (2021). Tendencias en el consumo de alcohol en adolescentes escolarizados en España (2010-2018). *Gaceta Sanitaria, 35*, 35–41.

Leggat, G., Livingston, M., Kuntsche, S., & Callinan, S. (2021). The development of drinking trajectories among australian young adults. *Journal of Studies on Alcohol and Drugs, 82*(2), 237–245.

Lintonen, T., Härkönen, J., Raitasalo, K., Härkänen, T., & Mäkelä, P. (2016). Decreasing adolescent drinking: Is there evidence of a continuation into future adult cohorts? APC analysis of adolescent drinking in Finland, 1983–2013. *Scandinavian Journal of Public Health, 44*(7), 654–662.

Livingston, M. (2014)Trends in non-drinking amongst Australian adolescents. *Addiction, 109*(6), 922–929.

Livingston, M., Callinan, S., Raninen, J., Pennay, A., & Dietze, P. M. (2018). Alcohol consumption trends in Australia: Comparing surveys and sales-based measures. *Drug and Alcohol Review, 37*, S9–S14.

Livingston, M., Callinan, S., Vashishtha, R., Yuen, W. S., & Dietze, P. (2022). Tracking the decline in Australian adolescent drinking into adulthood. *Addiction, 117*(5), 1273–1281.

Livingston, M., & Dietze, P. (2016). National survey data can be used to measure trends in population alcohol consumption in Australia. *Australian and New Zealand Journal of Public Health, 40*(3), 233–235.

Livingston, M., Raninen, J., Slade, T., Swift, W., Lloyd, B., & Dietze, P. (2016). Understanding trends in Australian alcohol consumption - an age, period, cohort model. *Addiction, 111*(7), 1203–1213.

Meng, Y., Holmes, J., Hill-McManus, D., Brennan, A., & Meier, P. S. (2014). Trend analysis and modelling of gender-specific age, period and birth cohort effects on alcohol abstention and consumption level for drinkers in Great Britain using the General Lifestyle Survey 1984–2009. *Addiction, 109*(2), 206–215.

National Health and Medical Research Council. (2009). *Australian guidelines to reduce health risks from drinking alcohol*. NHMRC. Retrieved 9 January 2025, from https://aci.health.nsw.gov.au/__data/assets/pdf_file/0014/212153/NHMRC-Alcohol-guidelines.pdf

New Zealand Ministry of Health. (2022). *Annual Data Explorer 2021/22: New Zealand Health Survey*. New Zealand Ministry of Health. Retrieved 9 January 2025, from https://minhealthnz.shinyapps.io/nz-health-survey-2021-22-annual-data-explorer/_w_85911c0a/#!/home

Norström, T., & Ramstedt, M. (2018). The link between per capita alcohol consumption and alcohol-related harm in Sweden, 1987–2015. *Journal of Studies on Alcohol and Drugs, 79*(4), 578–584.

Norström, T., & Svensson, J. (2014). The declining trend in Swedish youth drinking: Collectivity or polarization? *Addiction, 109*(9), 1437–1446.

Observatorio Espanol de las Dragas y las Addiciones. (2023). *Estadisticas 2022 - Alcohol, tabaco y drogas ilegales in Espana: Encuesta Sobre Alcohol y Drogas en Espana, 1995-2022 (Statistics 2022 - Alcohol, tobacco and illicit drugs in Spain: Survey on alcohol and drugs in Spain, 1995-2022)*. Observatorio Español de las Drogas y las Adicciones (OEDA). Retrieved 9 January 2025, from https://pnsd.sanidad.gob.es/profesionales/sistemasInformacion/informesEstadisticas/pdf/2022OEDA-INFORME.pdf

Oldham, M., Holmes, J., Whitaker, V., Fairbrother, H., & Curtis, P. (2018). Youth drinking in decline. The University of Sheffield. Retrieved 9 January 2025, from https://eprints.whiterose.ac.uk/136587/1/Oldham_Holmes_Youth_drinking_in_decline_FINAL.pdf

Pape, H., Rossow, I., & Brunborg, G. S. (2018). Adolescents drink less: How, who and why? A review of the recent research literature. *Drug and Alcohol Review, 37*, S98–S114.

Patrick, M. E., Schulenberg, J. E., Miech, R. A., Johnston, L. D., O'Malley, P. M., & Bachman, J. G. (2022). *Monitoring the Future Panel Study annual report: National data on substance use among adults ages 19 to 60, 1976-2021.* University of Michigan Institute for Social Research. Retrieved 9 January 2025, from https://monitoringthefuture.org/results/annual-reports/panel-study-annual-report-adults-1976-2021/

Patrick, M. E., Terry-McElrath, Y. M., Miech, R. A., Schulenberg, J. E., O'Malley, P. M., & Johnston, L. D. (2017). Age-specific prevalence of binge and high-intensity drinking among U.S. Young Adults: Changes from 2005 to 2015. *Alcoholism: Clinical and Experimental Research, 41*(7), 1319–1328.

Pickett, W., Molcho, M., Elgar, F. J., Brooks, F., De Looze, M., Rathmann, K., Ter Bogt, T. F., Gabhainn, S. N., Sigmundová, D., & de Matos, M. G. (2013). Trends and socioeconomic correlates of adolescent physical fighting in 30 countries. *Pediatrics, 131*(1), e18–e26.

Raitasalo, K., Simonen, J., Tigerstedt, C., Mäkelä, P., & Tapanainen, H. (2018). What is going on in underage drinking? Reflections on Finnish European school survey project on alcohol and other drugs data 1999–2015. *Drug and Alcohol Review, 37*(S1), S76–S84.

Room, R., & Mäkelä, K. (2000). Typologies of the cultural position of drinking. *Journal of Studies on Alcohol, 61*(3), 475–483.

Svensson, J. A., & Andersson, D.-E. (2016). What role do changes in the demographic composition play in the declining trends in alcohol consumption and the increase of non-drinkers among Swedish youth? A time-series analysis of trends in non-drinking and region of origin 1971-2012. *Alcohol and Alcoholism, 51*(2), 172–176.

Vashishtha, R., Livingston, M., Pennay, A., Dietze, P., MacLean, S., Holmes, J., Herring, R., Caluzzi, G., & Lubman, D. I. (2020). Why is adolescent drinking declining? A systematic review and narrative synthesis. *Addiction Research and Theory, 28*(4), 275–288.

Vashishtha, R., Pennay, A., Dietze, P., Marzan, M. B., Room, R., & Livingston, M. (2021). Trends in adolescent drinking across 39 high-income countries: Exploring the timing and magnitude of decline. *European Journal of Public Health, 31*(2), 424–431.

Wechsler, H., Dowdall, G. W., Davenport, A., & Castillo, S. (1995). Correlates of college student binge drinking. *American Journal of Public Health, 85*(7), 921–926.

White, V., & Williams, T. (2016). *Australian secondary school students' use of tobacco, alcohol, and over-the-counter and illicit substances in 2014*. Cancer Council Victoria. Retrieved 9 January 2025, from https://www.health.gov.au/resources/publications/secWondary-school-students-use-of-tobacco-alcohol-and-other-drugs-in-2014?language=en

World Health Organisation. (2018a). *Adolescent alcohol-related behaviours: Trends and inequalities in the WHO European Region, 2002–2014*. WHO Regional Office for Europe. Retrieved 9 January 2025, from https://www.who.int/europe/publications/i/item/9789289053495

World Health Organisation. (2018b). *Global status report on alcohol and health 2018*. WHO. Retrieved 9 January 2025, from https://www.who.int/publications/i/item/9789241565639

# 3

# Alcohol, Young Adults, and the New Millennium: Changing Meanings in a Changing Social Climate

Gabriel Caluzzi and Amy Pennay

**Abstract** Situated within a social generations framework, this chapter explores some of the conditions shaping an apparent decline in alcohol consumption among young people. The authors review the importance of a number of changing social conditions and what it means for alcohol consumption among young adults, including changing patterns of work and study, living arrangements, the digital boom, the importance of parents, and an apparent decrease in a range of other risky activities. The decline in young adult drinking is also contrasted against an apparent rise in mental health problems for young adults. The authors reiterate the need to consider long-term trends in alcohol consumption alongside broader social and structural factors, and provide suggestions for future areas of research.

Since the turn of the millennium, significant declines in drinking have been observed among young adults (a term covering the transitional

---

G. Caluzzi (✉) • A. Pennay
Centre for Alcohol Policy Research, La Trobe University, Melbourne, VIC, Australia
e-mail: G.Caluzzi@latrobe.edu.au; A.Pennay@latrobe.edu.au



D. Conroy, F. Measham (eds.), *Young Adult Drinking Styles*, Sustainable Development Goals Series, https://doi.org/10.1007/978-3-031-98528-7_3

period from adolescence to adulthood) in many high-income countries. In recent years, a wealth of research has been undertaken exploring these declines. This includes epidemiological, psychological, and sociological studies attempting to unpack these declines. What we have learned so far is complex; individual factors often have both 'push' and 'pull' effects on young people's drinking, are often interrelated, and occur within the broader social changes to young people's lives. Changing understandings of health and risk, new practices around parenting, leisure and technology, broad labour market shifts, and ways of doing 'young adulthood' have undoubtedly influenced the social role and meanings associated with alcohol. By drawing on sociological and empirical literature we argue for the importance of examining young adults' current drinking practices in high-income countries within the context of unique post-millennial developments.

## Understanding Young Adults: A Social Generations Perspective

We situate young adults' drinking in high-income countries within a social generations perspective. That is, we contend that young adults exist within socio-historical conditions that create generations of shared experiences and consciousness (see Mannheim, 1952 [1927]). For example, almost a quarter of the way through the twenty-first century, young adults are staying in education for longer, while 'traditional' transitions into work, family formation, and home ownership have become protracted often well into the late twenties and thirties, or abandoned altogether. While young adults face contemporary conditions that affect all other age groups—including economic precarity, climate crises, and other social challenges—they are more susceptible to social change, and more likely to experiment with different ways of living as a response (Woodman & Wyn, 2014). Sociologists have suggested young adults today are experiencing several unique conditions: precarious labour markets marked by job competitiveness, higher education levels, ubiquity of digital communications, greater pursuit of satisfying careers, difficulty building and maintaining intimate relationships, delayed family formation, and a diversification of lifestyles (Furlong & Cartmel, 2006; Woodman, 2016).

While generational patterns are not linear, universal, or deterministic, social generations theory is useful for thinking about the diversity of lifestyles young adults can now lead, and their shared experiences of fragmentation and social change. This approach is particularly relevant as globalisation and communications technology have forged a 'post-traditional cosmopolitan world' (Beck, 2000, p. 211) for young adults since the new millennium. One key feature of this world is the shift towards neoliberalism, and a subsequent emphasis on individualism, choice, and personal responsibility. As we will detail, these concepts are central to the generational changes that may be shifting the position of alcohol for young adults, including risk aversion and the changing nature of family, leisure, digital technology, and wellbeing.

## Decreasing 'Risky' Activities

Neoliberalism places the onus on individuals to 'manage risk', and there is good evidence to suggest that drinking is not the only risk practice that has declined, or is at least being delayed, for young adults in high-income countries. Age of learning to drive, socialising independent of parents, attending parties, dating, and having sex have also declined or been delayed for young adults across gender, socio-economic status, and ethnicities (Kann et al., 2016; Twenge, 2017). These have paralleled declines in drug use, as well as truancy, violence, and crime (Farrell et al., 2014; Vaughn et al., 2018). One theory is that because more contemporary young adults live in contexts with access to resources and parental support, they are more carefully planning out their lives, while avoiding risk and delaying 'adult' activities (Twenge & Park, 2019). Indeed, young abstainers tend to report greater academic engagement, parental cohesion, less propensity for risk, and having less substance-using peers (Vaughn et al., 2018). Even at a young age, young people can be conscious of how they spend their leisure time or 'free time', feeling obligated to be productive and think about their alcohol consumption (Caluzzi,

Pennay, MacLean et al., 2022). This suggests that young people are not only choosing to avoid risky activities but are also compelled by neoliberal imperatives to manage risk and think about the future. At the same time, many young adults face other ongoing forms of risk, such as insecure labour markets, economic downturns, climate crises, and, more recently, global pandemics.

The pressures to manage everyday risks—a seemingly inevitable feature of modern life—includes alcohol. In recent years, there has been an expansion of alcohol-related knowledge (often focused on harms) and heightened media coverage highlighting the negative effects of alcohol on young adults (Azar et al., 2014; Pennay et al., 2022). Such representations in media and popular discourse feed into associations between risk and alcohol, in turn encouraging self-regulation and responsibility. For example, recent studies have emphasised how young people view drinking alcohol as an increasingly risky activity requiring active management or avoidance (Ball et al., 2023; Caluzzi, Pennay, & MacLean, 2021; Pennay et al., 2023).

The risk aversion theory fits in with notions of delayed adulthood and postponement of risky practices; however, young adults also demonstrate more forward planning at a younger age than their generational predecessors (Wyn, 2016). This has led to the suggestion that young adults are exhibiting signs of earlier maturation, are becoming adult-like more quickly, and are more responsible and reflective than previous generations (Törrönen et al., 2019). Thus, it might not be that young people are avoiding risk, but rather are engaging with it differently. Indeed, it may be that many activities previously thought of as 'adult' (e.g., alcohol use, drug use, and other risk practices) have lost some of their connection to young adulthood, alongside alternative avenues for developing identity and independence.

## Parental Influence on Young Adults' Drinking

With its focus on individual responsibility, neoliberalism has been argued to shift responsibility for children's behaviour, success, and health firmly onto parents. Popular discourses (reinforced through education and media representations) promote the message that parents are expected to raise 'good' and productive children (Cook et al., 2023; Fargion, 2023). Alongside these shifting expectations of parental roles, delayed transitions to independence may also be changing young people's relationships with their parents. Indeed, with many young people spending more time in the family home and relying on parents for social and economic support for longer, the role of intergenerational familial relationships has become increasingly important, even as children transition into young adulthood. Longitudinal findings from Australian and Canadian studies indicate that since the late 2000s, family relationships have been reported as the most significant influence on the lives of young people (Wyn, 2011). Recent decades have seen a decline in the number of children parents have and an increase in the amount of time parents spend with their children (Sobotka & Toulemon, 2008). Related to this, some researchers have also noted a shift in parenting styles, which may have ramifications for young people's drinking (Chan et al., 2016; Scheffels et al., 2020; Törrönen et al., 2019).

On the one hand, young people's drinking has long been associated with rebellion against parents and previous generations (Johnson, 2013). If young people have less reason to symbolically 'rebel' against parents, so too might this impact their drinking styles. Indeed, it has been suggested that improved family cohesion, parent-child relationships, monitoring, and discipline have potentially contributed to declining alcohol use (Bhattacharya, 2016; Pape et al., 2018). Likewise, since traditional markers of independence (such as moving out) are also associated with increased autonomy, longer periods of economic constraint and delayed independence might also delay, or limit, consumption practices. For example, hedonistic consumption practices might become bounded by longer periods of dependence and increased familial supervision, limiting in a practical sense the time and space young adults have to 'let loose'.

On the other hand, one of the more consistent findings in research on declines in young adult drinking has suggested the importance of parents in monitoring, setting norms, and building closer relationships with their children (Pape et al., 2018; Vashishtha et al., 2019). Awareness of the role parents play in setting norms and expectations around alcohol use is also important. Parental permissiveness or strictness around alcohol is recognised as key to the development and shaping of drinking norms and practices in later life (Raitasalo & Holmila, 2017; Yap et al., 2017), including when and how parents introduce alcohol to young people. The neoliberal push towards 'competent parenting' (Cook et al., 2022) includes educational focus on delaying young people's alcohol initiation, increasing parental awareness of how they set drinking norms through policy changes and public health campaigns (e.g., secondary supply laws and education campaigns around parental modelling), and informal depictions of 'bad' parents in media representations of young people's drinking (Cook et al., 2023).

## The Digital Age

The incorporation of technology into the everyday lives of young adults has reshaped social worlds, fundamentally changing how young people understand themselves, connect with their social networks, and engage with broader cultural norms. As we have suggested, the impact of the digital age on young adults' drinking can be understood at the micro, meso, and macro levels (Caluzzi, Pennay, & Livingston, 2022). At the micro level, technologies like social media have become central to practices of identity work and performance (Goodwin & Griffin, 2017). Social media encourages curated presentations of health, style, and discipline, making social media's effect on alcohol consumption complicated. It may encourage drinking through positive alcohol narratives and photos (Supski et al., 2017) and there is some evidence to suggest a link between increased social media use and drinking (Larm et al., 2018; Pape et al., 2018). However, the link between alcohol and social media is likely to be mediated by social networks, as well as how individuals wish to portray themselves. In their neoliberal worlds, young adults may also be aware of the 'pedagogy of regret' that can accompany a night out (Brown & Gregg, 2012), with the idea that anyone (including parents, future employers, romantic interests, and friends) can survey social media content. Technologies also offer other ways of doing identity—for example, they can afford young men ways of expressing their masculinity through online gaming instead of alcohol consumption (Törrönen et al., 2019).

At the meso level, technologies can disrupt and transform the way young adults interact, connect with their social networks, and potentially drink with peers. The ability to socialise digitally can be done remotely and often at home, where young people are often still 'co-present' with their peers. With the Internet increasingly being used to initiate and maintain social relationships, both romantic and otherwise, the use of alcohol as a social lubricant may also be less necessary, and the imperative to find potential partners in licensed venues may have weakened. In contrast to busy entertainment precincts, technologies might provide young people with safer, more controlled, and cheaper alternatives to the night-time economy. Online gaming and increased access to networked media like streaming services have become meaningful, accessible, and pleasurable sources of social engagement for young adults. As credible pastimes, these may be replacing, or at least supplementing the role of alcohol. At the same time, digital technologies afford young people new ways to organise events and drinking contexts, meet up on a night out, create private networks and spaces to drink together, and, in general, greater opportunities to socialise (Caluzzi et al., 2023). Thus, the ways young adults coordinate their social activities (including drinking) is linked to the technologies that facilitate their interactions with people, locations, and various elements like transportation and alcoholic beverages.

At the macro level, digital technologies can also mediate cultural norms around alcohol. For example, social media sites also regularly expose their users to alcohol advertising, thus actively shaping discourses around alcohol normalisation and brand engagement, and raising questions about the 'intoxigenic' nature of digital spaces (Griffiths & Casswell, 2010). This commercialisation of alcohol is to some degree countered by health promotion campaigns, and the dissemination of information constructing alcohol as a hazard. Technologies have enabled also new cultural shifts, such as the online health and wellness movements and sobriety initiatives (Atkinson et al., 2023). Indeed, at the broader social and cultural level, it may be that digital technologies have fundamentally changed the way young adults live and interact—which may have deep-seated impacts on how they consume alcohol.

## The Link Between Mental Health and Alcohol

Despite general improvements in health, living conditions, life expectancy, and population-level affluence, mental health concerns continue to impact the wellbeing of many young adults in high-income countries. For young adults in the twenty-first century, internalising problems such as stress, anxiety, and depression have risen (Bor et al., 2014), as well as affective and emotional problems (Collishaw 2015). Because the relationship between alcohol and mental health is complex and often bi-directional (Hagell et al., 2012), it is important to explore the changing issues around mental health and its relationship with alcohol for young adults.

While many objective quality of life measures have improved, other culturally specific goals continue to shape perceptions of happiness. For example, stresses around body image, academic performance, career success, unstable employment conditions, and economic independence are all associated with psychological distress for young adults (West, 2016; Wyn et al., 2015). Indeed, neoliberalism puts the onus on individuals to manage health and wellbeing in the form of 'healthism'—pervasive discourses that privilege health, prescribe certain forms of beauty and consumption, and create pressures for young people to manage their health (Crawford, 1980). At the same time, worries about precarious and uncertain futures, for both themselves and the world, mean that stress and anxiety may also be more common features of the lives of contemporary young adults. Digital technologies are also implicated in changes to physical activity, sleep, social interactions, beauty and body image standards, online bullying and aggression, as well as creating accessible spaces for interaction, meaningful leisure pursuits, and new interfaces to support mental health.

This focus on health has been suggested as a reason for declines in young people's drinking (Caluzzi, MacLean et al., 2021). While it can provide positive benefits to wellbeing by enhancing confidence, sociability, and sense of belonging, it is also linked with well-known negative mental health outcomes including depression, stress, anxiety, and relationship problems (Newbury-Birch et al., 2009). Given the self-medicating properties of alcohol and its relationship with poorer mental health (Pedersen & von Soest, 2015), it might be expected that young adults would increase drinking if they face increased stresses in their lives. On the other hand, alcohol use might be avoided given its potential for disrupting productivity and diminishing mental health. Studies have shown that young people think about their physical and mental health in different ways than previous generations and draw on health as a reason to manage or reduce their drinking (Caluzzi, MacLean et al., 2021; Törrönen et al., 2021). The mounting evidence linking alcohol and mental health problems may be a connection that young adults are increasingly wary of. Now with new ways of socialising and immersion without alcohol, and greater emphasis on mental health awareness and self-care strategies, alcohol's previously established association with sociability and, by extension, social wellbeing may be changing.

At the same time, alcohol has been considered an important aspect of young people's social lives and wellbeing. Declines in young people's drinking have also not corresponded with increased engagement with other health behaviours (Fat et al., 2018; Vashishtha et al., 2021). Indeed, it may be that pressures placed on young adults to manage their lives, futures, and health in uncertain times might influence their relationship with alcohol, without necessarily enabling 'healthier lifestyles' (Caluzzi, Pennay, & MacLean, 2021). Thus, we may be witnessing a generation of young adults whose response to stress is to think about alcohol differently.

## Changing Lives, Changing Drinking Cultures

Alcohol, like other goods, is a cultural commodity tied to social status, individualism, choice, and identity. Historical trends highlight how broader societal and cultural reactions to alcohol can change over time according to sociohistorical context (Room et al., 2009). The effects of an increasingly connected and globalised world in diversifying culture, leisure pursuits, and access to information are all part of this context. For example, acculturation between traditional heavier and lighter drinking cultures may have had some impact on social norms around drinking

(Hoffmann et al., 2020; Rogne et al., 2019). Similarly, while gender norms associating alcohol and masculinity still exist, they are challenged by new ways of performing masculinity without alcohol and performing femininity with it (Demant & Törrönen, 2011; Törrönen et al., 2019). There also seems to be reduced acceptance of heavy drinking among young people (Ball et al., 2020) and young adults seem to demonstrate greater ambivalence towards losing control and drunkenness (MacLean et al., 2018).

The growth of no and low-alcohol alternatives highlights how the alcohol industry is seemingly accommodating the uptick of non-drinking among young people, enabling people to partake in drinking environments or situations while demonstrating responsibility and protection of their health (Nicholls, 2021). Alongside this, sobriety movements and initiatives that encourage young adults to challenge social norms around alcohol consumption have grown. Indeed, it seems that broader social shifts and more direct changes to alcohol-related norms among many young people have led to drinking cultures where light and non-drinking have become increasingly normalised, while heavy drinking has become, at least to some degree, denormalised (Caluzzi et al., 2022).

## Reflecting on Norms and Social Change

Building upon some of our theoretical discussions, we turn now to short reflections from interviews conducted with young adults in 2022. The young adults we talked to were participants in a longitudinal qualitative study examining the social practices and cultural norms related to alcohol among young people in Australia. When we first talked to them in 2018, they were aged 16–19 years old, and all identified as either abstainers or light drinkers (see Caluzzi et al., 2020). We then interviewed them two years later in 2020, and again in 2022 (La Trobe University ethics ID HEC19479). Each wave of interviews explored drinking patterns and attitudes towards alcohol, as well as technology use, health, relationships, and expectations for the future. Here, we draw on the most recent wave of interviews conducted in 2022, where the 36 participants interviewed were predominately in their early twenties. While the young people started as abstainers and light drinkers, drinking trajectories varied over time. Some maintained low levels of drinking or abstinence, some went through periods of experimentation and heavier drinking, and others gradually increased their drinking. We use selected excerpts to reflect on the ideas we have discussed above, and that reflect the many ways in which the role of alcohol might have changed for young adults. All excerpts presented use pseudonyms.

The young people we talked to had different living arrangements—some had moved out of home or were living at university campuses, and many still lived at home with their families. While most young people felt their drinking practices had become independent from their parents, several participants described continued cultural and religious expectations that influenced their drinking. Those living with their parents, in particular, maintained a degree of communication about their social lives. For example, Erica articulated how her parents' expectations continued to shape her views and practices around alcohol:

> *It kind of went without saying in our family that obviously you don't drink and drive under any circumstances. That would be a really stupid decision. I think my brother and I, I think would know that if we ever went to a party, especially if it was for a friend nearby, we're very comfortable just saying to our parents, instead of us Ubering home, can, as either myself or my sibling, go get the other sibling or can we have a lift from our parents or a friend or something like that. That has never really been an issue. (Erica, 21)*

Like many young people in our sample, Erica emphasised the risks associated with drink-driving, which were embedded in how her family communicated around alcohol. Moreover, because she was still living with her parents, she sometimes kept an open line of communication with them on a night out to help her get home.

Thinking about risks associated with alcohol, Yasmine reflected on her time at university (having recently left). Even though being at university brought opportunities for regular and heavy drinking, Yasmine felt there was a greater emphasis on risk, and the mitigation of risk, at university events.

*University clubs will hold events and they'll have people who are designated sober people to look after people, so I think maybe there's more awareness. You hear stories of people. Some things happen in bars. They're more conscious of the fact that things can go wrong. So, they're probably more aware and probably more restrictive because like, I don't want that to happen to me. (Yasmine, 21)*

As young people were beginning to leave university, opinions differed on how this change might affect drinking practices. Some young people talked about how the end of their time at university also signalled pressures and expectations around a competitive job market. Josh, who was highly career-focused when we talked to him, contrasted his time at university and the early stage of his career:

*…so there's the pressure to find a job and so going out has decreased compared to when it was 2020. Twenty years old, you're still in uni; people thinking about going out during the [semester] but I guess the adult responsibilities kick in for a lot of people so there are less opportunities. (Josh, 22)*

While some felt the shift to adult responsibilities limited opportunities for drinking, others felt that working more provided greater economic freedom to drink:

*Before, maybe I was a poor student at the time. So, I was like, I don't want to get a drink. But now because I have a job and I'm working, it's—yeah, I feel like alcohol is definitely more present, especially in that corporate workplace. (Yasmine, 21)*

Overall, young people talked about how alcohol held significance at points in time, such as being legally allowed to purchase it at 18 years old, within particular contexts such as at university, parties, or within some work industries (such as hospitality). But for the most part, for those who were drinking, it tended to be sporadic and event-oriented, rather than regular. One young person, Ella, suggested that regular drinking was part of a longer-term trajectory of stability, a reward for having one's life 'on track':

*Interviewer: So what age do you think that's [regular drinking] okay?*

> *Ella: Maybe not an age but like a point in life. Like maybe when you do have a stable job and family—stable family—at a point where you've got a career and a family and all that […] I just feel like if you haven't really got yourself sorted but yet you're still I'm going drink—to drink at least one every day, it just sounds like—it makes your lifestyle kind of look a bit bad. (Ella, 21)*

This reflection from Ella was limited to older adults. Among the young people we talked to, the stigma around young people's regular drinking, such as having one or two drinks a day, was much greater than that of heavier occasional drinking. Young people consistently described their drinking as 'social', and the social aspect of drinking as their main motivator (although some acknowledged this could change as they grew older).

When people detailed the link between alcohol and their social lives, there was a sense that alcohol was both embedded in the way young people socialised, but also restricted by the business of day-to-day lives. For example, Bec asserted:

> *People are just spending more time doing other things than getting tipsy. Doing what they like to do, hobbies and getting busy with work or uni assignments, catching up with people rather than getting tipsy. (Bec, 23)*

Similarly, Zak, who continued to abstain from alcohol for religious reasons, suggested that while alcohol remained highly normalised, the cultural diversity in Australia allowed for new and different drinking practices:

> *I feel like it's very accepted here. It's a cultural and societal norm. But in saying that, Australia is a very diverse and multicultural place. So for those that are fine with the current drinking culture […] but the fact that this country is so multicultural and diverse, I don't think there's an issue. Because those who want to drink will drink and those who don't want to drink won't drink. So it's very accepting of different views. (Zak, 21)*

Even though alcohol was intertwined with the ways and places that young people socialised within, heavy drinking was not always the norm. Yasmine, who was working in a bar on weekends when we last interviewed her, talked about how she felt there was less of an emphasis on alcohol in traditional drinking spaces where she spent time with friends and colleagues. She described people enjoying the spaces where alcohol was consumed, while not necessarily pursuing purposeful intoxication:

> *I think people want the vibe, but not everyone wants the drink. I think it's nice because it's like—bars are basically places to hang out with people but why does alcohol have to be a part of that? At the bar I do see a lot of people ordering—more people than I expect order just a Coke or just a Sprite, which I think is good. Or I'll have people at the bar say—because we're trying to—not up-sell but like, get a jug instead of a pint and they're like, no, I don't want to drink that much. I think people are becoming more aware of how much they want to drink. (Yasmine, 21)*

While mental health emerged as an important consideration in young people's drinking practices, there was also ambivalence about alcohol and mental health. For example, some young people we spoke to talked about alcohol helping alleviate some of their social anxiety. As Tom suggested, alcohol was still a tool among some young people to manage the emotional changes associated with 'growing up':

> *I have been privy to a lot of people who use alcohol to deal with their feelings and thoughts. Especially young adults, you know growing up, now being 20, 21. (Tom, 21)*

However, other young people also suggested they consciously managed or limited their drinking due to mental health concerns:

> *I have quite severe anxiety, so I just don't kind of—I try not to drink or do drugs or anything like that, just to take care of my mental health … Sometimes. Sometimes it helps deal with them, sometimes it exacerbates them. But I just kind of—yeah, I don't know. Because it's a bit unpredictable, I just stay away. (Yvonne, 20)*

Young people also described the variety of affordances of technology that influenced their drinking and non-drinking practices—particularly since digital technologies and social media were central tools for how they organised their social lives. When asked about drinking patterns in the future Garth projected how technologies could create new and immersive forms of entertainment that could transform drinking practices:

> *I think just with the way the world is and tech and everything, talks of the Metaverse, stuff like that, everything going online, digital, Web 3.0 [...] I think there'll probably be less drinking if everyone's in the Metaverse. In 10 years' time everyone just stuck in their rooms in a virtual reality AR, if you like, that would stimulate them. Yeah, maybe drinking would go down because people would find other forms of entertainment or escapism. Yeah, maybe, because I don't know, drinking companies might integrate that into the Meta, I don't even know. (Garth, 22)*

These reflections from young people in Australia highlight the varied but interrelated concepts that we have argued are central to the generational changes that have shifted the position of alcohol for young adults, including but not limited to, concern about risk, and the importance of family communication, leisure time, digital technology, diversity of lifestyles, and considerations around wellbeing for young people.

## What Does This Mean for Future Alcohol Consumption?

There are two broad perspectives we might consider when thinking about recent changes in young adult alcohol consumption, and what it might mean for future consumption. The first perspective assumes drinking rates change over time through processes of normalisation (marked by the relaxing of formal and informal controls) and corresponding problematisation (marked by the tightening of alcohol policies and increased stigma) (see Mäkelä et al., 1981). Thus, declines in drinking would occur as a societal reaction to the excesses of previous generations, and increases occur through 'generational forgetting' (Johnston et al., 2018). In this respect, high rates of drinking in the late 1990s and the subsequent 'demonising' of young adult drinking might be seen as a precipitant to the current decline. The 1990s saw an intersection of several public health concerns, including health, criminal activities, and other problems related to young people (Measham, 2006), allowing young adults to be pathologised and 'othered' as a risky subgroup. Focused sanctions and regulatory approaches that included taxes on pre-mixed drinks, lockout laws, secondary supply laws, minimum drinking ages, and targeted education campaigns all highlight efforts to address 'moral panics' (Cohen, 2011) around young adult drinking in the first decade of the 2000s. However, formal policy and legislative responses tend to lag behind informal social responses (such as collective pressures by communities and the media) (Room et al., 2009), and public health initiatives are as much symptoms of change as they are precipitators. Therefore, the problematisation of young adult alcohol use that occurred in the early 2000s may have encouraged a change in drinking styles and destabilised its normalised status, as it did with smoking in the late twentieth century.

The second perspective is that the current reduction in consumption represents a unique historical and social phenomenon. Declines might be part of a broader change in the way young adults are 'doing' or 'performing' young adulthood, and this may mean a more sustained change. As we have argued, structural shifts in education and labour markets have meant young people have had to adapt to insecure and flexible labour, longer time in education, declining tradition, individualisation, growing diversity of information and choice, and an expanding and globalised media. Young adults' struggle for autonomy has created new challenges that present practical limitations to consumption, as well as changes in how they might do leisure or 'do' young adulthood. Thus, the practice of being a young adult (and indirectly, the meanings attributed to alcohol) might be distinct from previous generations.

Because of the tangled and rapid nature of these social changes, what they mean for the future of alcohol consumption is unclear. Whether this constitutes a continuation of historical drinking trends, or a turning point for the place of alcohol in the lives of young adults requires time and ongoing theoretically informed investigation drawing not only on the alcohol and public health literature but also sociological studies of youth and young adulthood.

## Conclusion

Alcohol has historically been (and for many continues to be) a means of experiencing pleasure, time-out, enhancement, and excitement, while also providing a sense of belonging, celebration, and adulthood. However, today's generation of young adults more than ever must adapt to neoliberal conditions that emphasise individual responsibility and restraint. Policy, regulation, and media problematisation of alcohol use have coincided with a boom in new digital forms of consumption and alternative lifestyles, which is likely to have had a synergistic effect in changing alcohol use. Declines in alcohol use and other behaviours deemed risky may be part of a shift towards actively meeting neoliberal requirements around productivity at the cost of leisure time, and a potential decline in social wellbeing. This seems to have created an environment that opposes 'letting loose' and drunken comportment in favour of alternative lifestyles, new forms of consumption and entertainment, and new ways to achieve status and identity. Indeed, shifts in alcohol consumption may be symptomatic of changing lifestyles among young adults. We may be witnessing a reimagination of the types of activities and rituals that mark young adulthood in high-income countries, providing new ways of achieving adult identities, and changing the role of alcohol for young adults in a sustained and significant way.

## References

Atkinson, A. M., Matthews, B. R., Nicholls, E., & Sumnall, H. (2023). 'Some days I am a lunatic that thinks I can moderate': Amalgamating recovery and neo-liberal discourses within accounts of non-drinking among women active in the 'positive sobriety' community on Instagram in the UK. *International Journal of Drug Policy, 112*, 103937. https://doi.org/10.1016/j.drugpo.2022.103937

Azar, D., White, V., Bland, S., Livingston, M., Room, R., Chikritzhs, T., Durkin, S., Gilmore, W., & Wakefield, M. (2014). 'Something's brewing': The changing trends in alcohol coverage in Australian newspapers 2000–2011.

*Alcohol and Alcoholism, 49*(3), 336–342. https://doi.org/10.1093/alcalc/agt139

Ball, J., Edwards, R., Sim, D., Cook, H., & Denny, S. (2020). What explains the decline in adolescent binge-drinking in New Zealand? *International Journal of Drug Policy, 84*, 102826. https://doi.org/10.1016/j.drugpo.2020.102826

Ball, J., Pettie, M. A., Poasa, L., & Abel, G. (2023). Understanding youth drinking decline: Similarity and change in the function and social meaning of alcohol use (and non-use) in adolescent cohorts 20 years apart. *Drug and Alcohol Review*. https://doi.org/10.1111/dar.13685

Beck, U. (2000). *The brave new world of work*. Polity Press.

Bhattacharya, A. (2016). *Youthful abandon—Why are young people drinking less*. Report for Institute of Alcohol Studies.

Bor, W., Dean, A. J., Najman, J., & Hayatbakhsh, R. (2014). Are child and adolescent mental health problems increasing in the 21st century? A systematic review. *Australian & New Zealand Journal of Psychiatry, 48*, 606–616.

Brown, R., & Gregg, M. (2012). The pedagogy of regret: Facebook, binge drinking and young women. *Continuum, 26*(3), 357–369. https://doi.org/10.1080/10304312.2012.665834

Caluzzi, G., Fenton, L., Holmes, J., MacLean, S., Pennay, A., Fairbrother, H., & Törrönen, J. (2023). '90 per cent of the time when I have had a drink in my hand I'm on my phone as well': A cross-national analysis of communications technologies and drinking practices among young people. *New Media & Society*. https://doi.org/10.1177/14614448221150775

Caluzzi, G., Livingston, M., Holmes, J., MacLean, S., Lubman, D., Dietze, P., Vashishtha, R., Herring, R., & Pennay, A. (2022). Declining drinking among adolescents: Are we seeing a denormalisation of drinking and a normalisation of non-drinking? *Addiction, 117*(5), 1204–1212. https://doi.org/10.1111/add.15611

Caluzzi, G., MacLean, S., Livingston, M., & Pennay, A. (2021). "No one associates alcohol with being in good health": Health and wellbeing as imperatives to manage alcohol use for young people. *Sociology of Health & Illness, 43*, 493–509. https://doi.org/10.1111/1467-9566.13237

Caluzzi, G., MacLean, S., & Pennay, A. (2020). Re-configured pleasures: How young people feel good through abstaining or moderating their drinking. *International Journal of Drug Policy, 77*, 1–9. https://doi.org/10.1016/j.drugpo.2020.102709

Caluzzi, G., Pennay, A., & Livingston, M. (2022). How does technology influence young people's drinking? A complex relationship in need of innovation. *Addiction Research & Theory, 30*(4), 288–293. https://doi.org/10.1080/16066359.2021.2021402

Caluzzi, G., Pennay, A., & MacLean, S. (2021). Reflexive habitus and the new obligation of choice: Understanding young people's light drinking and alcohol abstinence. *Journal of Youth Studies, 24*(7), 886–900. https://doi.org/10.1080/13676261.2020.1778658

Caluzzi, G., Pennay, A., MacLean, S., & Woodman, D. (2022). No time for a 'time out'? Managing time around (non)drinking. *Sociology, 56*(1), 21–37. https://doi.org/10.1177/00380385211008370

Chan, G. C., Kelly, A. B., Connor, J. P., Hall, W., Young, R. M., & Williams, J. W. (2016). Does parental monitoring and disapproval explain variations in alcohol use among adolescents from different countries of birth? *Drug & Alcohol Review, 35*(6), 741–749. https://doi.org/10.1111/dar.12413

Cohen, S. (2011). *Folk devils and moral panics: The creation of the mods and rockers*. Taylor and Francis.

Collishaw, S. (2015). Annual research review: Secular trends in child and adolescent mental health. *The Journal of Child Psychology and Psychiatry, 56*(3), 370–393. https://doi.org/10.1111/jcpp.12372

Cook, M., Caluzzi, G., & Pennay, A. (2023). "Sober message to parents": Representations of parents in Australian News Media on youth drinking. *Contemporary Drug Problems, 50*(2), 254–268. https://doi.org/10.1177/00914509221147047

Cook, M., Pennay, A., MacLean, S., Dwyer, R., Mugavin, J., & Callinan, S. (2022). Parents' management of alcohol in the context of discourses of 'competent' parenting: A qualitative analysis. *Sociology of Health & Illness, 44*(6), 1009–1026. https://doi.org/10.1111/1467-9566.13475

Crawford, R. (1980). Healthism and the medicalization of everyday life. *International Journal of Health Services, 10*(3), 365–388. https://doi.org/10.2190/3h2h-3xjn-3kay-g9ny

Demant, J., & Törrönen, J. (2011). Changing drinking styles in Denmark and Finland. Fragmentation of male and female drinking among young adults. *Substance Use & Misuse, 46*(10), 1244–1255. https://doi.org/10.3109/10826084.2011.569965

Fargion, S. (2023). Representations of parenting and the neo-liberal discourse: Parents' and professionals' views on child-rearing practices in Italy. *Journal of*

*Family Studies, 29*(1), 188–204. https://doi.org/10.1080/13229400.2021.1905049

Farrell, G., Tilley, N., & Tseloni, A. (2014). Why the crime drop? *Crime and Justice, 43*(1), 421–490. https://doi.org/10.1086/678081

Fat, L. N., Shelton, N., & Cable, N. (2018). Investigating the growing trend of non-drinking among young people; analysis of repeated cross-sectional surveys in England 2005–2015. *BMC Public Health, 18*(1), 1090. https://doi.org/10.1186/s12889-018-5995-3

Furlong, A., & Cartmel, F. (2006). *Young people and social change*. McGraw-Hill Education.

Goodwin, I., & Griffin, C. (2017). Neoliberalism, alcohol and identity: A symptomatic reading of young people's drinking cultures in a digital world. In A. Lyons, T. McCreanor, I. Goodwin, & H. M. Barnes (Eds.), *Youth drinking cultures in a digital world: Alcohol, social media and cultures of intoxication* (pp. 16–30). Routledge.

Griffiths, R., & Casswell, S. (2010). Intoxigenic digital spaces? Youth, social networking sites and alcohol marketing. *Drug and Alcohol Review, 29*(5), 525. https://doi.org/10.1111/j.1465-3362.2010.00178.x

Hagell, A., Aldridge, J., Meier, P., Millar, T., Symonds, J., & Donmall, M. (2012). Trends in adolescent substance use and their implications for understanding trends in mental health. In A. Hagell & M. Rutter (Eds.), *Changing adolescence: Social trends and mental health* (pp. 117–150). Policy Press.

Hoffmann, S. H., Pisinger, V. S. C., Norredam, M., Tolstrup, J. S., & Thygesen, L. C. (2020). Does class proportion of students with non-Western origin in high schools affect drinking habits among ethnic Danish students? *Alcohol and Alcoholism*. https://doi.org/10.1093/alcalc/agaa069

Johnson, P. (2013). 'You think you're a rebel on a big bottle': Teenage drinking, peers and performance authenticity. *Journal of Youth Studies, 16*(6), 747–758. https://doi.org/10.1080/13676261.2012.744816

Johnston, L. D., Miech, R. A., O'Malley, P. M., Bachman, J. G., Schulenberg, J. E., & Patrick, M. E. (2018). *Monitoring the Future national survey results on drug use, 1975-2017: Overview, key findings on adolescent drug use*. Numerical/Quantitative Data; Reports – Research.

Kann, L., McManus, T., Harris, W., Shanklin, S., Flint, K., Hawkins, J., Queen, B., Lowry, R., Olsen, E. O.'. M., Chyen, D., Whittle, L., Thornton, J., Lim, C., Yamakawa, Y., Brener, N., & Zaza, S. (2016). Youth risk behavior surveillance—United States, 2015. *MMWR Surveillance Summary, 65*, 1–174.

Larm, P., Raninen, J., Åslund, C., Svensson, J., & Nilsson, K. W. (2018). The increased trend of non-drinking alcohol among adolescents: What role do internet activities have? *European Journal of Public Health, 29*(1), 27–32. https://doi.org/10.1093/eurpub/cky168

MacLean, S., Pennay, A., & Room, R. (2018). 'You're repulsive': Limits to acceptable drunken comportment for young adults. *International Journal of Drug Policy, 53*, 106–112. https://doi.org/10.1016/j.drugpo.2017.10.005

Mäkelä, K., Walsh, B., Sulkunen, P., Single, E., & Room, R. (1981). *Alcohol, society, and the state: I. A comparative study of alcohol control.* Addiction Research Foundation.

Mannheim, K. (1952 [1927]). The problem of generations. In *Essays on the sociology of knowledge* (pp. 276–322). Routledge.

Measham, F. (2006). The new policy mix: Alcohol, harm minimisation, and determined drunkenness in contemporary society. *International Journal of Drug Policy, 17*(4), 258–268. https://doi.org/10.1016/j.drugpo.2006.02.013

Newbury-Birch, D., Walker, J., Avery, L., Beyer, F., Brown, N., Jackson, K., Haighton, C., Mcgovern, R., Kaner, E., & Gilvarry, E. (2009). *Impact of alcohol consumption on young people: A systematic review of published reviews.* Report for the Department for Children, Schools and Families.

Nicholls, E. (2021). Sober rebels or good consumer-citizens? Anti-consumption and the 'enterprising self' in early sobriety. *Sociology, 55*(4), 768–784. https://doi.org/10.1177/0038038520981837

Pape, H., Rossow, I., & Brunborg, G. S. (2018). Adolescents drink less: How, who and why? A review of the recent research literature. *Drug and Alcohol Review, 37*(S1), S98–S114. https://doi.org/10.1111/dar.12695

Pedersen, W., & von Soest, T. (2015). Adolescent alcohol use and binge drinking: An 18-year trend study of prevalence and correlates. *Alcohol and Alcoholism, 50*(2), 219–225. https://doi.org/10.1093/alcalc/agu091

Pennay, A., Caluzzi, G., Livingston, M., & MacLean, S. (2023). Risk and restraint—The key to understanding the decreasing use of alcohol for young people in high income countries? *Drug and Alcohol Review.* https://doi.org/10.1111/dar.13709

Pennay, A., Cook, M., MacLean, S., Lubman, D. I., Dietze, P., Herring, R., Caluzzi, G., Vashishtha, R., & Livingston, M. (2022). Examining trends in the representation of young people and alcohol in Australian newspapers over twenty years (2000–2019). *International Journal of Drug Policy, 99*, 103461. https://doi.org/10.1016/j.drugpo.2021.103461

Raitasalo, K., & Holmila, M. (2017). Practices in alcohol education among Finnish parents: Have there been changes between 2006 and 2012? Drugs: Education. *Prevention and Policy, 24*(5), 392–399. https://doi.org/10.1080/09687637.2016.1183587

Rogne, A. F., Pedersen, W., & Bakken, A. (2019). Immigration and the decline in adolescent binge drinking. *Drug and Alcohol Dependence, 203*, 35–43. https://doi.org/10.1016/j.drugalcdep.2019.05.031

Room, R., Osterberg, E. S. A., Ramstedt, M., & Rehm, J. (2009). Explaining change and stasis in alcohol consumption. *Addiction Research & Theory, 17*(6), 562–576. https://doi.org/10.3109/16066350802626966

Scheffels, J., Buvik, K., Tokle, R., & Rossow, I. (2020). Normalisation of non-drinking? 15–16-year-olds' accounts of refraining from alcohol. *Drug and Alcohol Review, 39*(6), 729–736. https://doi.org/10.1111/dar.13084

Sobotka, T., & Toulemon, L. (2008). Overview Chapter 4: Changing family and partnership behaviour: Common trends and persistent diversity across Europe. *Demographic Research, 19*, 85–138. https://doi.org/10.4054/DemRes.2008.19.6

Supski, S., Lindsay, J., & Tanner, C. (2017). University students' drinking as a social practice and the challenge for public health. *Critical Public Health, 27*(2), 228–237. https://doi.org/10.1080/09581596.2016.1190001

Törrönen, J., Roumeliotis, F., Samuelsson, E., Kraus, L., & Room, R. (2019). Why are young people drinking less than earlier? Identifying and specifying social mechanisms with a pragmatist approach. *International Journal of Drug Policy, 64*, 13–20. https://doi.org/10.1016/j.drugpo.2018.12.001

Törrönen, J., Samuelsson, E., Roumeliotis, F., Room, R., & Kraus, L. (2021). 'Social health', 'physical health', and well-being: Analysing with bourdieusian concepts the interplay between the practices of heavy drinking and exercise among young people. *International Journal of Drug Policy, 91*, 102825. https://doi.org/10.1016/j.drugpo.2020.102825

Twenge, J. M. (2017). *IGen: Why today's super-connected kids are growing up less rebellious, more tolerant, less happy-- and completely unprepared for adulthood (and what this means for the rest of us)*. Atria Books.

Twenge, J. M., & Park, H. (2019). The decline in adult activities among U.S. Adolescents, 1976–2016. *Child Development, 90*(2), 638–654. https://doi.org/10.1111/cdev.12930

Vashishtha, R., Livingston, M., Pennay, A., Dietze, P., MacLean, S., Holmes, J., Herring, R., Caluzzi, G., & Lubman, D. (2019). Why is adolescent drinking declining? A systematic review and narrative synthesis. *Addiction Research & Theory, 28*(4), 275–288. https://doi.org/10.1080/16066359.2019.1663331

Vashishtha, R., Pennay, A., Dietze, P. M., & Livingston, M. (2021). Trends in adolescent alcohol and other risky health- and school-related behaviours and outcomes in Australia. *Drug and Alcohol Review, 40*(6), 1071–1082. https://doi.org/10.1111/dar.13269

Vaughn, M. G., Nelson, E. J., Oh, S., Salas-Wright, C. P., DeLisi, M., & Holzer, K. J. (2018). Abstention from drug use and delinquency increasing among youth in the United States, 2002–2014. *Substance Use & Misuse, 53*(9), 1468–1481. https://doi.org/10.1080/10826084.2017.1413392

West, P. (2016). Health in youth: Changing times and changing influences. In A. Furlong (Ed.), *Routledge handbook of youth and young adulthood* (pp. 327–338). Routledge.

Woodman, D. (2016). The sociology of youth and generations. In A. Furlong (Ed.), *Routledge handbook of youth and young adulthood* (pp. 20–26). Routledge.

Woodman, D., & Wyn, J. (2014). *Youth and generation: Rethinking change and inequality in the lives of young people*. SAGE Publications.

Wyn, J. (2011). The sociology of youth: A reflection on its contribution to the field and future directions. *Youth Studies Australia, 30*(3), 34–39.

Wyn, J. (2016). Educating for late modernity. In A. Furlong (Ed.), *Routledge handbook of youth and young adulthood* (pp. 91–98). Routledge.

Wyn, J., Cuervo, H., & Landstedt, E. (2015). The limits of wellbeing. In K. Wright & J. McLeod (Eds.), *Rethinking youth wellbeing: Critical perspectives* (pp. 55–70). Springer.

Yap, M., Cheong, T., Zaravinos-Tsakos, F., Lubman, D. I., & Jorm, A. (2017). Modifiable parenting factors associated with adolescent alcohol misuse: A systematic review and meta-analysis of longitudinal studies. *Addiction, 112*(7), 1142–1162. https://doi.org/10.1111/add.13785

# 4

# Shifting Tides: Life Transitions, High-Risk Drinking, and "Maturing Out"

Marjana Martinic

**Abstract** The transition from adolescence to adulthood is marked by changing roles and responsibilities, self-discovery, and boundary-testing. This journey is reflected in an evolving relationship with alcohol. It is generally accepted that high-risk drinking during this period is symbolic of experimentation with independence, eventually transitioning into a process of "maturing out" that results in drinking patterns more compatible with adult roles and responsibilities. Yet more recent research indicates that the drinking trajectory during this period is neither predictable nor necessarily sequential, but subject to considerable variation. Numerous individual and group factors, as well as broader cultural and societal shifts, play determining roles in its progression. Over recent decades, the timing of life stages, perceptions of appropriate roles and

This chapter builds on "Life Transitions into Adulthood and the Drinking Trajectory" by M. Martinic and A. Bigirimana, included in the first edition of this book.

M. Martinic (✉)
MM Science & Policy Advisors, LLC, Washington, DC, USA
e-mail: mmartinic@mm-spa.com

 
D. Conroy, F. Measham (eds.), *Young Adult Drinking Styles*, Sustainable Development Goals Series, https://doi.org/10.1007/978-3-031-98528-7_4

behaviors, and macro-level global trends have shifted and with them the trajectory of drinking from adolescence into adulthood. Drawing largely from the epidemiological literature, this chapter explores the role played by the many factors involved. They include gender, family and peer relationships, employment, and parenthood, as well as changing definitions and perceptions of adolescence and adulthood and the changing social saliency of drinking in the lives of some young people.

## Introduction

In industrialized Western countries, it is generally assumed that young people transition from adolescence into young adulthood between the ages of 18 and 25 years, a period typically marked by experimentation, self-discovery, and the testing of personal limits and societal boundaries (Arnett, 2000). Life transitions are marked by notable milestones that delineate the end of old and the beginning of new phases of life that are variously marked by formal education, employment, stable intimate relationships, and parenthood (Staff et al., 2014). Each brings new roles, responsibilities, and both individual and societal expectancies around appropriate and normative behavior (Pinquart & Borgolte, 2022).

The concept of the "drinking trajectory", first described within the context of binge drinking during the transition from late adolescence into early adulthood (e.g., Schulenberg et al., 1996), offers a developmental perspective on the evolution of drinking patterns. This evolution reflects the biological and psychological changes that take place during this period of development, as well as changing social roles (Brown et al., 2008; Arnett, 2000). It begins with the initiation of drinking, followed by an increase in frequency and intensity, usually as peer relationships become more salient (Demant & Järvinen, 2006; Herold & Frank, 2022). High-risk drinking patterns during this time are perceived as symbolic of boundary testing, newly found independence, and the adoption of adult behaviors. It is thought that when these risky patterns become incompatible with the responsibilities of adult life, they will eventually wane, stabilizing into more moderate, mature patterns of drinking. The concept of "maturing out" of high-risk drinking, first described by Winick

(1962), has become firmly entrenched in theory and research (e.g., Järvinen & Bom, 2019; Herold & Frank, 2022; Lee & Sher, 2018; Windle, 2020a).

Life transitions are generally assumed to be discrete and predictable, and to follow a defined order. However, closer scrutiny reveals that the transition from adolescence into adulthood, accompanying drinking behaviors, and the process of maturing out itself are neither clear-cut nor necessarily sequential. Life stages are variable and fluid. They may overlap, be delayed, or altogether absent, often making a clear delineation between the end of adolescence and onset of adulthood difficult. For some young people, maturing out of high-risk drinking may be an extended process, for others, it may never occur. Individual-level differences between and within groups determine the timing, sequence, and intensity of the trajectory and shape its accompanying drinking patterns. Macro-level societal shifts have changed the very definitions of adolescence and adulthood, challenging not only assumptions about stage-appropriate behaviors but also the social meaning of drinking itself. This chapter draws primarily from the epidemiological and quantitative literature for its discussion and analysis. The following section explores the factors that shape drinking trajectories, the importance of gender and peer relationships, and the place of drinking within the shifting boundaries of adolescence and adulthood.

## Navigating Transitions in Life and Drinking

Increased drinking is an expected hallmark of the transition into the stages of young adulthood (Patrick et al., 2020). Yet the road to "maturing out" is far from predictable. It varies across groups, cultures, and contexts, as does the order of transitional milestones. Variations also depend on both group-level variables and intra-individual differences. The weight of adult responsibilities offers only a limited explanation (Järvinen & Bom, 2019) and drinking patterns may reflect pressure to conform to societal expectations of stage-appropriate behavior.

In their research on US college students, for example, Hultgren et al. found that drinking initiation usually occurred during the first year of university, and that the odds of remaining a non-drinker decreased with each subsequent year (Hultgren et al., 2019). This coincides with observations by other authors (e.g., Pinquart & Borgolte, 2022) of a U-shaped relationship with drinking intensity and frequency during this period. But closer examination reveals distinct subcategories of drinkers who differ from each other in both drinking frequency and intensity, as well as when and even whether they transition between light and heavy drinking (Hultgren et al., 2019). High-risk drinkers were unlikely to move into lower-risk groups and maintained positive attitudes and expectancies about drinking. For most young adults, however, the actual increase in drinking was not significant, and other studies have shown that the patterns developed during this period often persist into adulthood without the need for maturing out (Windle, 2020a).

In higher-income Western societies, employment, stable intimate relationships, marriage, parenthood, and family life are often regarded as key drivers of maturing out of high-risk drinking (Staff et al., 2014). Closer scrutiny shows that the role of each of these life domains varies and depends on individual-level and societal factors. Some studies from high-income Western countries like the Netherlands, United States, and the United Kingdom have reported an inverse correlation between steady employment and heavy drinking (e.g., Bamberger et al., 2018; Mangot-Sala et al., 2022). This relationship appears strongest for the youngest age cohorts in their 20s (e.g., Morikawa et al., 2014). The type of employment itself also appears to be important, with research from the United States, China, and Japan reporting greater likelihood of maturing out among that those working in professional jobs than those in non-professional roles (Lee et al., 2022; Morikawa et al., 2014; Okui, 2021; Qian et al., 2018). Cohort drinking norms, a permissive drinking environment, and other factors associated with the workplace also shape the transition (Liu et al., 2023; Oesterle et al., 2023).

But maturing out does not always predictably follow employment. Geisner et al. (2018), for example, found that individual-level personality factors play an important role. Individuals with low impulse control were likely to maintain or even intensify the drinking patterns they acquired as adolescents, while those with higher control were more likely to mature out once they had stable employment. Other research has shown that high impulsivity and sensation-seeking are associated with overall lower odds of maturing out (e.g., Lee & Sher, 2018; Waddell et al., 2022).

The impact on maturing out of being in a committed relationship or being married has been explored. The "marriage effect" as a driver of reduced drinking has been identified across cultures and described in studies from the United States (e.g., Lee et al., 2022) and Switzerland (Kuntsche et al., 2016) to Nepal (Axinn et al., 2022) and China (Yang et al., 2020). Some authors have suggested that marriage and stable relationships may lead to dwindling peer interactions and a narrowed range of social contexts involving alcohol (Axinn et al., 2022; Windle & Windle, 2018). However, this relationship is neither universal nor consistent, with others reporting a direct correlation between marriage and increased alcohol use across different cultural settings, including Korea (Choe et al., 2018), Japan (Okui, 2021), and in some lower- and middle-income countries in Eastern Europe, Africa, Asia, and the Caribbean regions (Mutumba & Schulenberg, 2019). The timing of marriage may play a role, with a more pronounced impact on drinking in young adulthood but negligible for those in their 30s or older (Lee et al., 2022).

Of all life domains, parenthood is most consistently associated with maturing out (McKetta & Keyes, 2019), including in young adults with relatively heavy drinking patterns (Ahlström et al., 2001; Bowden et al., 2019). The effect has been described in cross-cultural research comparing Asia, Europe, Latin America, and Africa (Grittner et al. 2015; Qian et al., 2018). More detailed analysis suggests a central role for parental age and gender (Axinn et al., 2022; Kendler et al., 2019), with a more prominent effect in women (Grittner et al., 2015).

## Gender, Peers, and "Maturing Out"

Men and women have different relationships with drinking and gender plays a broader determining role in the overall maturing out trajectory. Across countries and cultures, men generally drink more than women (Peacock et al., 2018) and are often subject to different and more permissive social norms around consuming alcohol (discussed in greater detail by Bogren in this volume). Young men are likely to increase their drinking at an earlier age and to do so more significantly than young women. At the same time, they may mature out of high-risk drinking more quickly (Windle, 2020b). Over recent decades, the gender gap in drinking has narrowed, including among adolescents and young adults, according to international epidemiological surveys like the European School Survey Project on Alcohol and Other Drugs (ESPAD Group, 2020) and Health Behavior in School-aged Children (HBSC) (Charrier et al., 2024). Not only are more women and girls drinking than in previous generations, but they are drinking more heavily and are more likely to get drunk. According to the most recent HBSC findings, drinking prevalence among 15-year-old females is higher than among males in many countries including Sweden, Denmark, Spain, and the United Kingdom. US data show higher prevalence of drunkenness among female high-school students than among males (Patrick et al., 2022), while in Mexico past-month prevalence of heavy episodic drinking among adolescent girls rose three-fold between 2011 and 2016 (Instituto Nacional de Psiquitaría Ramon de la Fuente Muñiz (INPRFM) et al., 2017). The HBSC survey also reports significantly more drunkenness among young females than males, for example, in Spain and the United Kingdom (Charrier et al., 2024).

These changes in drinking habits also affect maturing out and may be explained in part by shifting views of femininity and normative female behavior. In most cultures, women's drinking has traditionally been stigmatized (e.g., Sudhinaraset et al., 2016). Studies report that women who align with more traditional norms of femininity that include modesty, humility, domestic values, and sexual fidelity are less likely to drink and to report heavy episodic drinking (Kaya et al., 2016; Mahalik et al., 2005). With increasing access to new work environments and social contexts in which women's drinking is acceptable and accepted, women are increasingly adopting both traditionally masculine and feminine norms in relation to their drinking, which translates into what they drink and where, as well as how much and how often they drink (Kaya et al., 2016). Hennell et al. (2023), for example, report that for young women in Britain, a "proper night out" involves both drinking and intoxication. Studies from Norway (Vandal & Dahl, 2021) and the United Kingdom (Nicholls, 2016) report an evolution in women's own views on gender norms around drinking, with greater emphasis on independence and pleasure, which reflect and are in turn reflected in changing societal gender norms. Mackiewicz (2015) suggests that intoxication within the context of entertainment is now an expected and normalized aspect of young women's social lives. Those who adopt traditionally more masculine norms may experience increased high-risk drinking and alcohol-related physical and mental health problems (reviewed in McCaul et al., 2019). The roles of gender, femininity, and masculinity are explored in more detail in Chap. 5 by Bogren, Hunt, and Petersen in this volume.

Drinking during specific life domains also shows gender-based differences. Full employment has been reported to reduce both the prevalence and frequency of heavy drinking in women across cultural contexts from Europe to Asia and Africa (Ahlström et al., 2001; Okui, 2021; Qian et al., 2018; Staff et al., 2014), but more recent research has found that women in higher-status careers, particularly where parity with men was greater (McKetta et al., 2023), drank more than those in lower-status jobs and those with less parity. This suggests that both the type of job and a woman's status within an organization are important.

Even the impact of parenthood on drinking appears to be gender dependent (McKetta & Keyes, 2019). In general, women are more likely to mature out of heavy drinking patterns earlier in parenthood than men. This process often begins in pregnancy and may reflect awareness of potential risks. While most resume their drinking after childbirth, they are likely to do so less heavily and frequently than men and also less heavily and frequently than before becoming parents (Bowden et al., 2019; Kendler et al., 2019). Yet the impact of parenthood on maturing out is not universal. While women's drinking may decline after childbirth, its subsequent intensity depends on the ages of their children. Those living with younger children are likely to reduce their drinking, but drinking often increases as these children age (e.g., Bowden et al., 2019; Kendler et al., 2019).

The impact of parenthood on men's drinking is, by all accounts, less significant than it is on women's drinking and may not reflect the same declines in consumption following the birth of a child (Borschmann et al., 2019). For example, the age of a resident child appears less of a factor in reducing paternal drinking (Borschmann et al., 2019; Kendler et al., 2019), and increased drinking has been reported to accompany parenthood among some men, particularly first-time fathers. The relationship appears to be modulated by educational level. Men with higher education are reportedly more likely to increase their drinking in fatherhood than those with less education (Leggat et al., 2021). No such difference in an educational effect was reported in women.

Across cultures, peers contribute to a "social ecology" in which favorable attitudes towards substance use may be normative and increase the likelihood of engaging in risky behaviors (Sanchez et al., 2023; Trucco, 2020), for example, as a way of fitting in. Much of the epidemiological and quantitative literature is devoted to the role of peers in drinking initiation, the adoption of heavy drinking patterns during adolescence, and in antisocial behavior (e.g., Brislin et al., 2021; Samek et al., 2016). Studies indicate a more significant role for peers in late adolescence (Samek et al., 2016). There is evidence that the selection of peers, rather than socialization itself, may be more closely related to drinking patterns established during this period, with young people selecting those with whom they share common interests and attitudes (reviewed in Sudhinaraset et al., 2016 McCaul et al., 2019). Among young women, the role of drinking may be particularly important in socialization (Nicholls, 2020).

The timing of maturing out may provide some insights into differences in individual trajectories. In their review, Lee and Sher point to different temporality in maturing out that appears to be related to different motives. Those who change their drinking in response to social pressure to adopt adult roles and responsibilities may be more likely to mature out at a younger age (Lee & Sher, 2018). Other factors may be more significant for those who mature out later. For some people, personality factors appear to play an important role (Littlefield et al., 2009). For others, transitioning out of heavy drinking reflects negative experiences and a recognition of the need to change behavior. Transitioning out may also be part of a natural trend that does not involve an extended maturing out process. As the next section will discuss, recent trends in life transitions and accompanying drinking patterns suggest that all three explanatory models and the very nature of maturing out merit further review. They should be viewed within the context of broader trends in maturing out of risky drinking (Tucker et al., 2021), as well as of other "adult" behaviors like driving a motor vehicle, going out with peers, dating, having sex, and working for pay (Ball et al., 2023; Twenge & Park, 2019).

## Stalled in Transition: A Role for Delayed Adulthood

The lack of a consistent and predictable transition out of heavy drinking may in part be rooted in the phenomenon of "delayed" adulthood that is becoming increasingly more common in Western societies, in particular. Many young people no longer adhere to previously expected timing and age ranges during which they move into "adult" roles (Hayford & Furstenberg, 2008). For some, adolescence, as defined by specific responsibilities and social roles, now extends into their early 30s or even their 40s (Lee & Sher, 2018).

Various explanations have been offered for this shift (Whitaker et al., 2023). They include economic conditions and downturns, a tightening job market in many countries, increasing cost of living and education, limited availability of affordable housing, and, more recently, the COVID-19 pandemic. Many young adults, notably in middle- and high-income countries, are increasingly likely to continue to live in the parental home and unable to live independently. A recent study in the United States found that over half of 18- to 25-year-olds were living with their parents and fewer than half were able to meet their own expenses. Four out of every five reported financial issues as their most significant life stressor (Leech et al., 2020). Another study found that among 23-year-olds over half had graduated from college, but only a third were fully employed, a third were living independently, and only 2 in 5 were in a committed relationship (Tucker et al., 2021). These findings are not unique to the United States and reflect a more widespread delay across life domains compared with the commonly expected sequence.

An important contributing factor is a change in some parts of the world in women's roles and an evolution in societal views about gender-appropriate behaviors and expectations about the progression of life stages. These changes have also affected the process of maturing out. Women are increasingly deferring marriage and parenthood to focus on education and professional attainment, delaying the transition into parental and family roles. According to UN data, across Europe, the mean maternal age at first birth has risen in every country since 2001 (United Nations Economic Commission for Europe (UNECE), 2023). Similar trends are reported elsewhere. In China, the mean maternal age rose from 27.1 to 29.7 years between 2010 and 2017 (Cao et al., 2022), while in Brazil, the proportion of first-time mothers younger than 20 years dropped by half between 2000 and 2021 and the proportion of those between 30 to 39 years increased by almost 60% (STATISTA, 2024). Women are no longer forced to choose between family and career, and motherhood no longer represents the inevitable end of professional life. While choices remain limited for many young women, options are increasingly available for those with the education and economic power to access them. Delayed life stages like marriage and childbearing are also coinciding with shifts in what is considered acceptable drinking behaviors for women, and the narrowing of the gender gap in drinking discussed earlier in this chapter.

A third macro-level shift that has contributed to an extended period of maturing out is the increasing number of young people abstaining from drinking alcohol. This trend has been reported in high- and middle-income countries across Europe, North America, and Australia (ESPAD Group, 2020; Vashishtha et al., 2021). Not drinking is increasingly a viable and accepted choice among groups for whom heavy drinking was previously normative behavior (Caluzzi et al., 2022). The sociodemographic profile of young abstainers in higher-income countries has been changing. Early abstainers are now more likely to be wealthier and healthier than their drinking peers, to perform better in school, and to be in full-time education or employment (Corre et al., 2023). Despite this increasing trend, risky drinking is still widely prevalent among young people across cultures, with many continuing to engage in goal-directed and purposeful intoxication (see Martinic & Measham, 2008).

Several explanations have been offered for the increasing trend in abstention across countries, and the topic is discussed in greater detail in Chaps. 8 and 9 in this volume. According to Scheffels et al. (2020), young abstainers fall into three groups. This taxonomy itself might offer clues about motivation. For some, abstaining is driven by perceptions of negative social norms around alcohol consumption, while for others abstaining is a reflection of disapproval of drinking by parents and peers, and greater acceptance of regulations and restrictions aimed at preventing youth drinking. For a third group, abstaining from drinking reflects the reluctance to lose control and increase exposure to risk, with drinking viewed as counterproductive for academic and athletic performance. Religiosity is another reason for abstaining from alcohol and not captured in Scheffels' classification. Strong religious beliefs and practices have been identified as a protective factor against both drinking initiation and heavy drinking, by extension determining whether there is even a need for maturing out (e.g., Russell et al., 2020). Research has linked the observed decline in drinking and increase in abstinence in some middle- and high-income countries to shifting demographics and multiculturalism resulting from increased immigration and the importance of cultural and religious sanctions and parental control on alcohol consumption among some immigrant groups (e.g., Creemers et al., 2017; Vasiljevic et al., 2021).

Interestingly, there is some indication that the general trend in abstention may be transient and confined to adolescence and young adulthood, with the prevalence of abstainers declining as cohorts age (Corre et al., 2023). Abstention as a transient developmental period in the drinking career supports the notion of a delay in maturing out, with initiation into drinking occurring at a later age and delaying the transitioning out process. As ever, these changes are not universally consistent and depend to a large degree on culture, religion, and contextual factors (Loy et al., 2021; Raninen et al., 2022). However, as the next section will attempt to show, the changes reflect broader shifts in the saliency and social symbolism of alcohol in the lives of young people and their journey into adulthood.

## The Transforming Significance of Drinking

There are likely many reasons for the changes in drinking patterns observed during the transition from adolescence into adulthood, some of them contradictory and pointing to variability and divergence in maturing out. A further and final explanation may be found in changes in the social saliency of drinking during transitional period between adolescence to adulthood, explored in greater detail in the chapters in Part IV of this volume.

Some have suggested that the symbolic value of alcohol as a marker of adulthood has changed significantly for young people and no longer plays a central role in the creation of social bonds and group identity (Raninen et al., 2022; Törrönen et al., 2019). Declining peer pressure to drink has been reported, along with increased importance of activities like academics and athletic performance, which are generally viewed as incompatible with drinking (Scheffels et al., 2020; Stevely et al., 2022; Törrönen et al., 2019). Adolescents may be placing greater value on productive downtime and on maintaining control, with heavy drinking (or any drinking) viewed as a negative behavior that is potentially damaging to both reputation and health (reviewed in Chap. 3 by Caluzzi and Pennay in this volume). It has been suggested that the maturation process of young people, at least in high-income countries, has become more individualized and responsible, with heavy drinking less likely to be viewed as compatible with personal, social, and developmental goals (Törrönen et al., 2019). Recent country-level data reporting declines in heavy episodic drinking and intoxication in higher-income countries would support this notion (e.g., ESPAD Group, 2020; WHO, 2024). There is less information available from lower-income countries about the extent and direction of trends or about potential explanations and underlying causes (Dumbili, 2023). Nonetheless, despite declining trends, prevalence of heavy and high-risk drinking patterns among young people remains high across countries, regardless of income group.

For many young people, the period of adolescence and early adulthood continues to be operative in establishing social cohesion and group identity (e.g., McCabe et al., 2018). Drinking, particularly heavy drinking, and associated rituals symbolize belonging to social groups and shared experiences (MacArthur et al., 2020). Conroy et al. describe a dilemma potentially facing those who do not engage in ritualistic and heavy drinking as part of the bonding experience (Conroy et al., 2021). Failure to join in heavy drinking as part of the peer experience may mean foregoing group identity and the building of relationships, with the prospect of negative social outcomes and marginalization for those choosing not to engage (Conroy et al., 2021; Demant & Järvinen, 2006; Gambles et al., 2022). Part of the dilemma also relates to the role of drinking in facilitating social interaction, which seems particularly important during the early stages of building relationships with peer groups.

A trend of declining unstructured in-person time spent with friends and peers has been reported over recent years in some countries, accompanied by a weakening of social interactions (e.g., Kannan & Veazie, 2023). For young people, there has been a concomitant shift to more frequent socializing online, changing the dynamics of social interactions and time spent in shared leisure activities. This has diminished the traditional role of alcohol as a social lubricant and as a central element of shared social experiences. A study from New Zealand reported that adolescents and young adults were increasingly likely to substitute online and digital interactions for face-to-face engagement and to spend less time socializing with friends or attending parties. When personal social interactions, including those involving alcohol, occurred, they were increasingly at home and in small groups, and less likely to involve getting drunk (Ball et al., 2023). At the same time, these trends, while encouraging abstinence, have reportedly led to shrinking social networks and curtailed interactions among young people across countries, particularly during the social isolation of the COVID-19 pandemic (e.g., Dragioti et al., 2022). The longer-term implications of this relatively recent development in the role of alcohol within the trajectory from adolescence to adulthood and what it means for "maturing out" remains to be explored and depends on how the trend continues.

## Conclusions

This chapter has attempted to provide an overview of the many factors that shape the maturing out trajectory for drinking during the transitional period from adolescence to adulthood. It can be concluded that the process is neither predictable nor immutable, but varies both across and within groups, influenced by broader societal shifts in the evolution of life transitions and even drinking itself. It attempts to offer a fresh look at the evidence, challenging the notion of a clearly defined or even sequential process.

The role of adult responsibilities and societal expectations of age-appropriate behavior is clearly not uniformly central to the drinking of among young people as they enter formal adulthood. Variability in both population level and individual factors play a determining role, as do peer influences, changing gender roles, and social and demographic trends like the phenomenon of "delayed adolescence" that have upended our understanding of the drivers of both heavy drinking and the process of maturing out.

The transition between adolescence and adulthood is a time when behaviors are established that last into adulthood. How the changes in what were previously considered to be "adult" roles and normative behaviors will affect long-term drinking patterns remains to be seen as current cohorts age. Few studies to date have examined longitudinal trends. Some early work on the new generations of adolescent abstainers suggests that they may catch up in early adulthood with previously established drinking prevalence, but possibly with a reduction in risky drinking and consumption levels (e.g., Larm et al., 2023).

While declining high-risk drinking among adolescents and young adults is a welcome change from a public health perspective, the inability to transition neatly from one life domain into another during the process of emerging adulthood with its expected milestones may bring its own problems. Those unable to move from one domain to another and those who transition simultaneously across different domains may experience broader problems and potentially increased risk of substance use and abuse. At the same time, these expectations and milestones themselves may be changing, better reflecting the reality of life transitions during this formative period.

Only time and more research will tell whether the observed shifts in both risky drinking and the process of maturing out are transient or whether they indicate broader and more lasting change. We can conclude, however, that these shifts reflect broader adjustments in perceptions and definitions of life stages, roles, and responsibilities. In a globalized world, such evolution in higher-income countries usually precedes similar trends in lower-income countries where changes may be more pronounced and their impact potentially greater. Understanding this evolution and its relationship with underlying factors and trends also creates new opportunities for prevention, education, and health literacy that extends beyond the boundaries of "just" drinking alcohol.

## References

Ahlström, S., Bloomfield, K., & Knibbe, R. (2001). Gender differences in drinking patterns in nine European countries: Descriptive findings. *Substance Abuse, 22*(1), 69–85.

Arnett, J. J. (2000). Emerging adulthood: A theory of development from the late teens through the twenties. *American Psychologist, 55*, 469–480.

Axinn, W. G., Banchoff, E., Cole, F., Ghimire, D. J., & Smoller, J. W. (2022). The transition to parenthood, opportunity to drink, drinking, and alcohol use disorder. *Drug and Alcohol Dependence, 241*, 109697.

Ball, J., Pettie, M. A., Poasa, L., & Abel, G. (2023). Understanding youth drinking decline: Similarity and change in the function and social meaning of alcohol use (and non-use) in adolescent cohorts 20 years apart. *Drug and Alcohol Review*. https://doi.org/10.1111/dar.13685

Bamberger, P. A., Koopmann, J., Wang, M., Larimer, M., Nahum-Shani, I., Geisner, I., & Bacharach, S. B. (2018). Does college alcohol consumption impact employment upon graduation? Findings from a prospective study. *Journal of Applied Psychology, 103*(1), 111–121.

Borschmann, R., Becker, D., Spry, E., Youssef, G. J., Olsson, C. A., Hutchinson, D. M., Silins, E., Boden, J. M., Moreno-Betancur, M., Najman, J. M., Degenhardt, L., Mattick, R. P., Romaniuk, H., Horwood, L. J., & Patton, G. C. (2019). Alcohol and parenthood: An integrative analysis of the effects of transition to parenthood in three Australasian cohorts. *Drug and Alcohol Dependence, 197*, 326–334.

Bowden, J. A., Delfabbro, P., Room, R., Miller, C., & Wilson, C. (2019). Parental drinking in Australia: Does the age of children in the home matter? *Drug and Alcohol Review, 38*(3), 306–315.

Brislin, S. J., Clark, D. A., Heitzeg, M. M., Samek, D. R., Iacono, W. G., McGue, M., & Hicks, B. M. (2021). Co-development of alcohol use problems and antisocial peer affiliation from ages 11 to 34: Selection, socialization and genetic and environmental influences. *Addiction, 116*(8), 1999–2007.

Brown, S. A., McGue, M., Maggs, J., Schulenberg, J., Hingson, R., Swartzwelder, S., Martin, C., Chung, T., Tapert, S. F., Sher, K., Winters, K. C., Lowman, C., & Murphy, S. (2008). A developmental perspective on alcohol and youths 16 to 20 years of age. *Pediatrics, 121*(Suppl 4), S290–S310.

Caluzzi, G., Livingston, M., Holmes, J., MacLean, S., Lubman, D., Dietze, P., Vashishtha, R., Herring, R., & Pennay, A. (2022). Declining drinking among adolescents: Are we seeing a denormalisation of drinking and a normalisation of non-drinking? *Addiction, 117*(5), 1204–1212.

Cao, J., Xu, W., Liu, Y., Zhang, B., Zhang, Y., Yu, T., Huang, T., Zou, Y., & Zhang, B. (2022). Trends in maternal age and the relationship between advanced age and adverse pregnancy outcomes: A population-based register study in Wuhan, China, 2010–2017. *Public Health, 206*, 8–14.

Charrier, L., van Dorsselaer, S., Canale, N., Baska, T., Kilibarda, B., Comoretto, R.I., Galeotti, T., Brown, J., & Vieno, A. (2024). A focus on adolescent substance use in Europe, central Asia and Canada. Health Behaviour in School-aged Children international report from the 2021/2022 survey. Volume 3. World Health Organization. Regional Office for Europe. https://iris.who.int/handle/10665/376573. License: CC BY-NC-SA 3.0 IGO.

Choe, S. A., Yoo, S., JeKarl, J., & Kim, K. K. (2018). Recent trend and associated factors of harmful alcohol use based on age and gender in Korea. *Journal of Korean Medical Science, 33*(4), e23.

Conroy, D., Morton, C., & Griffin, C. (2021). 'Maturing Out' as dilemmatic: Transitions towards relatively light drinking practices among UK University students. *British Journal of Health Psychology, 26*(3), 902–916.

Corre, T., Barrense-Dias, Y., & Surís, J.-C. (2023). The growing trend of young people abstaining from drinking alcohol: A literature review. *Substance Use & Misuse, 58*(1), 77–84.

Creemers, H. E., Spanakis, P., Delforterie, M. J., & Huizink, A. C. (2017). Alcohol use of immigrant youths in The Netherlands: The roles of parents and peers across different ethnic backgrounds. *Drug & Alcohol Review, 36*(6), 761–768.

Demant, J., & Järvinen, M. (2006). Constructing maturity through alcohol experience—Focus group interviews with teenagers. *Addiction Research and Theory, 14*(6), 598–602.

Dragioti, E., Li, H., Tsitsas, G., Lee, K. H., Choi, J., Kim, J., Choi, Y. J., Tsamakis, K., Estradé, A., Agorastos, A., Vancampfort, D., Tsiptsios, D., Thompson, T., Mosina, A., Vakadaris, G., Fusar-Poli, P., Carvalho, A. F., Correll, C. U., Han, Y. J., Park, S., Il Shin, J., & Solmi, M. (2022). A large-scale meta-analytic atlas of mental health problems prevalence during the COVID-19 early pandemic. *Journal of Medical Virology, 94*(5), 1935–1949.

Dumbili, E. W. (2023). Decline in youth drinking in high-income settings: Implications for public health in low-income countries. *International Journal of Drug Policy, 114*, 103975.

ESPAD Group. (2020). *ESPAD Report 2019. Results from the European School Survey Project on Alcohol and Other Drugs*. EMCDDA Joint Publications Publication Office of the European Union.

Gambles, N., Porcellato, L., Fleming, K. M., & Quigg, Z. (2022). "If you don't drink at university, you're going to struggle to make friends." prospective students' perceptions around alcohol use at universities in the United Kingdom. *Substance Use & Misuse, 57*(2), 249–255.

Geisner, I. M., Koopmann, J., Bamberger, P., Wang, M., Larimer, M. E., Nahum-Shani, I., & Bacharach, S. (2018). When the party continues: Impulsivity and the effect of employment on young adults' post-college alcohol use. *Addictive Behaviors, 77*, 114–120.

Grittner, U., Nemeth, Z., Kuntsche, S., Gaertner, B., & Bloomfield, K. (2015). What is the role of roles? Exploring the link between social roles and women's alcohol use in low-and middle-income countries. *International Journal of Alcohol and Drug Research, 4*(2), 139–149.

Hayford, S. R., & Furstenberg, F. F., Jr. (2008). Delayed adulthood, delayed desistance? Trends in the age distribution of problem behaviors. *Journal of Research on Adolescence, 18*(2), 285–304.

Hennell, K., Limmer, M., & Piacentini, M. (2023). A 'Proper night out': A practice theory exploration of gendered drinking. *Sociological Research Online, 28*(2), 355–372.

Herold, M. D., & Frank, V. A. (2022). Alcohol use and narratives of 'maturing out' in the transition to adulthood among young Danes. In T. Thurnell-Read & L. Fenton (Eds.), *Alcohol, age, Generation and the life course*. Palgrave Macmillan.

Hultgren, B. A., Turrisi, R., Cleveland, M. J., Mallett, K. A., Reavy, R., Larimer, M. E., Geisner, I. M., & Hospital, M. M. (2019). Transitions in drinking behaviors across the college years: A latent transition analysis. *Addictive Behaviors, 92*, 108–114.

Instituto Nacional de Psiquiatría Ramón de la Fuente Muñiz (INPRFM). (2017). *Encuesta nacional de consumo de drogas, alcohol y tabaco, ENCODAT 2016-2017: Reporte de alcohol*. INPRFM.

Järvinen, M., & Bom, L. H. (2019). 'Maturing out' as normative standard: Qualitative interviews with young adult drinkers. *Journal of Youth Studies, 22*(5), 678–693.

Kannan, V. D., & Veazie, P. J. (2023). US trends in social isolation, social engagement, and companionship - nationally and by age, sex, race/ethnicity, family income, and work hours, 2003–2020. SSM – Population. *Health, 21*, 101331.

Kaya, A., Iwamoto, D. K., Grivel, M., Clinton, L., & Brady, J. (2016). The role of feminine and masculine norms in college women's alcohol use. *Psychology of Men & Masculinity, 17*(2), 206–214.

Kendler, K. S., Larsson Lönn, S., Salvatore, J. E., Sundquist, J., & Sundquist, K. (2019). The impact of parenthood on risk of registration for alcohol use disorder in married individuals: A Swedish population-based analysis. *Psychological Medicine, 49*(13), 2141–2148.

Kuntsche, S., Astudillo, M., & Gmel, G. (2016). Social roles among recruits in Switzerland: Do social roles relate to alcohol use and does role change have an impact? *Addictive Behaviors, 54*, 59–63.

Larm, P., Hellström, C., Raninen, J., Åslund, C., Nilsson, K. W., & Giannotta, F. (2023). Do non-drinking youth drink less alcohol in young adulthood or do they catch up? Findings from a Swedish birth cohort. *European Journal of Public Health, 33*(4), 640–644.

Lee, M. R., & Sher, K. J. (2018). "Maturing out" of binge and problem drinking. *Alcohol Research, 39*(1), 31–42.

Lee, M. R., Yeung, E. W., Littlefield, A. K., Stephenson, A., Kady, A., Kwan, T., Chassin, L., & Sher, K. J. (2022). A life span developmental investigation of marriage and problem-drinking reduction. *Developmental Psychopathology, 36*, 1–11.

Leech, T. G., Jacobs, S., & Watson, D. (2020). Factors associated with binged during the transition into adulthood: Exploring associations within two distinct young adult age ranges. *Substance Abuse, 14*, 1178221820951781.

Leggat, G., Livingston, M., Kuntsche, S., & Callinan, S. (2021). Changes in alcohol consumption during pregnancy and over the transition towards parenthood. *Drug and Alcohol Dependence, 225*, 108745.

Littlefield, A. K., Sher, K. J., & Wood, P. K. (2009). Is "maturing out" of problematic alcohol involvement related to personality change? *Journal of Abnormal Psychology, 118*(2), 360–374.

Liu, S., Bamberger, P., Wang, M., Nahum-Shani, I., Larimer, M., & Bacharach, S. B. (2023). Behavior change versus stability during the college-to-work transition: Life course and the "stickiness" of alcohol misuse at career entry. *Personnel Psychology, 76*(3), 945–975.

Loy, J. K., Seitz, N.-N., Bye, E. K., Raitasalo, K., Soellner, R., Törrönen, J., & Kraus, L. (2021). Trends in alcohol consumption among adolescents in Europe: Do changes occur in concert? *Drug & Alcohol Dependence, 228*, 109020.

MacArthur, G. J., Hickman, M., & Campbell, R. (2020). Qualitative exploration of the intersection between social influences and cultural norms in relation to the development of alcohol use behaviour during adolescence. *BMJ Open, 10*(3), e030556.

Mackiewicz, A. (2015). *Four: Alcohol, young women's culture and gender hierarchies*. Policy Press.

Mahalik, J. R., Morray, E. B., Coonerty-Femiano, A., Ludlow, L. H., Slattery, S. M., & Smiler, A. (2005). Development of the conformity to feminine norms inventory. *Sex Roles, 52*(7–8), 417–435.

Mangot-Sala, L., Smidt, N., & Liefbroer, A. C. (2022). Disentangling the association between alcohol consumption and employment status: Causation, selection or confounding? *European Journal of Public Health, 32*(6), 926–932.

Martinic, M., & Measham, D. (Eds.). (2008). *Swimming with crocodiles. The culture of extreme drinking*. Routledge.

McCabe, S. E., Veliz, P., & Schulenberg, J. E. (2018). How collegiate fraternity and sorority involvement relates to substance use during young adulthood and substance use disorders in early midlife: A national longitudinal study. *Journal of Adolescent Health, 62*(3s), S35–s43.

McCaul, M. E., Roach, D., Hasin, D. S., Weisner, C., Chang, G., & Sinha, R. (2019). Alcohol and women: A brief overview. *Alcoholism: Clinical and Experimental Research, 43*(5), 774–779.

McKetta, S., & Keyes, K. M. (2019). Heavy and binge alcohol drinking and parenting status in the United States from 2006 to 2018: An analysis of nationally representative cross-sectional surveys. *PLoS Medicine, 16*(11), e1002954.

McKetta, S., Prins, S. J., Hasin, D., Patrick, M. E., & Keyes, K. M. (2023). Structural sexism moderates work and occupational risks for alcohol consumption and binge drinking among US women, 1989–2016. *Social Science & Medicine, 324*, 115878.

Morikawa, Y., Nakamura, K., Sakurai, M., Nagasawa, S. Y., Ishizaki, M., Nakashima, M., Kido, T., Naruse, Y., & Nakagawa, H. (2014). The effect of age on the relationships between work-related factors and heavy drinking. *Journal of Occupational Health, 56*(2), 141–149.

Mutumba, M., & Schulenberg, J. E. (2019). Tobacco and alcohol use among youth in low and middle income countries: A multi-country analysis on the influence of structural and micro-level factors. *Substance Use & Misuse, 54*(3), 396–411.

Nicholls, E. (2016). 'What on earth is *she* drinking?' Doing femininity through drink choice on the girls' night out. *Journal of International Women's Studies, 2*, 8.

Nicholls, E. (2020). 'I feel like I have to become part of that identity': Negotiating femininities and friendships through alcohol consumption in Newcastle, UK. *International Journal of Drug Policy, 81*, 102524.

Oesterle, S., Bailey, J. A., Catalano, R. F., Epstein, M., Evans-Whipp, T. J., & Toumbourou, J. W. (2023). Alcohol-tolerant workplace environments are a risk factor for young adult alcohol abuse on and off the job in Australia and the United States. *International Journal of Environmental Research in Public Health, 20*(18), 6725.

Okui, T. (2021). An analysis of predictors for heavy alcohol drinking using nationally representative survey data in Japan. *BMC Public Health, 21*(1), 359.

Patrick, M. E., Rhew, I. C., Duckworth, J. C., Lewis, M. A., Abdallah, D. A., & Lee, C. M. (2020). Patterns of young adult social roles transitions across 24 months and subsequent substance use and mental health. *Journal of Youth and Adolescence, 49*(4), 869–880.

Patrick, M. E., Schulenberg, J. E., Miech, R. A., Johnston, L. D., O'Malley, P. M., & Bachman, J. G. (2022). *Monitoring the Future Panel Study annual report: National data on substance use among adults ages 19 to 60, 1976–2021* (Monitoring the Future Monograph Series). Institute for Social Research, University of Michigan.

Peacock, A., Leung, J., Larney, S., Colledge, S., Hickman, M., Rehm, J., Giovino, G. A., West, R., Hall, W., Griffiths, P., Ali, R., Gowing, L., Marsden, J., Ferrari, A. J., Grebely, J., Farrell, M., & Degenhardt, L. (2018). Global statistics on alcohol, tobacco and illicit drug use: 2017 status report. *Addiction, 113*(10), 1905–1926.

Pinquart, M., & Borgolte, K. (2022). Change in alcohol outcome expectancies from childhood to emerging adulthood: A meta-analysis of longitudinal studies. *Drug & Alcohol Review, 41*(5), 1216–1225.

Qian, L., Newman, I. M., Yuen, L. W., Shell, D. F., & Xu, J. (2018). Variables associated with Alcohol consumption and abstinence among young adults in central China. *International Journal of Environmental Research and Public Health, 15*(8), 1675.

Raninen, J., Livingston, M., Holmes, J., Svensson, J., & Larm, P. (2022). Declining youth drinking: A matter of faith? *Drug and Alcohol Review, 41*(4), 721–723.

Russell, A. M., Yu, B., Thompson, C. G., Sussman, S. Y., & Barry, A. E. (2020). Assessing the relationship between youth religiosity and their alcohol use: A meta-analysis from 2008 to 2018. *Addictive Behaviour, 106*, 106361.

Samek, D. R., Goodman, R. J., Erath, S. A., McGue, M., & Iacono, W. G. (2016). Antisocial peer affiliation and externalizing disorders in the transition from adolescence to young adulthood: Selection versus socialization effects. *Developmental Psychology, 52*(5), 813–823.

Sanchez, M., Gonzalez, M. R., Fernandez, A., Barton, A., Diaz, V., & Wang, W. (2023). Sociocultural influences on alcohol expectancies in early adolescence: Findings from the ABCD study. *Health Psychology, 42*(12), 842–855.

Scheffels, J., Buvik, K., Tokle, R., & Rossow, I. (2020). Normalisation of non-drinking? 15-16-year-olds' accounts of refraining from alcohol. *Drug and Alcohol Review, 39*(6), 729–736.

Schulenberg, J., Wadsworth, K. N., O'Malley, P. M., Bachman, J. G., & Johnston, L. D. (1996). Adolescent risk factors for binge drinking during the transition to young adulthood: Variable- and pattern-centered approaches to change. *Developmental Psychology, 32*(4), 659–674.

Staff, J., Greene, K. M., Maggs, J. L., & Schoon, I. (2014). Family transitions and changes in drinking from adolescence through mid-life. *Addiction, 109*(2), 227–236.

STATISTA. (2024). Distribution of live births in Brazil from 2000 to 2021, by age group of the mother. Retrieved 11 January 2024, from https://www.statista.com/statistics/1327207/distribution-births-brazil-by-mother-age/#:~:text=In%202021%2C%2013.2%20percent%20of,pertained%20to%20this%20age%20group

Stevely, A. K., Vashishtha, R., Fairbrother, H., Fenton, L., Henney, M., Livingston, M., & Holmes, J. (2022). Are changes in attitudes towards school associated with declining youth drinking? A multi-level analysis of 37 countries. *European Journal of Public Health, 32*(3), 354–359.

Sudhinaraset, M., Wigglesworth, C., & Takeuchi, D. T. (2016). Social and cultural contexts of alcohol use: Influences in a social-ecological framework. *Alcohol Research, 38*(1), 35–45.

Törrönen, J., Roumeliotis, F., Samuelsson, E., Kraus, L., & Room, R. (2019). Why are young people drinking less than earlier? Identifying and specifying social mechanisms with a pragmatist approach. *International Journal of Drug Policy, 64*, 13–20.

Trucco, E. M. (2020). A review of psychosocial factors linked to adolescent substance use. *Pharmacology Biochemistry and Behavior, 196*, 172969.

Tucker, J. S., Rodriguez, A., Davis, J. P., Klein, D. J., & D'Amico, E. J. (2021). Simultaneous trajectories of alcohol and cannabis use from adolescence to emerging adulthood: Associations with role transitions and functional outcomes. *Psychology of Addictive Behaviors, 35*(6), 628–637.

Twenge, J. M., & Park, H. (2019). The decline in adult activities among U.S. adolescents, 1976-2016. *Child Development, 90*(2), 638–654.

United Nations Economic Commission for Europe (UNECE). (2023). Mean age of women at birth of first child. Retrieved 12 January 2024, from https://w3.unece.org/PXWeb/en/Table?IndicatorCode=34

Vandal, K., & Dahl, S. L. (2021). Maturing out of 'binge drinking': Young adult women's performance of age and gender in terms of transition. *Journal of Youth Studies, 24*, 1326–1339.

Vashishtha, R., Pennay, A., Dietze, P., Marzan, M. B., Room, R., & Livingston, M. (2021). Trends in adolescent drinking across 39 high-income countries: Exploring the timing and magnitude of decline. *European Journal of Public Health, 31*(2), 424–431.

Vasiljevic, Z., Svensson, R., & Shannon, D. (2021). Trends in alcohol intoxication among native and immigrant youth in Sweden, 1999-2017: A comparison across family structure and parental employment status. *International Journal of Drug Policy, 98*, 103397.

Waddell, J. T., Jager, J., & Chassin, L. (2022). Maturing out of alcohol and cannabis co-use: A test of patterns and personality predictors. *Alcoholism: Clinical and Experimental Research, 46*(8), 1603–1615.

Whitaker, V., Curtis, P., Fairbrother, H., Oldham, M., & Holmes, J. (2023). Young people's explanations for the decline in youth drinking in England. *BMC Public Health, 23*(1), 402.

Windle, M. (2020a). Maturing out of alcohol use in young adulthood: Latent class growth trajectories and concurrent young adult correlates. *Alcoholism: Clinical and Experimental Research, 44*(2), 532–540.

Windle, M. (2020b). Sex differences in substance use from adolescence to young adulthood: Tests of increases in emergent adulthood and maturing out in later young adulthood. *Drug and Alcohol Dependence, 207*, 107813.

Windle, M., & Windle, R. C. (2018). Sex differences in peer selection and socialization for alcohol use from adolescence to young adulthood and the influence of marital and parental status. *Alcoholism: Clinical and Experimental Research, 42*(12), 2394–2402.

Winick, C. (1962). Maturing out of narcotic addiction. *Bulletin on Narcotics, 14*(1), 1–7.

World Health Organization (WHO). (2024). *Global status report on alcohol and health and treatment of substance use disorders*. WHO.

Yang, X., Wang, S., & Eklund, L. (2020). Reacting to social discrimination? Men's individual and social risk behaviors in the context of a male marriage squeeze in rural China. *Social Science & Medicine, 246*, 112729.

# Part II

## Diversity in Young Adult Drinking

# 5

# Gender, Drinking, and Drunkenness: From Discourses of Gender Difference to Youthful Femininities and Masculinities

Alexandra Bogren, Geoffrey Hunt, and Margit Anne Petersen

**Abstract** Bogren and colleagues offer an outline of the complex and shifting gendered meanings attributed to young adults' drinking and drunkenness in the period between the 1990s and the present. Focusing on the shifts in meaning brought about by consumer society, postfeminism, and health risk approaches to alcohol, the chapter identifies four key discourses of young adults' alcohol consumption. These discourses in relation to femininity and masculinity among young adults are examined, using research on young adults' perspectives and the Swedish media as illustrative examples. As well as looking into problematizing and celebratory discourses of drinking, Bogren also draws attention to the

A. Bogren (✉)
School of Social Sciences, Södertörn University, Flemingsberg, Sweden
e-mail: alexandra.bogren@sh.se

G. Hunt • M. A. Petersen
Centre for Alcohol and Drugs Research, Aarhus University, Aarhus, Denmark
e-mail: gh.crf@psy.au.dk; map.crf@psy.au.dk



D. Conroy, F. Measham (eds.), *Young Adult Drinking Styles*, Sustainable Development Goals Series, https://doi.org/10.1007/978-3-031-98528-7_5

relation between drinking, gender, and class. The chapter concludes with a discussion of the tensions and contradictions involved in future research on alcohol, femininity, and masculinity among young adults.

## Introduction

Drinking and intoxication are deeply social events. They occur in specific contexts, where young adults socialize and in which they are subject to customs, social norms, rituals, expectations, and socially shared meanings. As such, drinking and becoming intoxicated are practices that young adults make sense of by drawing on their own and others' experiences, on self-representations and other content in social media, and on cultural representations such as advertising and mass media accounts. In many parts of the world, notions of gender are one of the most important interpretive resources young adults use to talk about and understand drinking and intoxication, and a key topic in advertising, mass media accounts, and self-representations of alcohol consumption.

In Northern European countries, drinking has been assigned gendered meanings throughout history. For example, in early sixteenth century England, nineteenth century Sweden, and twentieth century Denmark, heavy drinking was considered a threat to femininity, and temperance or very moderate drinking was the option that secured women moral status and respectability. However, heavy drinking among men was viewed as an affirmation of male bonding and solidarity (Enefalk, 2015; von Sperling, 2023; Warner, 1997). The association of alcohol with masculinity has persisted in the twentieth and twenty-first centuries, and extensive research has documented how heavy drinking in some all-male groups is perceived as a symbol of the drinker's status as "a real man," and is linked to other masculine practices, such as risk taking and aggressiveness (De Keseredy & Schwartz, 1993; Lemle & Mishkind, 1989).

However, recent societal shifts have introduced further layers of complexity to these earlier gendered meanings of drinking and intoxication. The further development of consumer society, the shift from third- to fourth-wave feminism, and an increasing health policy interest in risk groups, coupled with a growing concern among young adults about living a healthy life, have all had an impact on the forms and patterns of drinking viewed as socially acceptable. This chapter presents an overview of and discusses current international research on the gendered discourses of young adults' drinking in the context of some of these shifts, using examples primarily from Scandinavian and other Northern European and Western influenced societies. Broadly defined, discourses are culturally and historically specific ways of signifying the world or particular aspects of it. As they are neither inherently fixed nor stable, discourses shift over time within specific domains and contexts. In using research examples from different societies, we do not wish to collapse individual cultures. Instead, we aim to show that youth and gender researchers today are increasingly utilizing examples from different societies with a high degree of Westernization, which share similar discursive concerns about alcohol, femininities, and masculinities.

## Studying Gendered Discourses About Drinking and Drunkenness

Discourse is a complex and contested concept. It may refer to speech and discussion in general, to a specific verbal presentation of a topic, or to a historically contingent social system that produces ways of naming, understanding, and acting in relation to a phenomenon (e.g. drinking problems) within a certain type of institutionalized practice (e.g. biomedical science) (Titscher et al., 2000). Discursive research can involve the study of how broader patterns of discourse can be revealed from analysing textual data such as official documents, media representations, and organizational minutes, but also the study of how discourse unfolds in naturally occurring talk or interviews, and how discourse shapes identities and selves (Howarth, 2000). These different approaches tend to either see social actors as users of discourse, or to see subjectivity—and by way of extension, agency—as constituted in discourse (Bacchi, 2005). In this chapter, we adopt a synthetic approach that acknowledges that actors can use discourses and sometimes do so strategically, but that use is shaped by the cultural resources available to them and by the social context in which they are situated.

When young adults talk about gender in making sense of drinking practices or drunkenness, they are using gendered discourses. Researchers have increasingly begun to document how drinking and intoxication are coupled with a range of different masculinities and femininities and how these are performed and understood differently across class, ethnicity, age, and sexuality (Hunt & Antin, 2019). In this way, gendered discourses are not only about gender as a binary category (women/men, femininity/masculinity) but may also be about a set of different femininities and the ways in which they are performed, for example, by young and middle-age women. Thus, we adopt the position that discourses on alcohol and intoxication are gendered in different ways that may also change over time and suggest that in performing different femininities and masculinities, young adults are actively negotiating and using gendered discourses of drinking and drunkenness.

An ongoing discussion within research on gender and drinking is the extent to which notions of gender equality appear in discourses on alcohol consumption. In particular, public debate about alcohol has long been pre-occupied with the idea that gender equality has "gone too far" (Day et al., 2004; Jackson & Tinkler, 2007). From the 1990s to the 2020s, discourses of drinking in Scandinavia and elsewhere in northern Europe have been shaped by this criticism of gender equality and by the notion of postfeminism—the idea that gender equality is already achieved and therefore feminism is outdated (Gill, 2018; McRobbie, 2007). Within postfeminist discourse, agency and choice are central, and incorporated into a postfeminist sensibility where feminism is both celebrated and undone. Postfeminism has been connected to both the third- and fourth-wave feminism of the 1990s and 2010s (Rivers, 2017; Sternadori, 2019). This period had also seen a general cultural and political shift towards consumer culture and market liberalism (Measham & Brain, 2005), and a health policy interest in risk groups, especially young people and working-class women. In the alcohol and drugs field, a growing body of evidence from the 2020s also documents the importance of digital platforms in shaping young adults' understandings of the gendered risks and pleasures of drinking (Atkinson & Sumnall, 2016; Romo-Avilés et al., 2020; Vranken et al., 2023), as well as growing awareness and valuation of healthy lifestyles and non- or light drinking among young adults (Nicholls, 2021; Pennay et al., 2022).

Although many discourses, both past and contemporary, primarily treat alcohol and drug use as problematic and risky, others highlight the various pleasures and benefits people experience (Hunt & Antin, 2019; Thurnell-Read & Monaghan, 2023). While increasing attention is being paid to the fact that these categories are not always separable (Petersen et al., 2023), risk and pleasure are two broader societal discourses that people often draw on when they talk about gender and drinking.

## Risky Drinking: Gender and Risk in Policy and News Media Discourses of Young Adults' Alcohol Consumption

Official discourses found, for example, in governmental reports, policies, news reports, and statements by alcohol policy stakeholders, tend to emphasize the risks of drinking (Farrugia et al., 2022; Keane, 2017; Månsson & Bogren, 2014). A common objective is often to educate or warn the public about the downsides and dangers of alcohol. Earlier research shows that when gender is brought to the fore in these materials, it is often equated with women, for example, in describing women's brains and bodies as more biologically vulnerable to alcohol than men's (Bogren, 2011; Farrugia et al., 2022; Keane, 2017). The alcohol discourse within these accounts adopts a risk perspective which tends to present drinking and intoxication as riskier for women than for men. The discourse emphasizes biological differences and constructs alcohol consumption as a risk to women's physical appearance; a sexual risk (leading to sexually transmitted diseases and sexual victimization); a social risk (the risk of losing one's status and reputation); and a health risk (Abrahamsson & Heimdahl, 2010; Day et al., 2004; Keane, 2013; Lyons et al., 2006; Månsson & Bogren, 2014). A recent policy example of emphasizing biological differences can be seen in the recommendations by the Danish Ministry of Health, which up until 2022 recommended that women drink no more than 7 units of alcohol a week, while for men it was 14. A similar development had already taken place in the UK, where the Chief Medical Officer's Low Risk Drinking Guidelines up until 2016 had different recommendations for women and men and highlighted biological differences. An example of alcohol as a sexual risk appeared in the Swedish media debate in the early 2000s, where commentators argued that heavy drinking among young women was a sign of the problems of gender equality and might lead to sexual victimization (Bernhardsson & Bogren, 2012; Bogren, 2011). Similar parallels to this debate were visible in UK media representations of millennial young women's alcohol consumption in the 1990s and early 2000s, which were particularly targeted towards young working-class women who presumably "drank like men." Labelled "ladettes," they were described as "crude," "aggressive," and "sexually loose," their clothing, appearance, and ways of acting pathologized (Day et al., 2004; Griffin et al., 2013; Lyons et al., 2006; Skeggs, 2005). While public debates about young women's drinking during this period were not necessarily openly moralizing, they did highlight—and continue to do so—the various negative aspects of alcohol for young women in particular.

While focusing on women, some of the discourse did also construct men's drinking as a gendered risk and problem, most notably in policy and news discourses on alcohol and violence. For example, a number of articles in Swedish newspapers in the early 2000s described men's heavy drinking as a cause of violence in intimate relationships and as part of an accepted pattern of gender domination and "macho behaviour" in the sports world (Bogren, 2011). Yet unlike those focusing on young women, Swedish newspapers did not exhort young men to stop drinking "like lads" nor did they claim that heavy drinking among men was due to a misunderstanding of gender equality (Bogren, 2011). Similarly, in a recent comparative study of alcohol policy stakeholders in Australia, Canada, and Sweden, Farrugia et al. (2022) found that stakeholders from all three countries saw young men as key perpetrators—and victims—of violence in drinking contexts. However, instead of proposing policy responses focused on men and masculinities, the stakeholders advocated generic interventions (e.g. general restrictions of alcohol availability in different milieu), thereby de-gendering a possible solution. Atkinson et al. (2023) also found that women's magazines in the UK drew attention to alcohol's role in men's violence against women, however, the ways in which such stories were told deflected responsibility from the perpetrator to the effects of alcohol, and in so doing framed the problem as alcohol-related rather than a problem of men and masculinities (Moore et al., 2020).

Problem-oriented discourses on drinking and drug use have a long history, but the ways in which they problematize women's and men's drinking differ. Whereas important progress in the general norms, values, and discourses on women's alcohol and drug use have been made in the decades from the 1970s until today, women's *intoxication* is still often viewed more negatively than men's (Hunt & Antin, 2019). Today, this negative valuation is frequently framed within discourses of risk. Heavy drinking among young women tends to be associated with a broader repertoire of risks than heavy drinking among young men, and the perceived solutions to the problems of women's heavy drinking, but not men's, tend to emphasize gender. Yet despite the general dominance of problem-oriented risk discourses in public health policies of the twenty-first century, alternative discourses that highlight the pleasurable aspects of drinking and drunkenness nevertheless exist. While early studies on men's drinking did not explicitly address pleasure, there was an in-built assumption that male bonding was pleasurable. The same was not true of women's alcohol consumption. In criticizing previous research for focusing only or mostly on the negative aspects of women's drinking and drug use, feminist scholars in the 1990s argued that drinking and drug use among women should be conceptualized along a continuum that included normal and recreational consumption (Ettorre, 1992; Henderson, 1999; Measham, 2002). This shift in emphasis eventually generated more studies of the pleasurable aspects of drinking among women, and consequently, a majority of the research on discourses of gender and pleasurable drinking has focused on women and femininities.

## Pleasurable Drinking: Gender and Enjoyment in Advertising and Popular Media Discourses

In the 1990s and early 2000s, advertising and women's magazines in several Western-influenced societies primarily constructed drinking as a project of pleasure, liberation, and freedom of choice for women rather than as a gendered risk (Beccaria et al., 2018; Lyons et al., 2006; Månsson, 2014). These media outlets depicted women's drinking as trendy, cool, and professional, addressing the audience primarily as potential consumers (Lyons et al., 2006; Månsson, 2014). In the 2020s, this discourse of pleasurable drinking continues to be relevant but has also incorporated additional elements drawn from fourth-wave feminism, visible in alcohol marketing on digital platforms such as Facebook and Instagram where drinking is presented as a key component of traditional, postfeminist, *and* feminist femininities (Atkinson et al., 2022). As a part of this development, alcohol marketing seems to have moved away from sexualizing women (Törrönen & Juslin, 2013) and towards increasingly appropriating feminist and equality messages (Atkinson et al., 2022).

Discourses that conceptualize women's drinking as pleasurable do this in several ways. First, especially in commercial media from the early 2000s until today, drinking is portrayed as a form of pleasuring the self in relaxing, self-indulgent, and self-pampering practices (e.g. in photos of a colourful drink beside a bathtub filled with bubbles), images that echo the advertising of chocolate to female consumers (Atkinson et al., 2022; Månsson, 2014). In these portrayals, drinking is depicted as an escape from, or reward for, a hectic lifestyle and associated with women having time for themselves (Atkinson et al., 2022; Törrönen & Juslin, 2013).

Second, in women's magazines and alcohol advertising, female friendship is a key topic (Atkinson et al., 2022; Månsson, 2014). For example, in Swedish women's magazines in the early 2000s, drinking appeared as a pleasurable aspect of close friendships between women. Groups of women were portrayed as relaxing in an intimate and private sphere while sipping on wine or other alcoholic drinks. Again, alcohol is shown as a key ingredient in creating a gendered private space among a smaller group of "girlfriends" (Månsson, 2014). Similarly, in a study of alcohol brand marketing, Atkinson et al. (2022) found that female-targeted brands (e.g. wine and gin brands) used a language of feminized friendship ("bestie," "sisters," "queens") to promote bonding and group drinking among women. Similar gendered language was not used in male-targeted online posts (Atkinson et al., 2022).

Third, in the 1990s and 2000s, women's drinking was portrayed as pleasurable in the context of partying and fun (Lyons et al., 2006; Månsson, 2014; Törrönen & Juslin, 2013). In Swedish women's magazines, intoxication and wild partying were celebrated as popular activities where drinking represented an instrument for successfully becoming a fashionable and social person (Månsson, 2014). Similarly, UK women's magazines directed at the 18–25 age group repeatedly described the "goodtime girl" as a category that is professional, glamourous, and likes to party (Lyons et al., 2006). In a study of current alcohol commercials in the USA, Hall and Kappel (2018, p. 574) found that while the "party girl" is still a feature, "hotties" (women portrayed as "highly sexualized fantasy objects") and "bitches" (women who "undermine a man's freedom to enjoy erotic pleasures and bond with other men") are more common.

Rather than stressing biological differences between the male and female body, commercial discourses of pleasurable drinking among women emphasize femininity in behaviour and appearance. Via the portrayal of drinking as fashionable, cool, and professional, alcohol consumption is articulated as a sign of empowerment, entitlement, and choice (Atkinson et al., 2022; Månsson & Bogren, 2014). Empowerment, choice, style, and beauty are all central in both the postfeminist and the consumerist discourse of the time. Thus, in line with both postfeminist and consumerist discourse, many adverts and women's magazines represent postfeminist femininity as an identity display and a lifestyle choice for young adult women, a position they can cultivate through alcohol consumption. The extent to which sexualization or self-sexualization (intentionally engaging in activities to appear more sexually appealing, which may be used as a form of postfeminist empowerment with pleasurable aspects) is part of this postfeminist femininity is somewhat unclear, with the literature pointing in different directions (Atkinson et al., 2022; Hall & Kappel, 2018; Rodgers et al., 2019).

The cultural connections between pleasure and men's drinking are more implicit. Beyond generating masculine status, pleasure is always assumed to be part of men's alcohol consumption (Hunt & Antin, 2019). For example, in the early 2000s, representations of men's drinking in UK men's magazines directed at the 18–25 age group depicted men's nights out drinking as battles or adventures (Lyons et al., 2006). The adventure aspect suggests some elements of excitement and fun akin to a gendered, pleasurable experience—gendered because it was associated primarily with men's but not women's drinking. Moreover, in popular culture in the 2000s and 2010s, drinking was sometimes linked with "playboy" masculinity. Studying a smaller number of mainstream music videos, Lindsay and Lyons (2017) found that "playboys" were portrayed as "having the 'freedom' to consume alcohol and sex excessively and without repercussion" (Lindsay & Lyons, 2017, p. 9), and in this way linked men's drinking to a form of pleasure or hedonism, while women were portrayed as actively choosing and enjoying their characterization as "sex objects" who like to drink and party.

Having seen how official and commercial discourses position women's and men's drinking as risky and pleasurable, we now turn to the ways in which young adults themselves engage with these and other discourses in performing a range of different femininities and masculinities.

## Drinking Femininities: Gender and Intersectionality in Women's Discourses of Drinking and Drunkenness

Interview studies from the early 2000s and onwards consistently show that the opposing discourses of risky and pleasurable drinking reappear in many young women's narratives of alcohol, shaping their self-presentations and identity formation. For some young women, drinking is a normal and pleasurable part of everyday life, and essential to partying, but it also involves the risk of being positioned as "unfeminine," "slutty," or "bitchy" (Atkinson & Sumnall, 2016; Hutton, 2020; Pennay et al., 2022; Romo-Avilés et al., 2020). At the same time, researchers studying "new femininities" have noted that some young women re-appropriate negatively coded notions such as "slut" or "bitch," using them in an ironic sense and incorporating them into their own alternative femininities (Budgeon, 2013), and that tensions between idealized and problematized subjectivities are central to the challenges involved in achieving successful femininity today (Budgeon, 2013; Gill, 2007; Gill & Scharff, 2013). Young women negotiate these and other tensions, for example, between consumerism and environmentalism, in different ways, and in so doing, they perform different femininities as well as assign different femininities to others whom they talk about.

Alcohol and drug researchers have shown how, in discussing drinking, young adults attribute gendered problematic positions to others whose drinking they perceive as inappropriate (Griffin et al., 2013; Pennay et al., 2022). Such conceptions of proper and respectable drinking are also related to class, sexuality, age, and ethnicity/race. Above all, interview findings suggest that young adult middle-class women distinguish their own drinking from that of working-class women whom they assign as lacking respectability and taste and who display what is seen as an exaggerated "vulgar," distasteful, or "sexualized" femininity primarily through dress, make-up, and hairstyle (Griffin et al., 2013; Nicholls, 2018; Skeggs, 2005; Vaadal & Ravn, 2021). In such classed discourses of drinking, the meanings of hyperfemininity/emphasized femininity are contested—is it an ironic identity display, a form of pleasurable self-sexualization, or an expression of traditional femininity? Although emphasized femininity may be presented as a classless ideal in postfeminist discourse, research suggests that many young women themselves draw on classed discourses in identifying appropriate ways of performing this femininity. At the same time, studies point to the fact that for many young women looking "appropriately feminine" in nightlife drinking settings requires "the adoption of a more emphasised, exaggerated and—to an extent—(hetero) sexualised femininity than would be expected in other contexts" (Nicholls, 2017, p. 265). Investing in "sexy" femininity through dress and shoes allows straight women to "do heterosexual femininity," but may also allow lesbian women to "pass" as straight in nightlife drinking settings reducing the risk of homophobic abuse (Nicholls, 2017).

Some studies also suggest that discourses on appropriate, successful femininity in nightlife drinking settings vary across cultures. For example, Vaadal and Ravn (2021) show that for middle-class Norwegian women, rejecting excessive drinking is part of a "progressive" lifestyle where they construct their identities around successful careers, "classy" alcohol consumption patterns, "dressing up for other girls" instead of "dressing up for men," and an interest in environmental issues and gender equality. This mix of consumer-oriented discourses highlighting individuality and choice with discourses highlighting environmental concerns and gender equality might be related to differences in national gender cultures and the prominent role of gender equality discourse in Scandinavian societies (Vaadal & Ravn, 2021).

The studies discussed so far suggest that femininity is intersectional rather than monolithic. Young adults construct variations of femininity, or different femininities, in simultaneously navigating both gendered discourses about alcohol and norms and discourses of class, age, ethnicity, and sexuality. For example, acting appropriately according to one's age and ethnicity plays a key role in many young women's constructions of drinking femininities. Vaadal and Dahl (2021) found that a discourse of maturity was prominent among women in their mid- and late twenties, where the women talked about drinking as pleasurable primarily in controlled forms and as part of culinary enjoyment, rather than as related to the excessive intoxication they engaged in when they were younger. In this way, they were performing controlled, mature, and respectable middle-class femininities. Similarly, Pennay et al. (2022) found that maturity and "knowing one's limits," as expressed in patterns of light and moderate drinking, was central to young women's discourses of appropriate femininity in Sweden, Denmark, Australia, and the UK. In talking about maturity and drinking—whether it is heavy, moderate, light, or even non-drinking—women can both disidentify with other groups of women and men (e.g. who are not controlled or do not "know their limits") and achieve a set of different age-appropriate femininities. Furthermore, lighter drinking and non-drinking are not only relevant in the enactment of age-appropriate femininities, they are also key to Muslim and other ethnic minority young women's femininities. Research indicates that both risks and pleasures shape these young women's ways of relating to alcohol and that they manage these risks and pleasures in performing their own version of appropriate femininities (Baerndt, 2023; Pennay et al., 2022). For example, unlike commercial discourses that emphasize wild partying and heavy drinking as pleasurable, some young Muslim women in Denmark talked about being in control at a party as pleasurable (Baerndt, 2023)—a point of view they share with young women from minority ethnic backgrounds in other countries (Caluzzi et al., 2020).

As in commercial discourses of the pleasures of drinking, friendship and flirting are two prominent elements in young women's drinking femininities. Although the women in most studies value friendship highly, the way they talk about alcohol and friendship varies. Young women in the UK, for example, talked about alcohol as a key ingredient in a girl's night out, which helped them create space for socializing, dedicated "girl time," and fun (Nicholls, 2020; see also Pennay et al., 2022), whereas the slightly older Norwegian women in Vaadal and Dahl's (2021) study talked about drinking in a controlled manner as a practice that created intimacy with and expressed care for friends. For some young heterosexual women in Denmark, drinking and intoxication afford an opportunity to be more active and assertive in flirting and approaching potential partners or talking about sex (Bogren et al., 2022; Jensen & Hunt, 2020; Petersen et al., 2023), and for queer women and nonbinary individuals, intoxication may open up a space for exploring sex outside heteronormative expectations (Race et al., 2023).

While drinking can be incorporated in different ways into a range of different femininities as these studies suggest (cf. Measham, 2002), actively avoiding alcohol has also been described as linked to femininities centred around other activities, for example, healthy lifestyles, religion, or creative pursuits such as dance, photography, or film (Pennay et al., 2022). Moreover, for some young women, light or moderate drinking and sobriety may also be part of a risk-reducing strategy (Caluzzi et al., 2020; Pennay et al., 2022), for example, to avoid or manage the risk of sexual assault (Atkinson et al., 2023; Törrönen et al., 2019). The normalization of sexual violations in nightlife settings are important to young women in many contexts, prompting risk and personal safety discourses focused on ways to avoid men's sexual violence on a night out, such as having a drink limit while clubbing, guarding one's drink to avoid drink spiking, and avoid accepting a drink from a stranger (Romo-Avilés et al., 2020; Petersen et al., 2023).

These studies imply that young adult women are active in managing self-positioning and attempt to orient towards preferred positions, but also that their drinking is constrained by others' reactions and by the widespread official discourses that problematize their drinking. The positions young women inhabit may be contradictory and shift over time. The studies also indicate that media debaters' views of the motives behind women's drinking are much too narrowly conceived.

## Drinking Masculinities: Gender and Intersectionality in Men's Discourses of Drinking and Drunkenness

In the wake of feminist research on the emergence of "new laddism" in the 1990s, alcohol and drug researchers too began to explore performances of "laddish" identity among men. "New laddism" involved a culture that developed among often working-class but sometimes also middle-class men in response to felt oppression by a purportedly dominant "political correctness" and feminist politics in society (Jordan et al., 2022). Interview studies in the alcohol and drugs field found that some groups of men embrace a "laddish" identity in nightlife spaces, where heavy drinking—sometimes to the point of vomiting and passing out—casual sex, and loud and boisterous behaviour are celebrated (Dempster, 2011; Hennell et al., 2023; Thurnell-Read, 2013; Törrönen & Roumeliotis, 2014). Others, however, see heavy "laddish" drinking as an inauthentic front or adopt more egalitarian masculinities centred around moderate drinking (Dempster, 2011; de Visser & McDonnell, 2012; Törrönen & Roumeliotis, 2014). Studies document how violence and fights between men in the night-time drinking environment is a concern for young men themselves, prompting support between male friends and efforts to deescalate confrontations (Duncan et al., 2022). Recently, research has also identified how young adults draw on a discourse of lad culture to connect hypermasculinity to "pack mentality" in men's sports teams, "macho" drinking cultures, and various forms of sexual aggression, distancing themselves from such laddish identities (Jordan et al., 2022). Even young men who self-identify as laddish distance themselves from what they see as the nastiest aspects of laddishness such as abuse and sexual harassment aimed at women, while acknowledging that being in a group of men pushing them to cross those boundaries would make it more difficult not to do so (Jeffries, 2020).

Research further shows that the construction of certain drinks or drinking practices as "unmanly" shapes young adults' views of drinking. For example, both young men and women can be sceptical of men who do not drink and evidence from UK interview research has suggested that male non-drinkers may encounter pressure for them to "man up" (Conroy & de Visser, 2013). However, being viewed as "unmanly" in drinking contexts could also be counterbalanced by investing in masculine capital in other domains (e.g. having a muscular physique) (Conroy & de Visser, 2013; de Visser & McDonnell, 2013). Along similar lines, research suggests that non-drinking young men organize their masculinities around sport, desire for a "strong" physical appearance, or gaming (Pennay et al., 2022). Furthermore, class plays a part in the construction of what is viewed as "manly" alcohol consumption patterns, and hence in the performance of different class-based drinking masculinities. For example, a study comparing Finland, Italy, and Sweden suggests that educated middle-class men dis-identify with traditional masculine beverages and drinking styles in favour of "refined" practices such as wine drinking, while less educated men exclude what they perceive as feminine practices from their repertoire (Törrönen, Rolando, & Beccaria, 2017).

Friendship and flirting are key aspects of masculinities and drinking as well. Sports, alcohol, partying, and banter was part of the social "glue" that created deeper friendship bonds among a group of UK university students (Jeffries, 2020), and in Denmark, Herold and Hunt (2020) found that to play around and have fun, for example, in playful fights with male-identified friends, was one way to accomplish pre-party masculinity. Drinking in the company of friends was also common in Instagram posts among Spanish young adult men (Cerdán-Torregrosa et al., 2022). For Australian men, "drinking with the boys" could facilitate deeper friendship bonds, homosocial intimacy, and emotional support and like young men in the UK, they talked about caring for their friends on a night out (Duncan et al., 2022; Hennell et al., 2023; Wilkinson & Wilkinson, 2020). However, discourses and practices of care were constrained and complicated by the fact that the men in two of these studies also valued individual autonomy, independence, and self-reliance, and therefore care was circumscribed by the expectation that their friends would preferably control themselves (Duncan et al., 2022; Hennell et al., 2023).

Flirting and drinking among young adult men is often associated with performances of laddish or hypermasculinity, as discussed above. However, recent research has also found that young adult men in Denmark (Petersen et al., 2022) and the USA (Hirsch & Khan, 2020; Hunt et al., 2022) partly construct their drinking masculinities around a fear of being accused of rape—a concern that also reappears among some young adult men in our ongoing research on intoxication and sexual violence in Sweden.

These studies imply that there appears to be some similarities in notions of alcohol and masculinities across different Western-influenced cultures, for example, in the extent to which heavy drinking is tied to performances of a certain type of hypermasculinity. However, research also testifies to the contextual and local variations in how these masculinities are performed in practice.

## Discussion and Future Research Agenda

Despite men's disproportionate involvement in alcohol consumption and alcohol-related harms across many parts of the world (Duncan et al., 2022), research on gender in the alcohol and drugs field was long dominated by a problem lens that primarily highlighted the negative aspects of (young) women's drinking and drunkenness (Hunt & Antin, 2019). While research has partly shifted its focus, as a consequence of a growing literature on the broader social aspects and pleasures of women's drinking, in popular culture and everyday discourse women's intoxication is still often viewed more negatively than men's (Hunt & Antin, 2019). If historically middle-aged or older drunken women were considered more unacceptable (Waterson, 2000), today younger drunken women are viewed as more problematic and this uneven focus is reproduced in large shares of the existing research. Studies of young men's drinking have followed a different trajectory. Some of the early research on alcohol and masculinity was based in studies of work cultures, including the drinking practices of fishermen, stevedores, and coal miners (Mars, 1987). Current research is instead centred on young men and youth cultures. Since the 1990s, scholars have increasingly examined "the varied and problematic ways in which men attempt to approximate ideals of masculinity through drinking events, for example, by engaging in risk taking, "disorderly" drinking, and displays of aggression and intimidation (Duncan et al., 2022, p. 47). Lately, "inclusive masculinities" incorporating men's caring and supportive practices in drinking contexts have gained more attention as part of an attempt to nuance accounts of "laddish" or otherwise problematic masculinities (Duncan et al., 2022; Hennell et al., 2023; Wilkinson & Wilkinson, 2020). Consequently, some scholars suggest that drinking masculinities may be diversifying (Lyons & Kersey, 2020) or that multiple drinking masculinities exist side-by-side, none of them clearly dominating over the others (Törrönen & Roumeliotis, 2014).

Overall, research indicates that both femininities and masculinities of drinking are formed in a field of tensions between the risks and pleasures of alcohol. Some young women see themselves as strong and independent consumers but also identify with feminist femininities, others avoid alcohol crafting a femininity focused on healthy eating and wellness (Pennay et al., 2022; Vaadal & Ravn, 2021). Indeed, some of our ongoing research shows that some women do both at the same time (Petersen et al., 2023). For some young men, sports are the basis for constructing non-drinking masculinities. However, research on body building suggest that some men utilize other legal substances, such as steroids, to achieve the necessary form (Monaghan, 1999). While for others, it is closely tied to laddish drinking (Jeffries, 2020; Pennay et al., 2022). Diversity across class, age, ethnicity/race, and sexuality further complicates this picture. For example, cultures of drinking, intoxication, and masculinity are significantly different among Latino and African-American gangs (Hunt et al., 2005).

However, we still lack knowledge about the relation between these drinking practices and ideals and wider social change in women's and men's lives. Furthermore, given gender differences in access to power and opportunity in wider society, and in many different substance use contexts (Miller & Carbone-Lopez, 2015), the social processes of identity formation are likely to be different for women and men, as well as to be shaped by other intersecting forms of social categorization. Although research on masculinities and drinking is growing, many issues are still unexplored. For example, future studies might critically examine, as Duncan et al. (2022) did, the nature and extent of men's caring practices on a night out (such as looking out for friends who were drunk, "rescuing" women from unwanted attention, or diffusing physical conflicts), analysing not only potentially positive aspects but also the constraints, exclusions, and power dynamics such practices may involve (see also Hunt et al., 2005). Similar critical and in-depth analyses of the meanings and power dynamics involved in such varied practices as sports, gaming, and playful fights might reveal key insights about "healthy masculinities" more broadly conceived—whether they involve alcohol or not. Another relevant aspect to explore is the extent to which some men benefit from "lad culture" without themselves investing in explicit performances of laddish masculinity. For example, research on sexual harassment and violence against women on campus suggests that men lose "lad points" and hence status among "the lads" if they attempt to stop a guy from perpetrating violence, and that actively avoiding intervention could be part of such complicit masculinities (Jordan et al., 2022). In this way, it may be a benefit to some men's masculinity to not speak up against violence towards women even if they aren't generally behaving in a "laddish" way themselves. The hegemonic position of "laddish masculinity" in many college and partying contexts further suggests that alcohol and drug research needs to examine the hierarchy of masculinities (Carrigan, Connell & Lee, 1985; Messerschmidt, 2019)—how relative status, authority, and gendered power is distributed among men, and the social consequences of this distribution.

Since the 1990s, feminist sociocultural research on gender and alcohol has expanded. Within this specific subfield, femininities have been more extensively explored than masculinities, but there is nevertheless a lack of accounts that explicitly theorize both masculinity and femininity. For example, with regard to femininity, gender scholars are currently beginning to examine "rigid femininities," how to conceptualize feminine power, and in what ways vulnerability can act as a powerful mode of resistance (Hoskin & Blair, 2022). Some of these issues are also important to explore in relation to alcohol and drugs. Furthermore, apart from noting that drinking and sober masculinities and femininities are diverse, one may ask how the set of different masculinities and femininities that scholars have identified are related to one another. For example, are some gendered narratives of drinking primarily accessible to young men and women, as research on the constructions of maturity and drinking suggests? What are the similarities and differences between drinking femininities and masculinities performed by cisgender young adults and those performed by trans or non-binary young adults (Hunt et al., 2019)?

Other research could usefully explore drinking and drug use in relation to place to guide understanding of why "particular narratives of gender or particular ways of performing or 'doing' gender [are] more or less available within the life situations" of different groups of individuals within different social settings (Miller & Carbone-Lopez, 2015, p. 698).

Finally, on a methodological level, scholars need to address the difficulty of producing research that does not primarily react to or mirror media and everyday accounts of gendered drinking practices. An important tension for researchers here is to decide whether, and to what extent, this difficulty can or should be resisted or accommodated. Indeed, addressing this tension may help guide understanding of why gendered representations, norms, and discourses of drinking may change at different rates and in different ways to ongoing patterns of change in young adult drinking practices.

## References

Abrahamsson, M., & Heimdahl, K. (2010). Gendered discourse in Swedish national alcohol policy action plans 1965–2007: Invisible men and problematic women. *Nordic Studies on Alcohol and Drugs, 27*(1), 63–86.

Atkinson, A., Matthews, B., Nicholls, E., & Sumnall, H. (2023). 'Some days I am a lunatic that thinks I can moderate': Amalgamating recovery and neoliberal discourses within accounts of non-drinking among women active in the 'positive sobriety' community on Instagram in the UK. *International Journal of Drug Policy, 112*, 103937.

Atkinson, A., Meadows, B., Ross-Houle, K.-M., Smith, C., & Sumnall, H. R. (2023). Magazines as contradictory spaces for alcohol messaging: A mixed method content and thematic analysis of UK women's magazine representations of alcohol and its consumption. *Drugs: Education, Prevention and Policy, 30*(5), 474–485.

Atkinson, A., Meadows, B. R., Emslie, C., Lyons, A., & Sumnall, H. R. (2022). 'Pretty in Pink' and 'Girl Power': An analysis of the targeting and representation of women in alcohol brand marketing on Facebook and Instagram. *International Journal of Drug Policy, 101*, 103547.

Atkinson, A., & Sumnall, H. (2016). 'If I don't look good, it just doesn't go up': A qualitative study of young women's drinking cultures and practices on Social Network Sites. *International Journal of Drug Policy, 38*, 50–62.

Bacchi, C. (2005). Discourse, discourse everywhere: Subject agency in feminist discourse methodology. *Nordic Journal of Women's Studies, 13*(3), 198–209.

Baerndt, M. (2023). *Dilemmas of youth drinking: Young Muslim women's experiences within the Danish youth alcohol culture*. Aarhus University, Centre for Alcohol and Drug Research.

Beccaria, F., Rolando, S., Törrönen, J., & Scavarda, A. (2018). From housekeeper to status-oriented consumer and hyper-sexual imagery: Images of alcohol targeted to Italian women from the 1960s to the 2000s. *Feminist Media Studies, 18*(6), 1012–1039.

Bernhardsson, J., & Bogren, A. (2012). Drink sluts, brats, and immigrants as others: An analysis of Swedish media discourse on gender, alcohol and rape. *Feminist Media Studies, 12*(1), 1–16.

Bogren, A. (2011). Gender and alcohol: The Swedish press debate. *Journal of Gender Studies, 20*(2), 155–169.

Bogren, A., Hunt, G., & Petersen, M. A. (2022). Rethinking intoxicated sexual encounters. *Drugs: Education, Prevention and Policy, 30*(1), 31–41.

Budgeon, S. (2013). The contradictions of successful femininity: Third-wave feminism, postfeminism and 'new' femininities. In R. Gill & C. Scharff (Eds.), *New femininities: Postfeminism, neoliberalism, and subjectivity* (pp. 279–292). Palgrave Macmillan.

Caluzzi, G., MacLean, S., & Pennay, A. (2020). Re-configured pleasures: How young people feel good through abstaining or moderating their drinking. *International Journal of Drug Policy, 77*, 102709.

Carrigan, T., Connell, B., & Lee, J. (1985). Toward a new sociology of masculinity. *Theory and Society, 14*(5), 551–604.

Cerdán-Torregrosa, A., La Parra-Casado, D., & Vives-Cases, C. (2022). "If you do not fit in with the stereotype, they eat you alive": Discourses of masculinities and their reflections in young Spanish men's health. *Qualitative Health Research, 32*(2), 225–237.

Conroy, D., & de Visser, R. (2013). Man up! Discursive constructions of non-drinkers among UK undergraduates. *Journal of Health Psychology, 18*(11), 1432–1444.

Day, K., Gough, B., & McFadden, M. (2004). Warning! Alcohol can seriously damage your feminine health. *Feminist Media Studies, 4*(2), 165–183.

De Keseredy, W. S., & Schwartz, M. D. (1993). Male peer support and woman abuse: An expansion of DeKeseredy's model. *Sociological Spectrum, 13*(4), 393–413.

de Visser, R., & McDonnell, E. (2012). That's OK. He's a guy: A mixed-methods study of gender double-standards for alcohol use. *Psychology & Health, 27*(5), 618–639.

de Visser, R., & McDonnell, E. (2013). Man points: Masculine capital and young men's health. *Health Psychology, 32*(1), 5–14.

Dempster, S. (2011). I drink, therefore I'm man: Gender discourses, alcohol and the construction of British undergraduate masculinities. *Gender and Education, 23*(5), 635–653.

Duncan, T., Roberts, S., Elliott, K., Ralph, B., Savic, M., & Robards, B. (2022). "Looking after yourself is self-respect": The limits and possibilities of men's care on a night out. *Contemporary Drug Problems, 49*(1), 46–63.

Enefalk, H. (2015). Alcohol and femininity in Sweden c. 1830–1922: An investigation of the emergence of separate drinking standards for men and women. *Substance Use & Misuse, 50*(6), 736–746.

Ettorre, E. (1992). *Women and substance use.* Red Globe Press.

Farrugia, A., Moore, D., Keane, H., Ekendahl, M., Graham, K., & Duncan, D. (2022). Noticed and then forgotten: Gender in alcohol policy stakeholder responses to alcohol and violence. *Qualitative Health Research, 32*(10), 1419–1432.

Gill, R. (2007). Critical respect: The difficulties and dilemmas of agency and "choice" for feminism. *European Journal of Women's Studies, 14*(1), 69–80.

Gill, R. (2018). Post-postfeminism? New feminist visibilities in postfeminist times. In J. Keller, J. Littler, & A. Winch (Eds.), *An intergenerational feminist media studies*. Routledge.

Gill, R., & Scharff, C. (Eds.). (2013). *New femininities: Postfeminism, neoliberalism, and subjectivity*. Palgrave Macmillan.

Griffin, C., Szmigin, I., Bengry-Howell, A., Hackley, C., & Mistral, W. (2013). Inhabiting the contradictions: Hypersexual femininity and the culture of intoxication among young women in the UK. *Feminism & Psychology, 23*(2), 184–206.

Hall, G., & Kappel, R. (2018). Gender, alcohol, and the media: The portrayal of men and women in alcohol commercials. *The Sociological Quarterly, 59*(4), 571–583.

Henderson, S. (1999). Drugs and culture: The question of gender. In N. South (Ed.), *Drugs: Culture, controls, and everyday life* (pp. 36–48). Sage.

Hennell, K., Limmer, M., & Piacentini, M. (2023). A 'proper night out': A practice theory exploration of gendered drinking. *Sociological Research Online, 28*(2), 355–372.

Herold, M., & Hunt, G. (2020). Drinking comfortably? Gender and affect among Danish pre-partiers. *International Journal of Drug Policy, 81*, 102522.

Hirsch, J., & Khan, S. (2020). *Sexual citizens: Sex, power and assault on campus*. W.W. Norton.

Hoskin, R. A., & Blair, K. L. (2022). Critical femininities: A 'new' approach to gender theory. *Psychology & Sexuality, 13*(1), 1–8.

Howarth, D. (2000). *Discourse*. Open University Press.

Hunt, G., & Antin, T. (2019). Gender and Intoxication: From masculinity to intersectionality. *Drugs: Education, Prevention & Policy, 26*(1), 70–78.

Hunt, G., Antin, T., Sanders, E., & Sisneros, M. (2019). Queer youth, intoxication and queer drinking spaces. *Journal of Youth Studies, 22*(3), 380–400.

Hunt, G., MacKenzie, K., & Joe-Laidler, K. (2005). Alcohol and masculinity: The case of ethnic youth gangs. In T. M. Wilson (Ed.), *Drinking cultures: Alcohol and identity* (pp. 225–254). Berg.

Hunt, G., Sanders, E., Petersen, M. A., & Bogren, A. (2022). Blurring the line: Intoxication, gender, consent and sexual encounters among young adults. *Contemporary Drug Problems, 49*(1), 84–105.

Hutton, F. (2020). *Cultures of intoxication*. Palgrave Macmillan.

Jackson, C., & Tinkler, P. (2007). Ladettes and modern girls: Troublesome young femininities. *Sociological Review, 55*(2), 251–272.

Jeffries, M. (2020). 'Is it okay to go out on the pull without it being nasty?': Lads' performance of lad culture. *Gender and Education, 32*(7), 908–925.

Jensen, M. B., & Hunt, G. (2020). Young women's narratives on sex in the context of heavy alcohol use: Friendships, gender norms and the sociality of consent. *International Journal of Drug Policy, 81*, 102526.

Jordan, A., Anitha, S., Jameson, J., & Davy, Z. (2022). Hierarchies of masculinity and lad culture on campus: "Bad guys", "good guys", and complicit men. *Men and Masculinities, 25*(5), 698–720.

Keane, H. (2013). Healthy adults and maternal bodies: Reformulations of gender in Australian alcohol guidelines. *Health Sociology Review, 22*(2), 151–161.

Keane, H. (2017). Female vulnerability and susceptible brains: Gendered discourses of addiction. *Social History of Alcohol and Drugs, 31*, 126–139.

Lemle, R., & Mishkind, M. E. (1989). Alcohol and masculinity. *Journal of Substance Abuse Treatment, 6*(4), 213–222.

Lindsay, S., & Lyons, A. (2017). Pour it up, drink it up, live it up, give it up: Masculinity and alcohol in pop music videos. *Men and Masculinities, 21*(5), 624–644.

Lyons, A., Dalton, S., & Hoy, A. (2006). Hardcore drinking: Portrayals of alcohol consumption in young women's and men's magazines. *Journal of Health Psychology, 11*(2), 223–232.

Lyons, A., & Kersey, K. (2020). Alcohol and intoxication. In F. Hutton (Ed.), *Cultures of intoxication*. Palgrave Macmillan.

Månsson, E. (2014). Drinking as a feminine practice: Post-feminist images of women's drinking in Swedish women's magazines. *Feminist Media Studies, 14*(1), 56–72.

Månsson, E., & Bogren, A. (2014). Health, risk and pleasure: The formation of gendered discourses on women's alcohol consumption. *Addiction Research & Theory, 22*(1), 27–36.

Mars, G. (1987). Longshore drinking, economic security and union politics in Newfoundland. In M. Douglas (Ed.), *Constructive drinking*. Routledge.

McRobbie, A. (2007). Top girls? *Cultural Studies, 21*(4–5), 718–737.

Measham, F. (2002). "Doing gender"—"doing drugs": Conceptualizing the gendering of drugs cultures. *Contemporary Drug Problems, 29*(2), 335–373.

Measham, F., & Brain, K. (2005). Binge drinking, British alcohol policy and the new culture of intoxication. *Crime, Media, Culture, 1*(3), 262–283.

Messerschmidt, J. W. (2019). The salience of "hegemonic masculinity". *Men and Masculinities, 22*(1), 85–91.

Miller, J., & Carbone-Lopez, C. (2015). Beyond doing gender: Incorporating race, class, place and life transitions into feminist drug research. *Substance Use & Misuse, 50*(6), 693–707.

Monaghan, L. (1999). Challenging medicine? Bodybuilding, drugs and risk. *Sociology of Health and Illness, 21*(6), 707–734.

Moore, D., Duncan, D., Keane, H., & Ekendahl, M. (2020). Displacements of gender: Research on alcohol, violence and the night-time economy. *Journal of Sociology, 57*(4), 860–876.

Nicholls, E. (2017). Dulling it down a bit: Managing visibility, sexualities and risk in the night time economy in Newcastle, UK. *Gender, Place & Culture, 24*(2), 260–273.

Nicholls, E. (2018). *Negotiating femininities in the neoliberal night-time economy: Too much of a girl?* Springer International Publishing.

Nicholls, E. (2020). 'I feel like I have to become part of that identity': Negotiating femininities and friendships through alcohol consumption in Newcastle, UK. *International Journal of Drug Policy, 81*, 102524.

Nicholls, E. (2021). Sober rebels or good consumer-citizens? Anti-consumption and the 'enterprising self' in early sobriety. *Sociology, 55*(4), 768–784.

Pennay, A., Törrönen, J., Herold, M., Fenton, L., MacLean, S., Caluzzi, G., Fairbrother, H., Frank, V., Samuelsson, E., & Holmes, J. (2022). "There's a lot of stereotypes going on": A cross-national qualitative analysis of the place of gender in declining youth drinking. *International Journal of Drug Policy, 108*, 103827.

Petersen, M. A., Bogren, A., & Hunt, G. (2023). Ambiguous encounters: Young women's expectations and experiences with intoxicated sexual relations in Danish nightlife. *Young - Nordic Journal of Youth Research, 31*(5), 175–183.

Petersen, M. A., Borup, S., Schröder, S., Bogren, A., & Hunt, G. (2022). Alkohol er med til at komplicere unge mænds forståelse af egne og andres seksuelle grænser. *STOF, 42*, 50–57.

Race, K., Pienaar, K., Murphy, D., & Lea, T. (2023). 'Uninhibited play:' The political and pragmatic dimensions of intoxication within queer cultures. In G. Hunt, T. Antin, & V. Frank (Eds.), *Routledge handbook of intoxicants and intoxication*. Routledge.

Rivers, N. (2017). *Postfeminism and the arrival of the fourth wave*. Palgrave Macmillan.

Rodgers, K., Hust, S. J. T., Fitts Willoughby, J., Wheeler, J., & Li, J. (2019). Adolescents' sex-related alcohol expectancies and alcohol advertisements in magazines: The role of wishful identification, realism, and beliefs about women's enjoyment of sexualization. *Journal of Health Communication, 24*(4), 395–404.

Romo-Avilés, N., García-Carpintero, M., & Pavón-Benítez, L. (2020). Not without my mobile phone: Alcohol binge drinking, gender violence and technology in the Spanish culture of intoxication. *Drugs: Education, Prevention & Policy, 27*(2), 154–164.

Skeggs, B. (2005). The making of class and gender through visualizing moral subject formation. *Sociology, 39*(5), 965–982.

Sternadori, M. (2019). Situating the fourth wave of feminism in popular media discourses. In M. Marron (Ed.), *Misogyny and media in the age of Trump*. Rowman & Littlefield.

Thurnell-Read, T. (2013). 'Yobs' and 'snobs': Embodying drink and the problematic male drinking body. *Sociological Research Online, 18*(2), 3.

Thurnell-Read, T., & Monaghan, M. (2023). *Intoxication: Self, state and society*. Palgrave Macmillan.

Titscher, S., Meyer, M., Wodak, R., & Vetter, E. (2000). *Methods of text and discourse analysis*. Sage.

Törrönen, J., & Juslin, I. (2013). From genius of the home to party princess: Drinking in Finnish women's magazine advertisements from the 1960s to the 2000s. *Feminist Media Studies, 13*(3), 463–489.

Törrönen, J., Rolando, S., & Beccaria, F. (2017). Masculinities and femininities of drinking in Finland, Italy and Sweden: Doing, modifying and unlinking gender in relation to different drinking places. *Geoforum, 82*, 131–140.

Törrönen, J., & Roumeliotis, F. (2014). Masculinities of drinking as described by Swedish and Finnish age-based focus groups. *Addiction Research & Theory, 22*(2), 126–136.

Törrönen, J., Roumeliotis, F., Samuelsson, E., Kraus, L., & Room, R. (2019). Why are young people drinking less than earlier? Identifying and specifying social mechanisms with a pragmatist approach. *International Journal of Drug Policy, 64*, 13–20.

Vaadal, K., & Dahl, S. (2021). Maturing out of 'binge drinking': Young adult women's performance of age and gender in times of transition. *Journal of Youth Studies, 24*(10), 1326–1339.

Vaadal, K., & Ravn, S. (2021). It feels like life is narrowing: Aspirational lifestyles and ambivalent futures among Norwegian 'top girls'. *Sociology, 55*(6), 1135–1150.

von Sperling, A. (2023). *Fulde liv. Hvordan kvinder har drukket og er blevet set på imens*. Informations Forlag.

Vranken, S., Murru, S., & Beullens, K. (2023). "Boys are allowed to be drunk": Exploring gender norms in adolescents' alcohol references across different social media platforms and message types. *Journal of Drug Issues*. https://doi.org/10.1177/00220426231163791

Warner, J. (1997). The sanctuary of sobriety: The emergence of temperance as a feminine virtue in Tudor and Stuart England. *Addiction, 92*(1), 97–111.

Waterson, J. (2000). *Women and alcohol in social context*. Palgrave.

Wilkinson, S., & Wilkinson, C. (2020). Young men's alcohol consumption experiences and performances of masculinity. *International Journal of Drug Policy, 81*, 102550.

# 6

# Navigating Drinking Cultures Among Muslim Young Adults: An Overview of Relevant Literature and Findings from a Danish Study Concerning Experiences of Young Muslim Women

Marie Fjellerup Bærndt and Vibeke Asmussen Frank

**Abstract** A reluctance to investigate religious explanations for the non-use of alcohol, combined with the widespread assumption that Muslims are abstinent, has contributed to Muslims' invisibility in alcohol research. Drawing on the literature on young adult Muslims and alcohol consumption, we have two interconnected errands: Firstly, we present the most common themes in the literature, and secondly we revisit these themes in light of findings from a recent research project on young adult Muslim women in Denmark. Zooming in on the dilemmas of being Muslim and growing up in societies where alcohol is highly integrated in young

M. F. Bærndt (✉)
VIVE, The Danish Center for Social Science Research, Aarhus, Denmark
e-mail: mafb@vive.dk

V. A. Frank
Research Center for Social Marginalisation, VIA University College, Aarhus, Denmark
e-mail: VFRA@via.dk



D. Conroy, F. Measham (eds.), *Young Adult Drinking Styles*, Sustainable Development Goals Series, https://doi.org/10.1007/978-3-031-98528-7_6

people's social life, we focus on issues that affect both youth life among peers and family/community life and, not least, how they are often interconnected. We show the complexities in the relationship between young adult Muslims and alcohol consumption and discuss how these are related to broader difficulties of merging a Muslim identity with another (national) identity. Finally, we argue that it is central to apply approaches that sensitively point to differences and similarities among and between different groups of young adults to make the results recognizable, which is necessary if we want to improve policy and prevention initiatives.

The study of minorities and their drinking experiences is important. It is a way to recognize that the position of alcohol is understood in numerous ways that find different meanings among different individuals. Some minorities are more unlikely research subjects than others. This is the case for Muslims and especially Muslims living in non-Muslim countries.

In many European countries, alcohol consumption levels among young adults are high. Drinking to intoxication is a widespread norm and a meaningful and prevalent way to access different groups and communities. Young people in Denmark have some of the highest alcohol use levels compared to their peers in Europe. Drinking is central in their formation of sociality, they start drinking at an early age, and being drunk is a goal (Frank et al., 2020a; Herold & Kolind, 2022). However, young people in many Western countries are exhibiting a growing interest in drinking less and being sober curious, a trend that has caught the interest of public health professionals, politicians, and media (Pennay et al., 2018). Despite these two contradictory tendencies, which are also found in Denmark, the conversation about abstinence and alcohol consumption rarely reaches central groups who are known to support abstinence, such as many religious minorities, among them Muslims. In this chapter, we focus on Muslim young adults and their rather unexplored but important approach to abstinence and alcohol consumption.

A general assumption about Muslims is that they do not drink alcohol, because the Quran and other Islamic texts condemn consumption of alcohol and being drunk as *haram* (Mallik et al., 2021). Alcohol consumption was not outright prohibited in Islam from the beginning but "went from a behavior that was tolerated, then discouraged, then forbidden, then strongly forbidden" (Michalak & Trocki, 2006, p. 531).

Alcohol is considered an intoxicant that "befogs the mind", leads to other haram behaviors, and is broadly disapproved among Muslims (ibid., p. 529). The assumption that Muslims do not drink alcohol includes Muslim immigrants and their descendants in countries, for example, Australia, Denmark, and the UK, where alcohol and alcohol consumption are social imperatives and drinking cultures are widespread, particularly among young people (e.g., Griffin et al., 2013; McKay et al., 2009; Herold & Frank, 2022).

However, Muslims do not necessarily follow religious rules and regulations to the letter (Matthee, 2014). Religious historians, anthropologists, and sociologists highlight the difference between religious texts and everyday practices of a religion, and that local cultures and traditions might be as—or even more—important than following religious doctrines (Eller, 2021; Ernst, 2020; Morris, 2006). Historically, production and consumption of alcohol have existed in most Muslim majority countries (Thurnell-Read & Monaghan, 2023), and contemporary empirical studies show that alcohol is consumed in Muslim majority countries (Al-Ansari et al., 2016; Kamela et al., 2016; Chegeni et al., 2020), although this literature is sparse (AlMarri & Oei, 2009). Other studies have shown that alcohol use is prevalent among Muslims living in Muslim-minority countries (Pannu et al., 2009), and some researchers point to the acculturation of Muslims into alcohol cultures as a cause of a generational increase in consumption (Mir, 2014).

In other words, we cannot unequivocally conclude that Muslims do not drink alcohol. Perceptions and experiences vary significantly, both across Muslim majority countries and within Muslim minority communities (Michalak & Trocki, 2006), which underscores the importance of being careful with assumptions when investigating the connections between drinking, abstinence, and being Muslim. The perception that Muslims are abstinent has made them unlikely research subjects in social science alcohol research and caused a lack of research on alcohol consumption among Muslims in general and among Muslims in non-Muslim majority countries in particular. Here, we focus on young adult Muslims and the apparent paradox of being Muslim and growing up in societies where alcohol is part of the national culture and alcohol consumption is integrated in young people's social life, for instance, in relation to friendship (MacLean, 2016; Thurnell-Read, 2016; Conroy & MacLean, 2019), youth culture (McCreanor et al., 2013; Järvinen & Room, 2017), ideas of age and maturity (Herold & Frank, 2022; Demant & Järvinen, 2006), and gendered norms (De Visser & McDonnell, 2012; Frank et al., 2020a; Pennay et al., 2022). The chapter explores evidence that illustrates the array of dilemmas that young Muslims in general, and young Muslim women in particular, have to navigate.

The chapter consists of two parts. First, we present three major themes in the literature on the subject: (1) harmful gossip as a social control mechanism in drinking contexts, (2) Islam as a culture of abstinence, and (3) racism, othering, and exclusion of young Muslims in drinking settings. Second, we focus on young Muslim women and discuss three additional themes based on data from a study conducted by the first author of this chapter (see Bærndt & Kolind, 2021; Bærndt & Frank, 2022; Bærndt, 2023a, 2023b): (1) the inherent dilemmas in their experiences with youth drinking cultures concerning national identity and belonging, (2) social inclusion and exclusion, and (3) Muslim drinking stories. Finally, we discuss the importance of incorporating diversity and intersectionality in youth alcohol research to make the knowledge relatable for more young people in a multifaceted and differentiated world.

## Dominant Themes in the Literature on Young Muslims and Alcohol

The three themes mentioned above are not clear cut but overlapping. As we unfold them, we include studies that focus on Muslims as well as ethnic minority youth in general, since they often include young people with a Muslim background.

### Community Gossip and Self-Discipline as Examples of Social Control

Social control as an in-group mechanism that strongly urges group members to behave in certain ways is a prevalent theme in the literature. An example is community gossip about alcohol consumption and its consequences. Bradby (2007), in her study among British Asians, including Muslims, found that particularly female drinking was disapproved of, and the few young Muslim women in her study who did drink alcohol, did so secretly. Furthermore, young Muslim women, more than young men, were concerned about malicious gossip, because harm to their reputation was almost impossible to erase and could lead to social ostracism or limited marriage prospects (see also Mirdal, 2006; Waltorp, 2015). The consequences thus seem to be harsher for young Muslim women, whereas young Muslim men can compensate their damaged reputation, for instance if their parents hold a decent position in the community. Consequently, young Muslim women constrain their behavior more than men do, and some even resort to begging or intimidating their friends if they fear that stories of alcohol use will be passed on to their families (Bradby, 2007).

Community gossip is often linked to the way many young Muslim women experience an ever-present potential for being under surveillance (Valentine et al., 2010). Young Muslims who go out often have "a sense that the eyes of the community are always on the street", which means that some young Muslims who want to drink instead exercise self-discipline and feel compelled to abstain. Community gossip and fear of sanctions contribute further to feelings of shame and embarrassment in connection with parties and alcohol consumption. Douglass et al. (2022), in their study among young migrants and ethnic minorities in Australia, found that their participants saw self-control as both important and as a two-edged sword: It grows both from the pressure to avoid being the topic of community gossip and the pressure to be perceived as hardworking and productive to be accepted in Australian society. The pressure to be seen as a model minority was present at home, at work, and in education, and they worked hard to not be seen as problematic (Douglass et al., 2022). Coming across as the best version of yourself is therefore a strategy among young Muslim men and women when they go out. Being in control rather than losing control is broadly considered more pleasurable among many ethnic minority and Muslim youth in contrast to norms of controlled loss of control among many majority young people growing up in cultures of intoxication (Measham, 2004).

While social control mechanisms in general can include different acts of self-disciplining (e.g., manners, clothing style, or curfew) stemming from a sense of being observed and sanctioned, it seems that social control in the literature on alcohol and alcohol consumption among Muslims is especially related to gossip. This relates to the next theme on Islam as a culture of abstinence.

## Islam as a Culture of Abstinence

In this second theme, the research literature focuses explicitly on Islam as a culture of abstinence, where community values provide directions for the individual and sanction those who deviate. Valentine et al. (2010) found that values of religiously motivated abstinence could generate physical discomfort and emotions of disgust and repulsion toward alcohol among the British Pakistani young adults and adults who participated in their study, even though they did not drink alcohol. One central point made by Valentine et al. (2010) is that even though not all their participants are abstinent, growing up in families and/or communities with a culture of abstinence poses certain dilemmas for drinkers and abstainers alike. Other researchers argue that studies of Muslims and alcohol consumption have relied too heavily on orthodoxy and text rather than lived experience, and that research has been too sober and blind to the diversity in experiences with and perceptions of alcohol consumption among Muslims (Ahmed, 2016). These critical voices are not based on empirical research but on a more theoretical position that religious doctrines can be practiced in very different ways in everyday lives (ibid.).

We know that the expectation that everyone drinks alcohol can be troublesome for abstainers in general (Bannister et al., 2025), but Muslim abstainers face specific problems in quite different settings, like at work and sports events. Arifeen (2020) describes the particular difficulties abstinent Muslim women encounter at certain workplace events where drinking is expected. Within the confines of a workplace, all employees feel obligated to participate, and abstinent Muslim women therefore do difficult emotional work in order to be present and still risk feeling socially excluded and stigmatized. In a different setting, Fletcher and

Spracklen (2014) show that ritualized drinking of alcohol after amateur cricket matches is a way of socializing that can be excluding. British Pakistani Muslim cricket players risk being socially excluded if they do not participate and may be perceived as enacting a typical Muslim behavior whereby they exclude themselves.

The increasing scholarly interest in abstinence as a cultural phenomenon among young people and adults typically does not include a focus on religious background or practices as a reason for abstaining. The quantitative literature that examines young people abstaining from alcohol in societies where drinking is a social imperative mentions religion in a generalized form as a reason for abstaining. Qualitative studies on abstinence from alcohol among young people only sporadically mention religion as a reason for abstaining, for example, as culturally sanctioned (Conroy & de Visser, 2014, 2015), or not at all (Frank et al., 2020b). Dotinga (2005) find that respondents with a Moroccan or Turkish—and therefore most often Muslim—background in the Netherlands are underrepresented in quantitative research on alcohol consumption because, the authors argue, they are reluctant to participate because of the Islamic ethics against alcohol. The lack of detailed knowledge about abstinence among Muslim minority youth in general—also in the literature on abstinence—is perhaps a result of a biased focus on Muslims as non-drinkers due to religious doctrines. While many Muslim communities can be characterized as cultures of abstinence in relation to alcohol, we miss out on the diversity of practices that exist among different groups of Muslim minority youth if we forget to investigate these communities further. The third and last theme concerns community and societal aspects of being Muslim and drinking alcohol.

## Racism, Othering, Exclusion: Social Spaces and Alcohol Consumption

The third and last theme in the literature concerns studies that are more indirectly linked to alcohol consumption among young adult Muslims, focus on common settings for alcohol consumption, and center on racism, othering, and exclusion of ethnic minority youth, including Muslims.

The literature on nightlife venues shows that ethnic minorities, particularly ethnic minority men, are rejected at the entrance (Søgaard, 2017; May & Chaplin, 2008). Bouncers (i.e., security guards in licensed venues) play a key role in regulating the nightlife, and their policing of accessibility tends to reproduce ethnic divisions and inequalities (Søgaard, 2017). Many venues have their own entry requirements, which materialize as more or less subtle forms of discrimination based on age, appearance, social class, gender, ethnicity, and sexuality (Hobbs et al., 2003).

In, for example, Germany, the Netherlands, and the UK, discrimination of ethnic minorities at the door of popular clubs or the lack of or exclusion of ethnic music in mainstream nightlife have contributed to the creation of ethno-parties organized by and for one single ethnic minority (Boogarts, 2008; Huq, 2007). Some see the emergence of separate clubbing scenes as a threat to social cohesion since it reflects a growing tendency toward division rather than a more multicultural party scene. However, as Boogarts (2008) argues in her empirical study of the Turkish party scenes of Amsterdam and Rotterdam, the threat precedes the ethno-parties as many young ethnic minorities feel they are pushed out of mainstream nightlife. They prefer the ethno-party scene where they can dance to the music they want and come together with co-ethnics with whom they share feelings of understanding, sameness, and belonging and who do not ask questions about religion or (non-) drinking of alcohol.

In the next part of the chapter, we expand on the three themes by introducing results from a study among young adult Muslim women conducted in Denmark by the first author. The results are published in Bærndt (2023a), Bærndt and Frank (2022), and Bærndt and Kolind (2021) and form the backbone of a PhD dissertation (2023b) funded by Aarhus BSS.

## Three Additional Themes from a Study of Alcohol Consumption Among Young Muslim Women in Denmark

The study conducted by the first author was based on interviews with 32 young Muslim women aged 16–34 (mean age 23) and included abstainers as well as regular consumers of alcohol. The first author was in her early thirties at the time of the interviews, she belongs to the ethnic majority, is non-Muslim, and has a middle-class, urban background. Most of the women in the study were urban and well educated. The interviews contained material relating to social control, religious abstinence, and racism roughly matching the dominant themes in the literature referenced above, but study findings introduced and developed the following additional themes: (1) concerns about different ways of belonging including national identity; (2) experiences of exclusion from family as well as Danish peers; and (3) how the telling of drinking stories is contextually different for young Muslim women than generally referenced in the literature. All themes are presented within a framework of a Danish youth drinking culture.

### Dilemmas of Belonging: Feelings of Belonging and National Identity

In *Dilemmas of belonging: Young Muslim women in the Danish youth alcohol culture* (Bærndt & Frank, 2022), we presented findings from the study that suggested how drinking practices often play a central role in the formation of social relations and in deciding who belongs to a particular group or even nation, and who does not. Alcohol and drinking alcohol are thus intertwined with feelings of belonging, also to a broader national community (Grønkjær et al., 2011). Some Danish research has emphasized that drinking can be a way to "do" Danishness, and drinking can help consolidate your Danish national identity (Grønkjær et al., 2011; Simonsen, 2016). This implies that not only is light drinkers and abstainers' ability to have fun questioned in these specific contexts, so is their Danish identity. Our study shows that young adult Muslim women often find themselves caught between two sets of expectations, norms, and values, where it is considered Danish to drink and Muslim to be abstinent (Bærndt & Frank, 2022). In our interpretation, the social imperative to drink to belong is likely felt more intensely by young Danes who have connections across cultures, religions, or countries.

Our findings also show that being Muslim in Denmark is not only linked to abstinence but also associated with several persistent prejudicial, negative, and unwanted stigmas and tropes, such as the oppressed Muslim woman and the Muslim terrorist or patriarch. Since the first groups of Muslim immigrants arrived in Denmark in the 1960s as so-called "guest workers" (i.e., economic migrants), being Muslim has generally become a marker of the opposite of being Danish (Rytter & Pedersen, 2014). With this point of departure, we explored how young Muslim women in Denmark were challenged, within the context of a specific social occasion (a party), in their sense of belonging to both a Danish and a Muslim identity. Many of them felt that there was less space to navigate if they were too obvious Muslim women in party contexts and consequently generally toned down being Muslim. Naeemah (16 years old, Palestinian background, lower secondary school) describes how many of her friends strategically take off their headscarf at parties, and that she does not wear the Muslim headscarf but carries a necklace with the hand of Fatima when she goes out (Bærndt & Frank, 2022). The headscarf in particular is associated with a Muslim identity in a recognizable and visible way (Korteweg & Yurdakul, 2014), while the hand of Fatima is less identifiable and a more discrete or toned down Muslim marker.

Findings from our publication are in line with other recent studies (e.g., Douglass et al., 2022) where ethnic minority young adults can feel pressure to tone down central aspects of their identity to fit in and be a "model minority". We found that toning down being Muslim complicated many young Muslim women's feelings of belonging. Many strived to navigate between their family (and Muslim community) and their youth life (including an alcohol culture) without choosing one over the other. This ambition often left them feeling uneasy and uncomfortable, particularly when their surroundings demanded contradictory things from them. Our participants described the challenge and, ultimately, impossibility of merging a Muslim identity with a youth identity of drinking and/or partying. Rasha (23 years old, Syrian background, student nurse): "When I was in tenth grade I was like 'well, I am not a Muslim' because you must be a good Muslim. You must be like this and that, and I was not. I did not feel I was Muslim if I was drinking and partying" (Bærndt & Frank, 2022, p. 31).

Our work suggested that young women are taught and experience that their identities as Muslim and Danish are incompatible and that it is impossible to practice both sides simultaneously. Esra (24 years old, Turkish background, social work student): "I have been missing a lot in my earlier life. At one time, I think I even had like an identity crisis. I could not figure out who I was as a person. I sort of lacked someone with whom I could identify" (ibid., 2022, p. 31). The difficulties of bridging a Muslim and a Danish identity thus meant that many young women experienced what might be understood as a crisis of identity. Particularly those young Muslim women who were in their identity-formative years in upper secondary school lacked someone to identify with.

For a few women in the study, the attempt to merge contradictory norms and values was too difficult, and they opted out of the Danish (youth alcohol) culture altogether. Another way to reconcile their sometimes conflicting identities as Muslim and Danish was in their personal interpretation of Islam and by choosing what kind of Muslim they wanted to be; for instance believing that drinking a glass of white wine was acceptable in their understanding of their Muslim identity (Bærndt & Frank, 2022).

Results from our work presented in this section highlight that the parallel associations between alcohol and a Danish identity and abstinence and a Muslim identity makes it complicated to achieve a sense of belonging as a young adult Muslim woman. The inherent opposition between the two identities intensifies dilemmas in regard to belonging to Danish youth as a young Muslim woman.

## Young Muslim Women Navigating Social Inclusion and Exclusion in Youth Drinking Spaces

Another publication from the study presents interview data concerned with the social inclusion and exclusion of young Muslim women in drinking contexts (Bærndt & Kolind, 2021). It is well established that youth living in drinking cultures who drink moderately or abstain often risk social marginalization (Frank et al., 2020b; Nicholls, 2019; Parder, 2018). This suggests that young Muslim women who abstain would be at risk of exclusion in a youth context. Bærndt and Kolind (2021) found that many young Muslim women, abstinent as well as drinkers, found the Danish youth drinking culture excluding. For both groups, it seemed that being excluded because you are Muslim became more pronounced with the advent of parties in their young teenage years. Sila Nur (24 years old, Turkish background, social work student): "I felt that it went downhill when the parties started … [when she was 14 years old]" (Bærndt & Kolind, 2021, p. 4). Sila Nur, who was abstinent, describes a division between her and her ethnic Danish classmates that was caused by a combination of being left out by her classmates and her own withdrawal. Her experiences are shared by many participants who did drink alcohol, which suggests that the Danish youth drinking culture enhances ethnic and religious exclusion, regardless of the young women's drinking habits.

Yara (23 years old, Syrian and Iraqi background, nursing student) consumed alcohol regularly and found it unpleasant to be singled out as being a better Muslim: "They [ethnic Danes] typically say, 'Oh, we want more of your kind,' like, really, they say that. That is such a standard thing to say for Danes" (Bærndt & Kolind, 2021, p. 5). It seemed impossible, for drinkers and abstainers alike, to avoid being singled out as different and as part of a problematic and stereotypical Muslim community, and it was a continuous struggle for many of the women to be comfortable at parties.

The different ways they negotiated and experienced inclusion and exclusion was not delimited to their life among peers and the normalized Danish drinking culture. It is worth noting that the youth drinking culture affected their position negatively in their families too. It seemed to enhance or actualize gendered ideals in their families, and several women experienced more conflicts around subjects concerned with drinking and partying. Jamilah (29 years old, Palestinian background, medical student) began to participate in parties secretly and developed crafty strategies to avoid confrontations on the subject by her family. She had two separate calendars on her phone; one with her actual social plans and another with fictitious work shifts and innocent friend visits. She would go out but tell her parents that she was "working at the hospital or I am spending the night at a [friend's house]" (Bærndt & Kolind, 2021, p. 6). She had harmless pictures in stock from work or study activities to show her parents if they seemed suspicious. Jamilah thus incorporated her education and her use of technology in her everyday life to work against the social control that was triggered by her use of alcohol and participation in parties.

Ultimately, the different and intricate ways in which young Muslim women experience exclusion related to participation in parties and/or use of alcohol contribute to feelings of (possible) exclusion from their family/ Muslim community as well as Danish society. This suggests that they are particularly exposed in a way that demands their attentiveness if they want to navigate smoothly in the Danish youth alcohol culture.

## Muslim Drinking Stories

The final publication from the study explores drinking stories among young Muslim women in Denmark (Bærndt, 2023a). The findings relate to the significance of having a double audience (one Muslim, one Danish) in terms of how drinking stories or narratives are constructed. The findings are connected to the literature on drinking stories (i.e., stories told by people in the aftermath of consuming alcohol together) in the research field of youth alcohol drinking (e.g., Workman, 2001; Tutenges & Rod (2009); Cullen, 2011; Sandberg et al., 2019). Much can be gained by looking at cultural phenomena that are usually performed by the majority (such as telling drinking stories) and replacing "the usual suspects" (young white men) with a minority group (young Muslim women). A minority perspective reveals the unequal distribution of having story-worthy experiences and a voice within youth communities and in society more broadly.

Telling stories is existential and something we all engage in, for example, to make meaning of life (Jackson, 2002). The literature on drinking stories suggests that despite the lack of meaning or coherence in drinking behaviors, even clumsiness, accidents, vomit, urine, nudity, sex, lawbreaking, and pranks can become meaningful through the telling of drinking stories (Sandberg et al., 2019). Drinking stories can work as scripts for behavior—regardless of how problematic the behavior might be—and are part of how we construct social reality (Workman, 2001; Vaynman et al., 2020; Fleetwood, 2014). However, when investigating drinking stories, we should be particularly sensitive to the possible absences, silences, and audiences because they are part of the discourse and DNA of drinking stories (Fleetwood, 2014). This is exactly what the first author did when she investigated how young Muslim women navigate and accommodate a Muslim and a Danish audience (Bærndt, 2023a). Several of the young women in her study were conscious of the audience and strategically directed the right details to the proper one. This suggests that not all stories are meant for any audience. Asra (29 years old, Palestinian background, medical student) happily shares stories of parties and intoxication. However, her family is unaware of her party experiences, and Asra is certain that they would sanction her and react harshly if they knew. Therefore, when someone takes her picture while she and her friends are drunk and dancing and sends it to her brother with the text: "Is that not your sister?", it puts a damper on Asra's party spirit. "It simply ruined too much", she explained (Bærndt, 2023a, p. 110). Having two conflicting audiences thus affects how drinking stories are constructed. Asra's story is characteristic of Muslim drinking narratives in the way fun and pleasure are interrupted by something serious that disqualifies the story as a drinking story (Fleetwood, 2014). In addition, Bærndt (2023a) found that many events from drinking settings are never retold. For instance, Casho (23 years old, from Somalia, public health student) shares a story she has never told before about a party in upper secondary school six years ago. Her father and brother reacted strongly when they discovered her whereabouts, and she almost broke down in the girls' restroom while they kept calling and texting her. She knew she was in "deep trouble" and her father was angry and violent when he picked her up (Bærndt, 2023a, p. 111). Bærndt (2023a) suggests that storytellers and listeners must have some level of shared references or sameness for the stories to be told and become drinking stories and that telling them is a way "to celebrate one's sameness with others in a group" (ibid., p. 114).

Based on our discussions of relevant literature and illustrations from our own analyses, it seems that otherwise story-worthy events can have serious consequences for some individuals. When we explore narratives about drinking and partying, it is evident that there are inequalities at stake that stem from differences in social positions such as gender, family, and religious background and these differences determine which drinking stories come to life and how (Cullen, 2011; Bærndt, 2023a). Particularly in drinking and partying contexts, it is difficult for the young women in our study to control which information is shared with whom. One way to achieve an increased sense of control is to participate in small private parties where everyone agrees not to take pictures (Bærndt & Frank, 2022). The parties the young women participate in and the stories shared in that connection are not for everyone to hear or understand.

In sum, the results describe a tangible manifestation of inequality and that, more generally, a focus on diversity can reveal new facets of otherwise known territory, such as drinking stories. Seeing the stories through the eyes of young Muslim women suggests that other minority perspectives would also convey new knowledge about drinking stories specifically and young adult drinking generally.

## Conclusion

The focus of this chapter was twofold: (1) to introduce the existing literature on alcohol consumption among Muslim young adults living in non-Muslim countries where alcohol plays an important role in youth life, and (2) discuss three publications and selections of data and results from a Danish study on young Muslim women who navigate a youth alcohol culture.

Both the existing literature and the Danish study show that young Muslims' relationship with alcohol is complex, the differences between religious texts and everyday practices of Islam are tangible and real, and there is no one singular answer to questions in this regard. To the contrary, Muslim young adults relate to alcohol in diverse ways, even though alcohol is officially haram. Muslim young adult women's relationship with alcohol depends on contextual factors, such as national and local settings, and differences in identity positions, for example, ethnic background, age, and family migration history. The intersections between these aspects of young Muslim identities are a focal point here, and diversity among Muslims broadly speaking contributes to differences in their alcohol approaches.

There is thus a central question concerning Muslim diversity that calls for approaches that sensitively consider differences in Muslims' use of alcohol. We argue that an intersectional orientation is worthwhile because it turns our attention toward social positions or identities that might explain different experiences and inequality in certain settings. Here, we have focused on gender and religious background and on how young Muslim women face certain challenges and exclusions that are qualitatively different from those of both young Muslim men and majority young adults in Denmark. The study also reveals differences between the young women, including their different ways of being Muslim in the context of national and international understandings of Islam (e.g., as being in opposition to being Danish). However, not everything is about Islam, and it is important to explore questions and answers that lie beyond assumptions attached to Muslim identities. For instance, the results from the Danish study included here indicate important similarities between the experiences of young Muslim women and young majority women when it comes to the contradictions and dilemmas that are foregrounded. The young women's Muslim communities largely consider female drinking disreputable, which is how female drinking has historically been viewed. Masculinity is traditionally related to excess in drinking, while femininity is related to constraint in Denmark (Eriksen, 1999; Frank et al., 2020a) and other Western countries (Hutton et al., 2013; Pennay et al., 2022). In present times, many women feel that they face contradicting demands when they drink, such as performing a femininity that is respectable and restrained but at the same time is liberated and sexually available (Griffin et al., 2013). The results thus point to differences and similarities between minority and majority, particularly in terms of femininity and respectability. The intersection of gender, youth, and alcohol in the case of young Muslim women to some degree push other differences, for example, ethnicity and religion, to the back seat. This might not be the case if the research subject were young Muslim men.

In sum, acknowledging diversity in youth alcohol research would make results recognizable for more young people, which is necessary if we want to improve policy and prevention initiatives. Rather than reinforce stereotypes about binge-drinking and overly intoxicated young people, diversity can help demonstrate that some young people have alternatives to youth cultures of heavy drinking. It will be interesting to see future research that explores whether growing groups with alternative drinking behavior will affect the intoxication orientation of many young adults in Denmark and other Western countries. This chapter has discussed Muslim minorities in drinking cultures, a clearly marginalized and underrepresented group in the alcohol field. The findings can nuance our understandings of this particular group and young adult drinking more broadly and highlight similarities and differences in relation to the majority of young people, who find themselves in clearly different positions in society. It is therefore important and worthwhile to consider diversity and differences in general, for instance concerning gender, class, sexuality, ethnic and religious background, and lifestyle identifications. We would like to see alcohol research do just that and imagine that it would change the field for the better.

## References

Ahmed, S. (2016). *What is Islam? The importance of being Islamic*. Princeton University Press.

Al-Ansari, B., Thow, A. M., Day, C. A., & Conigrave, K. M. (2016). Extent of alcohol prohibition in civil policy in Muslim majority countries: The impact of globalization. *Addiction, 111*(10), 1703–1713.

AlMarri, T. S., & Oei, T. P. (2009). Alcohol and substance use in the Arabian Gulf region: A review. *International Journal of Psychology, 44*(3), 222–233.

Arifeen, S. R. (2020). British Muslim women's experience of the networking practice of happy hours. *Employee Relations, 42*(3), 646–661.

Bærndt, M. F. (2023a). "Then someone takes my picture…" and other disrupted (drinking) stories: Constructing narratives about alcohol and intoxication among young Muslim women in Denmark. *Drugs, Habits and Social Policy, 24*(2), 104–116.

Bærndt, M. F. (2023b). *Dilemmas of youth drinking. Young Muslim women's experiences within the Danish youth alcohol culture*. PhD dissertation, Aarhus BSS, Aarhus University, Centre for Alcohol and Drug Research.

Bærndt, M. F., & Frank, V. A. (2022). Dilemmas of belonging: Young Muslim women in the Danish youth alcohol culture. *Nordic Studies of Alcohol and Drugs (NAD), 40*(1), 22–23.

Bærndt, M. F., & Kolind, T. (2021). Drinking and partying among young Muslim women: Exclusion in the context of a normalized youth drinking culture. *The International Journal of Drug Policy, 93*, 103170.

Bannister, E., Conroy, D., & Piacentini, M. (2025). Non-drinkers and Non-drinking: A Review, A Critique and Pathways to Policy. In Conroy, D. & Measham, F. (eds.) Young adult drinking styles. Current Perspectives on Research, Policy and Practice, 2nd edition. Palgrave Macmillan.

Boogarts, S. (2008). Claiming your place at night: Turkish dance parties in The Netherlands. *Journal of Ethnic and Migration Studies, 34*(8), 1283–1300.

Bradby, H. (2007). Watch out for the Aunties! Young British Asians' accounts of identity and substance use. *Sociology of Health & Illness, 29*(5), 656–672.

Chegeni, M., Kamel Khodabandeh, A., Karamouzian, M., Shokoohi, M., Abedi, L., Khalili, M., & Sharifi, H. (2020). Alcohol consumption in Iran: A systematic review and meta-analysis of the literature. *Drug and Alcohol Review, 39*(5), 525–538.

Conroy, D., & de Visser, R. (2014). Being a non-drinking student: An interpretative phenomenological analysis. *Psychology & Health, 29*(5), 536–551.

Conroy, D., & de Visser, R. (2015). The importance of authenticity for student non-drinkers: An interpretative phenomenological analysis. *Journal of Health Psychology, 20*(11), 1483–1493.

Conroy, D., & MacLean, S. (2019). Friendship and alcohol use among young adults: A cross disciplinary literature review. In D. Conroy & F. Measham (Eds.), *Young adult drinking styles: Current perspectives on research, policy and practice* (pp. 153–171). Palgrave Macmillan.

Cullen, F. (2011). The only time I feel girly is when I go out': Drinking stories, teenage girls, and respectable femininities. *International Journal of Adolescence and Youth, 16*(2), 119–138.

De Visser, R. O., & McDonnell, E. J. (2012). 'That's OK. He's a guy': A mixed-methods study of gender double-standards for alcohol use. *Psychology & Health, 27*(5), 618–639.

Demant, J., & Järvinen, M. (2006). Constructing maturity through alcohol experience – Focus group interviews with teenagers. *Addiction Research & Theory, 14*(6), 589–602.

Dotinga, A. (2005). *Drinking in a dry culture. Alcohol use among second-generation Turks and Moroccans: Measurements and results*. PhD dissertation, Erasmus University Rotterdam.

Douglass, C. H., Block, K., Eghrari, D., Horyniak, D., Hellard, M. E., & Lim, M. S. C. (2022). "You have to drink with a little bit of shame": Alcohol and other drug use among young people from migrant and ethnic minority backgrounds in Melbourne, Australia. *Journal of Ethnicity in Substance Abuse, 23*(2), 340–364.

Eller, J. D. (2021). *Introducing anthropology of religion: Culture to the ultimate*. Routledge.

Eriksen, S. (1999). Alcohol as a gender symbol. *Scandinavian Journal of History, 24*(1), 45–73.

Ernst, W. (Ed.). (2020). *Alcohol flows across cultures: Drinking cultures in transnational and comparative perspective*. Routledge.

Fleetwood, J. (2014). A feminist, narrative analysis of drinking stories. *The International Journal of Drug Policy, 25*(3), 351–352.

Fletcher, T., & Spracklen, K. (2014). Cricket, drinking and exclusion of British Pakistani Muslims? *Ethnic and Racial Studies, 37*(8), 1310–1327.

Frank, V. A., Herold, M. D., Antin, T., & Hunt, G. (2020a). Gendered perspectives on young adults, alcohol consumption and intoxication. *International Journal of Drug Policy, 81*, 102780.

Frank, V. A., Herold, M. D., Schrøder, S., Bjønness, J., & Hunt, G. (2020b). Legitimizing and negotiating abstinence: Young adults' narratives about practicing situational and long term abstinence in Denmark. *International Journal of Drug Policy, 81*, 102655.

Griffin, C., Szmigin, I., Bengry-Howell, A., Hackley, C., & Mistral, W. (2013). Inhabiting the contradictions: Hypersexual femininity and the culture of intoxication among young women in the UK. *Feminism & Psychology, 23*(2), 184–206.

Grønkjær, M., Curtis, T., De Crespigny, C., & Delmar, C. (2011). Acceptance and expectance: Cultural norms for alcohol use in Denmark. *International Journal of Qualitative Studies on Health and Well-Being, 6*(4), 8461.

Herold, M. D., & Frank, V. A. (2022). Alcohol use and narratives of 'maturing out' in the transition to adulthood among young Danes. In T. Thurnell-Read & L. Fenton (Eds.), *Alcohol, age, generation and the life course* (pp. 103–125). Springer International Publishing.

Herold, M. D., & Kolind, T. (2022). Young people's alcohol use is still strongly related to social inclusion. *Addiction, 117*, 1216–1217.

Hobbs, D., Hadfield, P., Lister, S., & Winlow, S. (2003). *Bouncers. Violence and Governance in the Nighttime Economy*. Oxford University Press.

Huq, R. (2007). *Beyond subculture: Pop, youth and identity in a postcolonial world*. Routledge.

Hutton, F., Wright, S., & Saunders, E. (2013). Cultures of intoxication: Young women, alcohol, and harm reduction. *Contemporary Drug Problems, 40*(4), 451–480.

Jackson, M. (2002). *The politics of storytelling: Violence, transgression, and intersubjectivity*. Museum Tusculanum.

Järvinen, M., & Room, R. (Eds.). (2017). *Youth drinking cultures*. Routledge.

Kamela, D., Vanderplasschen, W., Vindevogel, S., & Derluyn, I. (2016). The role of religion in alcohol consumption and demand reduction in Muslim majority countries (MMC). *Addiction, 111*(10), 1716–1718.

Korteweg, A. C., & Yurdakul, G. (2014). *The headscarf debates: Conflicts of national belonging*. Stanford University Press.

MacLean, S. (2016). Alcohol and the constitution of friendship for young adults. *Sociology, 50*(1), 93–108.

Mallik, S., Starrels, J. L., Shannon, C., Edwards, K., & Nahvi, S. (2021). "An undercover problem in the Muslim community": A qualitative study of imams' perspectives on substance use. *Journal of Substance Abuse Treatment, 123*, 108224.

Matthee, R. (2014). Alcohol in the Islamic Middle East: Ambivalence and ambiguity. *Past & Present, 222*, 100–125.

May, R. A. B., & Chaplin, K. S. (2008). Cracking the code: Race, class, and access to nightclubs in Urban America. *Qualitative Sociology, 31*(1), 57–72.

McCreanor, T., Lyons, A., Griffin, C., Goodwin, I., Moewaka Barnes, H., & Hutton, F. (2013). Youth drinking cultures, social networking and alcohol marketing: Implications for public health. *Critical Public Health, 23*(1), 110–120.

McKay, J., Emmison, M., & Janine, M. (2009). Lads, larrikins and mates: Hegemonic masculinities in Australian beer advertisements. In L. A. Wenner & S. J. Jackson (Eds.), *Sport, beer, and gender: Promotional culture and contemporary social life* (pp. 163–179). Peter Lang Publishing.

Measham, F. (2004). The decline of ecstasy, the rise of 'binge' drinking and the persistence of pleasure. *Probation Journal. The Journal of Community and Criminal Justice, 51*(4), 309–326.

Michalak, L., & Trocki, K. (2006). Alcohol and Islam: An overview. *Contemporary Drug Problems, 33*(4), 523–562.

Mir, S. (2014). *Muslim American women on campus* (Undergraduate Social Life and Identity). The University of North Carolina Press.

Mirdal, G. M. (2006). Changing idioms of shame: Expressions of disgrace and dishonour in the narratives of Turkish women living in Denmark. *Culture & Psychology, 12*(4), 395–414.

Morris, B. (2006). *Religion and anthropology: A critical introduction.* Cambridge University Press.

Nicholls, E. (2019). 'I feel like I have to become part of that identity': Negotiating femininities and friendships through alcohol consumption in Newcastle, UK. *International Journal of Drug Policy, 81*, 102524.

Pannu, G., Zaman, S., Bhala, N., & Zama, R. (2009). Alcohol use in South Asians in the UK. *BMJ, 339*, b4028.

Parder, M.-L. (2018). What about just saying "no"? Situational abstinence from alcohol at parties among 13–15 year olds. *Drugs: Education, Prevention and Policy, 25*(2), 189–197.

Pennay, A., Holmes, J., Törrönen, J., Livingston, M., Kraus, L., & Room, R. (2018). Researching the decline in adolescent drinking: The need for a global and generational approach. *Drug Alcohol Review, 37*(suppl. 1), 115–119.

Pennay, A., Törrönen, J., Herold, M. D., Fenton, L., MacLean, S., Caluzzi, G., Fairbrother, H., Frank, V. A., Samuelsson, E., & Holmes, J. (2022). "There's a lot of stereotypes going on": A cross-national qualitative analysis of the place of gender in declining youth drinking. *International Journal of Drug Policy, 108*, 103827.

Rytter, M., & Pedersen, M. H. (2014). A decade of suspicion: Islam and Muslims in Denmark after 9/11. *Ethnic and Racial Studies, 37*(13), 2303–2321.

Sandberg, S., Tutenges, S., & Pedersen, W. (2019). Drinking stories as a narrative genre: The five classic themes. *Acta Sociologica, 62*(4), 406–419.

Simonsen, K. B. (2016). Ghetto-society-problem: A discourse analysis of nationalist othering. *Studies in Ethnicity and Nationalism, 16*(1), 83–99.

Søgaard, T. F. (2017). Ethnicity and the policing of nightclub accessibility in the Danish night-time economy. *Drugs: Education, Prevention and Policy, 24*(3), 256–264.

Thurnell-Read, T. (2016). Identity, friendship and sociality. In T. Kolind, B. Thom, & G. Hunt (Eds.), *The SAGE handbook of drug and alcohol studies: Social science perspectives* (pp. 337–351). SAGE.

Thurnell-Read, T., & Monaghan, M. (2023). Intoxication, ethnicity, faith and nation. In T. Thurnell-Read & M. Monaghan (Eds.), *Intoxication: Self, state and society* (pp. 221–237). Springer International Publishing.

Tutenges, S., & Rod, M. H. (2009). 'We got incredibly drunk … it was damned fun': Drinking stories among Danish youth. *Journal of Youth Studies, 12*(4), 355–370.

Valentine, G., Holloway, S., & Jayne, M. (2010). Contemporary cultures of abstinence and the nighttime economy: Muslim attitudes towards alcohol and the implications for social cohesion. *Environment and Planning, 42*(1), 8–22.

Vaynman, M. J., Sandberg, S., & Pedersen, W. (2020). Locker room talk': Male bonding and sexual degradation in drinking stories. *Culture, Health & Sexuality, 22*(11), 1235–1252.

Waltorp, K. (2015). Keeping cool, staying virtuous: Social media and the composite habitus of young Muslim women in Copenhagen. *MedieKultur: Journal of Media and Communication Research, 31*(58), 49–67.

Workman, T. A. (2001). Finding the meanings of college drinking: An analysis of fraternity drinking stories. *Health Communication, 13*(4), 427–447.

# 7

# The Implications of Resource Scarcity, a National Lockdown, and a Global Pandemic on Alcohol Use, Mental Health, and Experiences of Intimate Partner Violence Among Young Adults in Low- and Middle-Income Countries: The Case of Uganda

Amanda P. Miller, Stephen Mugamba, and Susan M. Kiene

**Abstract** The COVID-19 pandemic profoundly impacted the global economy and public health, with lockdowns and stay-at-home orders bringing life to a halt. Evidence from high-income countries with social safety nets, such as sick leave and social welfare relief, indicates increased alcohol use during lockdowns. Drivers of alcohol use, such as intimate partner violence and depression, also increased globally as individuals were isolated at home, often with their abuser. While poverty and food

A. P. Miller (✉) • S. M. Kiene
School of Public Health, San Diego State University, San Diego, CA, USA
e-mail: apmiller@sdsu.edu; skiene@sdsu.edu

S. Mugamba
Africa Medical and Behavioral Sciences Organization (AMBSO), Hoima, Uganda



D. Conroy, F. Measham (eds.), *Young Adult Drinking Styles*, Sustainable Development Goals Series, https://doi.org/10.1007/978-3-031-98528-7_7

insecurity rose globally, the economic impact was greater in lower- and middle-income countries (LMIC), where most are employed in the informal sector and lack social safety nets. In Uganda, school closures persisted for 22 months, forcing many young adults to move home and put their lives and education on hold. In this context, patterns of alcohol use during the pandemic were diverse, influenced by economic insecurity, societal shutdowns, and alcohol availability. This chapter explores how mental health and alcohol use were affected during the pandemic, focusing on young adults in LMICs. Uganda, with its high alcohol consumption per capita among young adults and stringent lockdowns, provides a key case study. We conclude with recommendations for how LMICs can better address alcohol use and mental health in future public health crises.

## Introduction

In March 2020, governments around the world employed a variety of approaches to respond to the COVID-19 pandemic, which had an unprecedent impact on the global economy and public health. These included lockdowns and stay-at-home policies to curb the spread of the virus. Severity and haste of these response measures varied; in Uganda, a country with 1.3 intensive care unit beds per one million people (Atumanya et al., 2020), and a mechanical ventilator-to-population ratio of 0.23 ventilators per 100,000 people (Craig et al., 2020), the response was swift and far reaching. To prevent spread, Uganda, along with nine other countries in sub-Saharan Africa, instituted a national lockdown (Najmul et al., 2020). During the pandemic, two separate stay-at-home orders were put in place. The first ran from March through May of 2020 while the second was implemented from June to July of 2021 (during a resurgence). However, many of the measures extended beyond these periods. Restrictions in Uganda included school closures, non-essential business closures (including bars, restaurants, and other nightlife venues, which partially limited access to liquor), discontinuation of all public transportation and as the case rates intensified, “all non-essential” vehicles as well, suspension of public gatherings, border closings, and a national curfew (Uganda MOH, 2020). The night curfew, which required all businesses to close by 7 pm, was in place continuously from March 2020 through January 2022. Despite these stringent lockdown measures, alcohol sale for personal consumption at home was not banned. Because Uganda's public health infrastructure would not support a high volume of hospitalizations, COVID-19 restrictions were strictly enforced by the Local Defense Unit (LDU), an armed community-policing group that gained a reputation for frequently using excessive force to compel residents to comply (Human Rights Watch, 2020; Semakula, 2020). This led to high levels of obedience to social distancing measures, greatly assisting Uganda in preventing the spread of COVID-19 but leaving many of Uganda's 44 million citizens socially isolated and without a source of income.

As typically seen in low- and middle-income countries (LMICs), the informal economy (defined as the production of goods and services outside of the formal (taxed) economy) is where most Ugandans earn their livelihood. Three-quarters of all Ugandans earn their income from the informal economy, with a greater proportion of women (85%) and youth (92%) being employed informally (Andreou & Dayton, 2018). Many informal businesses shuttered their doors entirely during the COVID-19 lockdown; in instances where people continued to operate their business, income generation was severely diminished due to loss of purchasing power, challenges in paying bills, loss of clientele, transportation restrictions, and curfews, which meant early closure of businesses that resulted in supply chain issues (Wandera et al., 2023). A quarter of people employed in the formal sector were also impacted financially by the pandemic, with 10% losing all of their income and 14% of those who remained employed had their incomes reduced (McNabb et al., 2023).

In this chapter, we explore mental health (MH) and alcohol use in LMICs in the context of the COVID-19 pandemic with a focus on the experiences of young adults (aged 18–30 years). We have used Uganda, a country with a high burden of disease attributable to alcohol use and depression prior to the pandemic, as a case study and give recommendations for how LMICs can better prepare to address these issues in future public health crises. Of note, with a median age of 16.3 years (UN DESA, 2022), Uganda has one of the youngest age structures globally (median global age: 30.3 years), due to high fertility rates (total fertility rate of 4.6 in 2021 (The World Bank, 2022)), early childbearing (24% of women have their first child between 15 and 19 years (Uganda MOH, 2022)), and limited access to and utilization of effective contraception, especially among married couples. Therefore, while work presented here may not have been conducted exclusively among young adults, most study participants (and in fact, most of Uganda's citizens) fall into this demographic.

## Historical and Global Context

Evidence suggests a complicated relationship between public health crises and alcohol use, with two primary scenarios suggested in the case of COVID-19; an increase in use among populations disproportionately impacted by the pandemic, or an overall decrease in use due to restrictions on alcohol access and affordability (Rehm et al., 2020). Although there was heterogeneity in the effect of the COVID-19 pandemic on patterns of alcohol use, evidence from several high-income countries (HICs) with social safety nets (e.g., offering sick leave, disability, social welfare relief) indicate an increase in alcohol use during lockdowns (Grossman et al., 2020; Sallie et al., 2020; Weerakoon et al., 2021). A recent systematic review found that while overall alcohol use reduced in some HICs, others experienced increases in heavy episodic drinking, defined as having consumed >60 grams or more of pure alcohol (equivalent to six standard drinks) on at least one occasion in the past 30 days, and increases in the proportion of people with problematic alcohol use (Sohi et al., 2022). The review authors concluded that three factors may explain these results: (1) COVID-19 restrictions may have served as a deterrent for social drinking, (2) economic crises stemming from the pandemic may have had a bidirectional impact on use, with some drinking to cope and others no longer being able to afford alcohol, and (3) the increase of MH issues related to the pandemic and lockdown may have led to an increase in heavy episodic drinking (Sohi et al., 2022). There is also evidence that persons who engage in heavy episodic drinking or have alcohol use disorder increased their use, suggesting that these individuals may have been disproportionately affected (Boschuetz et al., 2020). Drivers and sequelae of hazardous alcohol use, such as intimate partner violence (IPV) (Wyckoff et al., 2023) and depression also increased globally as individuals were isolated at home, often with their abuser (Ahmadimazhin et al., 2021; Kourti et al., 2021; Sun et al., 2023), underscoring the web of interrelated public health issues that emerged in the context of the pandemic and pandemic-related measures.

Among young adults, a global review found an initial decrease in alcohol use in the early stages of the COVID-19 pandemic (2020), followed by a rebound one year later (2021) (Hussong et al., 2023). This reduction was primarily attributed to reduced access under pandemic restrictions. Several studies also found that college age young adults who moved home during the pandemic reduced their use when they returned to their parent's residence (Ryerson et al., 2021; Sokolovsky et al., 2021). In contrast, MH of adolescents and young adults deteriorated, with depression, anxiety and psychological distress all increasing (Kauhanen et al., 2023). Despite these divergent MH and alcohol consumption trends, a more granular look at the data tells a different story. For example, one US study found that pandemic-related social isolation among young people was directly related to anxiety, which in turn was directly related to increased severity of alcohol use. This demonstrates the interrelated nature of MH and substance use and again suggests that some populations may have been disproportionately impacted by the pandemic (Horigian et al., 2021). However, research from LMICs has been limited and therefore under-represented (or entirely absent, e.g., Sohi et al., 2022) from the reviews described above and the extant literature more broadly.

## Mental Health and Substance Use in Uganda Prior to the Pandemic

While just over half (53%) of Ugandans engage in alcohol use, the majority who do so engage in heavy episodic drinking (HED) (57%; HED is defined as consuming ≥6 standard drinks on at least one occasion in the past 30 days) (WHO, 2018a). HED is even more common among persons aged 15–19 years with a prevalence of 61% (WHO, 2018a). Patterns of alcohol use in Uganda are also gendered with men being more likely to drink alcohol and engage in HED. For example, among persons aged 15–19 years who report any alcohol use, HED is more than twice as prevalent among men than women (71% vs 35%) (WHO, 2018a). A robust evidence base suggests substantial public health, social and economic costs attributable to alcohol use in Uganda. Alcohol use ranks as the fifth highest risk factor contributing to disability-adjusted-life-years (a combined morbidity and mortality metric) in Uganda (IHME, n.d.). Extant literature also suggests that alcohol-use is associated with economic insecurity and excessive spending among certain populations in Uganda, such as fisherfolk, a population largely comprised of young adult men (Breur et al., 2019; Kiene & Tumwesigye, 2025).

Despite the tremendous burden of communicable diseases in Africa, depression is also a significant public health issue, and is the leading cause of years lived with disability (YLD, a standardized morbidity metric) on the continent (IHME, 2017). With a prevalence of 30.6% (Kaggwa et al., 2022), 16% of all YLD in Uganda prior to the pandemic were attributable to depression (IHME, 2017). Furthermore, depression is both a risk factor for and sequalae of substance use, with the two frequently co-occurring (Fergusson et al., 2009; Pacek et al., 2013). Alcohol use and depression have also been associated with HIV risk behavior (Lundberg et al., 2011; Zablotska et al., 2009) and poor outcomes throughout the HIV care continuum, making them critical factors in addressing the HIV epidemic and meeting Joint United Nations Programme on HIV/AIDS (UNAIDS) targets (Barrera et al., 2013; Miller, Pitpitan, et al., 2021b; Williams et al., 2016). Alcohol use and depression are also both associated with experiences of IPV (Zablotska et al., 2009), which further increases HIV risk through unsafe condom use practices (WHO, 2004) and forced sex (WHO, 2004).

Most African governments devote <1% of their budget to MH services (Molodynski et al., 2017). Uganda's MH care system, like many LMICs, is severely underfunded. Consequently, there is a shortage in trained MH service providers, with 1.4 MH workers per 100,000 people. Compared with a global average of 9 MH workers per 100,000 (WHO, 2015), it is unsurprising that an estimated 75% of persons experiencing mental disorders in LMICs do not receive any evidence-based treatment (Evans-Lacko et al., 2018). Collectively, MH and substance use were prevalent and under-resourced public health issues in Uganda prior to the pandemic.

## Theoretical Impact of Lockdown Measures on Mental Health, Substance Use, and Wellbeing

Pandemics and other large-scale public health crises are stressful life-disrupting events, which can increase risk for mental disorders, distress, and substance use through several causal pathways (see Fig. 7.1). For example, when exposure to stressful situations is prolonged, such stress can erode resilience and self-efficacy, reducing access to adaptive (healthy) coping strategies (e.g., seeking social support) (Jalloh et al., 2018; Luo et al., 2020; Pfefferbaum & North, 2020) and increase engagement in maladaptive (unhealthy) strategies (such as alcohol use) (Britton, 2009; Hasking et al., 2011). Further, uncertainty around the direct impact of

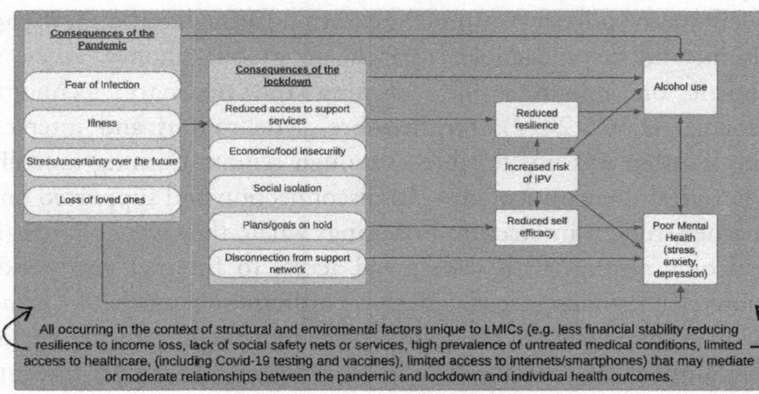


**Fig. 7.1** Conceptual model of the pandemic's influence on alcohol use and mental health

both the pandemic (i.e., on one's health) and lockdown (i.e., on economic security) may adversely impact MH through increased stress and anxiety (Khan et al., 2020; Muller et al., 2020; Wu et al., 2021). Critically, all of these pandemic sequelae occur in context. While the conceptual model presented here is relevant in a variety of settings, there were very real differences in the impact of "stay-at-home" orders in lower-resourced settings.

While poverty and food insecurity increased in HICs as well, the economic impact of the pandemic was more severe in LMICs. For example, the proportion of Ugandans living below the national poverty line (equivalent to living on $0.88 to $1.04 USD a day) increased by three percentage points between 2018 and 2021 (from 18.7% to 21.9%) (World Bank, 2023). It is worth nothing that this poverty line is well below the international poverty line ($2.15 USD a day), leading to poverty estimates that understate the severity of economic insecurity in Uganda both prior to and after the pandemic. Furthermore, differences in access to the Internet and computers meant that "working from home" or "learning from home" were not options for most in lower-resourced settings. In Uganda, school closures persisted for nearly 2 years (fully or partially closed for more than 83 weeks—the longest closure globally), forcing many young adults to move home and completely put their lives (and pursuit of a degree) on hold. While the Government of Uganda made efforts to support continued education through radio, newspaper, television, and downloadable curricula on mobile phones, access was dependent on resources (i.e., owning the necessary technology) (Datzberger et al., 2022). Furthermore, synchronous and interactive remote learning was not feasible. Although remote learning modalities were not ideal, they mitigated social disconnection and supported ongoing teacher-student interaction in settings where they were offered (i.e., high-income settings with widespread access to Internet and personal computers) (Betthäuser et al., 2023). Furthermore, much of Uganda's work force completely lost the ability to generate income during the lockdown (Suubi et al., 2022), leading to economic and food insecurity. Uganda's government provided food satchels to address rising food insecurity, but anecdotal reports indicate that these satchels did not sufficiently address the shortages (Devereux, 2021).

The lockdown also may have affected men and women differently, specifically through increased risk of IPV under the stringent stay-at-home order (Akina Mama Wa Afrika, 2020; Alupo, 2020). Evidence from prior infectious disease outbreaks in LMICs (e.g., Ebola outbreaks in West Africa and Zika outbreaks in the Dominican Republic) indicate women are disproportionately impacted by public health measures that restrict mobility and lead to isolation (Cepeda et al., 2017; O'Brien & Tolosa, 2016). Our own prior work in Uganda suggests that stress over finances is a leading driver of partner conflict in this setting (Miller et al., 2024; Miller, Ddaaki, et al., 2021a; Miller, Ziegel, et al., 2021c). In the context of job loss and economic insecurity, alcohol use may lead to disagreements, increased aggression, and high potential for IPV (Foran & O'Leary, 2008). For those experiencing IPV, the stay-at-home order frequently meant increased time isolated with perpetrators. A global body of literature (Aguero, 2021; Kgaugelo, 2020; Sharma & Borah, 2020; WHO, 2021), including research in sub-Saharan Africa specifically (Consolata & Fredrick, 2020; Mahmud & Riley, 2021; Miller et al., 2022; Ojeahere et al., 2022; Sileo et al., 2023), suggests that the COVID-19 lockdown measures were associated with increased incidence of IPV. In Uganda, where IPV is prevalent and limited resources to address violence existed prior to the pandemic, stay-at-home orders may have exacerbated violence and further limited access to necessary resources.

## Pandemic Impact

In mid-2020, we conducted a study to explore how the COVID-19 pandemic and initial lockdown impacted women's MH, alcohol use, and experiences of IPV. Given lockdown restrictions, data were collected via a telephone survey between June and August of 2020 as part of the Africa Medical and Behavioral Sciences Organization (AMBSO) Population Health Surveillance (APHS) longitudinal open cohort study, which has been described in detail previously (Miller, Ziegel, et al., 2021c; Mugamba et al., 2022). In brief, APHS is an open cohort study conducted across six communities in the districts of Hoima and Wakiso in Uganda. Residents between the ages of 13 and 80 years who provide informed consent (parental consent and assent for minors) and reside in the study communities are eligible to participate. The COVID-19 phone survey was conducted in the three study communities located in Wakiso district. Data were collected on general sociodemographic and health measures, as well as depression (measure using the nine-item Patient Health Questionnaire, PHQ-9 (Kroenke et al., 2001)), anxiety (measured using the Coronavirus Anxiety Scale (Lee, 2020)), alcohol use (measured using the AUDIT-C (Bush et al., 1998)), changes in alcohol use (retrospective assessment using the question, "How have your drinking behaviors changed during the COVID-19 pandemic? Would you say your alcohol use has increased, decreased, or remained the same?"), changes in experiences of IPV, and two self-reported measures of adaptive healthy coping skills—perceived self-efficacy (Center on Gender Equity and Health, 2020; Schwarzer & Jerusalem, 1995) and resilient coping (Center on Gender Equity and Health, 2020; Sinclair & Wallston, 2004)—that were modified to specifically address lockdowns.

Median age of participants (n=556) was 30 (inter-quartile range (IQR) 24–42) and most resided in rural or semi-urban communities (91%); 16% reported hazardous alcohol use (AUDIT-C ≥3) while 9% had PHQ-9 scores (≥5) indicative of potentially clinically significant depressive symptoms (Miller, Ddaaki, et al., 2021a). Most participants reported changes in their alcohol use since the pandemic began, with 60% reporting decreased use and 3% reporting increased use (Miller, Ddaaki, et al., 2021a). This is consistent with the trend observed in another Uganda-based study where 76% of persons reported decreased alcohol use during the lockdowns (Beesiga et al., 2023). We also asked about changes in experiences of IPV victimization among those who had reported recent IPV at the prior APHS study visit (~6 months earlier). Nearly half of women reported that physical (44%) and verbal (48%) IPV had increased in their relationship since the start of the pandemic, while one-fifth (21%) reported an increase in sexual IPV (Miller, Ddaaki, et al., 2021a). Women reporting recent experiences of IPV had significantly higher depressive symptom scores, higher anxiety symptom scores, and lower perceived generalized self-efficacy than those reporting no violence (Miller, Ddaaki, et al., 2021a). In models adjusted for age, marital status, employment, education level, and community type, we found that those reporting recent hazardous alcohol use had four times greater odds of reporting recent experiences of physical IPV (adjusted OR = 4.06; 95% CI = 1.65-10.02; p=0.0024) (Miller, Ddaaki, et al., 2021a). Other variables that had been significant in unadjusted models such as depressive and anxiety symptoms, and self-efficacy were no longer significant in adjusted models, suggesting that alcohol use was more predictive of recent IPV than the other MH and well-being variables of interest.

The prevalence of depressive symptoms observed in our sample was lower than levels reported during data collection in prior APHS rounds (a year prior) using the same measure (9% vs 29.2%). Two possible explanations for this are that participants may have been under-reporting over the phone (Miller, Ddaaki, et al., 2021a) and there may have been non-response bias, with depressed individuals being less likely to participate. A recently published meta-analysis comparing depression prevalence in Uganda before and during the pandemic tells a different story, with depression increasing from 29.3% prior to the pandemic to 48.1% during the pandemic (Kaggwa et al., 2022). A July 2020 online survey among university students (n=321) in Uganda found exceedingly high levels of depression, anxiety, and stress during the lockdown with prevalence of 80.7%, 98.4%, and 77.9%, respectively (Najjuka et al., 2021). In adjusted models, male respondents had three times greater odds of reporting depression than females (adjusted OR = 2.97 95% CI1.61—5.48, P=0.001) (Najjuka et al., 2021). This finding is notable because it undermines pre-pandemic gendered patterns of MH. In Uganda, ideals around hegemonic masculinity mean that MH disorders can be viewed as a weakness, undermining help-seeking among men. At the time of the survey, all universities in Uganda were closed and many students had returned home to their parents (Najjuka et al., 2021). Loss of freedom and a sense of stagnation in their journey toward financial independence may have differentially impacted men; especially if these are valued aspects of masculinity.

Given the cross-sectional nature of the study, we were unable to disentangle the temporality between relationships observed, but the literature suggests that experiences of IPV, alcohol use, and MH are bidirectionally related. Participants engaging in hazardous use may have had a reduced ability to de-escalate conflict, increasing risk of violence (McKinney et al., 2010). Women experiencing violence may have been using alcohol as a maladaptive coping mechanism (Khantzian, 1997). Such relationships are also frequently cyclical, with alcohol use often preceding experiences of IPV, which can in turn lead to increased alcohol use to cope (Kantor & Straus, 1989; Øverup et al., 2015). Similarly, alcohol use can serve as a form of self-medication to cope with ongoing depression and longitudinal work has linked alcohol use disorder to subsequent major depressive disorder (Edwards et al., 2014; Lasserre et al., 2022; Li et al., 2020; Pedrelli et al., 2016). Our findings from this community-based sample of women were consistent with findings from a separate contemporaneous body of qualitative work we conducted in a different region of Uganda among persons who engage in heavy alcohol use.

Prevalence of heavy alcohol use among persons living with HIV in Uganda is high (Magidson et al., 2019), and alcohol use is a risk factor for poor HIV care and treatment outcomes, making it an important modifiable risk behavior in this population (Miller, Pitpitan, et al., 2021b; Rehm et al., 2017). The Drinkers Intervention to Prevent Tuberculosis (DIPT) was a randomized, 2×2 factorial trial of an incentive-based alcohol use/medication adherence intervention among persons co-infected with HIV and TB who engage in hazardous alcohol use (Lodi et al., 2021). We conducted a qualitative sub-study with 32 DIPT participants and their intimate partners to understand how the intervention and pandemic impacted their relationship dynamics and experiences of IPV (Miller et al., 2024). In one-on-one interviews, several female partners reported increased experiences of IPV during the pandemic and this violence was frequently attributed to the economic impact of the lockdown and being confined to their homes (Miller et al., 2024). Both male and female participants described stress and anxiety related to economic insecurity leading to conflict (Miller et al., 2024). Among those who indicated they had reduced or stopped their alcohol use during the pandemic, lack of money to purchase alcohol was often described as a motivating reason. Taken together with the findings above, these results suggest the pandemic's influence on alcohol use may have adhered more to the predicted path of reduction due to contextual limitations on access and affordability (Rehm et al., 2020). Still, in some instances participants described continuing to drink despite the financial burden it had on their family, which resulted in further marital conflict (Miller et al., 2024). In addition, we would expect some underreporting around alcohol use in this sample due to social desirability bias, especially given ongoing participation in the DIPT study at the time of data collection.

Use of objective measures of alcohol use, such as the biomarker, phosphatidylethanol (PEth), is one way to remove bias introduced through self-reported measures and obtain more accurate estimates of alcohol use. A recently published longitudinal analysis of PEth measured changes in alcohol use prior to and during the pandemic among 200 persons living with HIV residing in Uganda who reported current alcohol use revealed that levels of biomarker confirmed unhealthy alcohol use did not decline during the period the lockdown was in place compared to pre-pandemic levels (Asiimwe et al., 2023). This was true despite the fact that drinking in bars did decline, suggesting that some folks who continued to consume hazardous amounts of alcohol adjusted patterns of use to do so in private spaces while the lockdown was in place (Asiimwe et al., 2023). While median age in this sample was older at 39 years (IQR 32–45), age was not significantly associated with biomarker measured hazardous use in unadjusted or adjusted models.

## Lessons Learned for Public Health Planning

These findings suggest that in Uganda, patterns of alcohol use during the pandemic were heavily impacted by the socioeconomic consequences of the lockdown. While loss of income and other contextual factors (e.g., closure of public drinking venues) may have served as a deterrent for some, alcohol use among individuals with more problematic drinking patterns persisted and may have been exacerbated in the context of the lockdown. Post-pandemic, alcohol use in Uganda continues to be a major public health issue. WHO estimates from 2023 indicate that per capita consumption in Uganda has rebounded beyond pre-pandemic levels (9.5 liters per year in 2016) to 12.21 liters per year, which is roughly two times the global average and the highest estimate in the WHO Africa region (WHO, 2018b, 2023). On average, men consume about 19.93

liters of pure alcohol annually, while women consume 4.88 liters, underscoring the severity of gendered difference in patterns of drinking (WHO, 2023). These numbers indicate that any reductions that may have occurred due to COVID-19 related circumstances has dissipated. Therefore, it is important to scale up access to evidence-based alcohol harm reduction and treatment services to not only prepare for future pandemics, but also to address pre-existing substance use healthcare needs and adapt with secular trends.

Findings regarding the impact of the pandemic on depression in Uganda tell a simpler story: the pandemic and lockdown led to challenging circumstances which increased mental distress, stress, anxiety, and depression across study samples. While longitudinal data on the impact of the pandemic on depression in Uganda is lacking, a prospective cohort study conducted across eight LMICs prior to, during, and after the pandemic suggests that while MH was affected most severely in the early months of the pandemic (when most lockdowns were in place), the impact lingered, with aggregate levels of depression remaining higher than pre-pandemic levels (Aksunger et al., 2023). While numerous factors likely contributed to the increase in mental disorders, primary factors identified included being confined to the house and economic uncertainty. Longitudinal data from LMICs shows a stronger link between MH decline and strict lockdown measures, rather than the actual number of COVID-19 cases. For women, increased risk for and experiences of IPV also adversely impacted MH with stress, depression, feelings of hopelessness, and unplanned/mistimed pregnancies being the most reported health sequalae among survivors of IPV in African countries during COVID-19 (Ansah et al., 2023). The 20% spike in unplanned pregnancies among Ugandan teenagers during the pandemic is particularly concerning and may be attributable to school closures (UNICEF, 2021). In future public health crises, addressing risk factors like economic hardship and improving access to violence reporting systems and resources in LMICs are crucial for supporting victims of violence.

**Specific recommendations include:**

1. **Ministries of Health must apply lessons learned from the COVID-19 pandemic and the social and economic impact of**

**COVID-19 pandemic responses and advocate with counterparts in Ministries of Education, Finance, and Social Development for greater coordination in pandemic preparedness planning.** Wholistic coordinated and collaborative public health planning must balance and consider social determinants of health and costs for mental and behavioral health in the same way it responds to and plans for infectious diseases. For example, school and university closures should be implemented based on cost-benefit analysis (accounting for transmission countermeasures) and with definitive timelines for reopening. Further, steps should be taken to better equip LMICs to support remote learning when it is needed in the future, including universal free wireless Internet access and coverage that can reach remote areas.

2. **LMICs must mitigate the socioeconomic burden of future pandemics through multipronged social protections programs**. Uganda did distribute food parcels, but more robust programs were implemented elsewhere in Africa including vertical shock response (increasing funds provided to existing beneficiaries), horizontal shock response (expansion of cash transfer program to include newly eligible households), establishment of new temporary cash transfer programs, utility subsidies and waivers (e.g., electrical), tax relief, unemployment benefits, food transfers, and social solidarity funds (Devereux, 2021). South Africa offers an example of a particularly robust social assistance response. In addition to offering unemployment insurance to those in the formal sector and topping off existing social assistance grants, South Africa established COVID-19 Special Relief of Distress grants to vulnerable populations and persons employed in the informal sector, expanding assistance to six million additional citizens (Gronback et al., 2022). Establishment of similar policies in Uganda that can reach the many employed in the informal economy may help to reduce both mental distress and experiences of IPV.
3. **Alcohol policies and regulations put in place during future pandemics must be comprehensive and responsive to segments of the population that are most in need of regulating their use** (e.g., those that engage in HED). We agree with Uganda's public health messaging approach to reducing access, by closing venues where individuals previously gathered to consume alcohol (as a means of preventing

COVID-19 transmission). In line with the lessons learned from a WHO policy brief of COVID-19 related alcohol policies of seven other African nations (WHO, 2022), we advocate for supplementary measures that account for the massive unregulated alcohol market in Uganda, the popularity of homebrews, and the fact that individuals who have problems regulating their use may see their drinking exacerbated when the social aspect of use is removed. Such approaches can include limiting alcohol sales for home consumption, tackling illegal sales, and investing in research to monitor the effects of alcohol legislation on consumption (to support evidence-based policies) (WHO, 2022).

4. **Mental health and substance use resources must be improved to support those interested in receiving them.** This will require the scale-up of sustainable evidence-based programming and the introduction of services that can accommodate remote delivery. Given that MH conditions are frequently co-occurring and many share symptoms and biopsychosocial properties, there is growing evidence that transdiagnostic dimensional approaches to addressing MH issues may be more suitable than diagnosis-specific approaches aimed at treatment of a single condition. The Common Elements Treatment Approach (CETA) is an evidence-based transdiagnostic intervention developed specifically for use in LMICs (Murray et al., 2014) with demonstrated effectiveness in 14 LMICs (Bogdanov et al., 2021; Bolton et al., 2014; Murray et al., 2018, 2020; Weiss et al., 2015). Investment in integration of this type of approach in Uganda could ensure greater access to psychosocial support services in future pandemics. Still, if a stay-at-home order is in place, such in-person counseling would become inaccessible. Given the increased coverage of smart phones in Uganda and other lower resourced settings, remotely delivered services for those that wish to stop drinking or need MH counseling could greatly increase access to social support.
5. **Funding for evidence-based violence prevention programs must be bolstered, expanding access to programming and shelter services, and engaging community stakeholders to ensure alignment with community preferences and needs.** Uganda relies on a referral system supported by government facilities and NGO providers to deliver gender-based violence programming. These programs were

underfunded prior to the pandemic with limited availability in remote rural regions (WHO, 2020). During the first national lockdown, such services were deemed non-essential, and programs shuttered. This was also the case in other African countries, including Nigeria, South Africa, and Kenya (John et al., 2023; Roy et al., 2021). These programs must be classified as essential for future humanitarian crises to avoid breaks in service delivery. To our second point, persisting gender norms and attitudes that uphold gender inequity and condone violence against women present challenges in shifting individual attitudes, beliefs, and behaviors around IPV and there is evidence globally that progress toward gender equitable norms deteriorated under pandemic circumstances (Nnyombi et al., 2022; UN WOMEN, 2022). Several successful evidence-based interventions, in Uganda and LMICs more broadly, that have reduced IPV among women in Uganda (Abramsky et al., 2014; Leight et al., 2023; Wagman et al., 2015) have focused on norm shifting through community mobilization and sensitization to reduce social acceptability of IPV and engage community in shifting norms around violence against women. Uganda requires government support and funding for widespread implementation of such programming. To make these types of interventions "pandemic proof", efforts should also address gaps in digital literacy/technology to expand prevention delivery and reporting methods and develop programs to ensure continued service delivery during future lockdowns.

## Conclusions

The COVID-19 pandemic impacted MH and patterns of substance use, globally disrupting the lives of an entire generation of young adults, but context and pandemic response played a critical mediating role. Mental and behavioral health preparedness (as well as preparedness for upstream drivers of poor MH and substance use, such as violence, social isolation, and economic uncertainty) are as critical to public health planning as infectious disease preparedness. The alternative is an incomplete public health response that includes policies that temper one public health threat only to exacerbate several others.

## References

Abramsky, T., Devries, K., Kiss, L., Nakuti, J., Kyegombe, N., Starmann, E., Cundill, B., Francisco, L., Kaye, D., Musuya, T., Michau, L., & Watts, C. (2014). Findings from the SASA! Study: A cluster randomized controlled trial to assess the impact of a community mobilization intervention to prevent violence against women and reduce HIV risk in Kampala, Uganda. *BMC Medicine, 12*(1), 122. https://doi.org/10.1186/s12916-014-0122-5

Aguero, J. M. (2021). COVID-19 and the rise of intimate partner violence. *World Development, 137*, 105217. https://doi.org/10.1016/j.worlddev.2020.105217

Ahmadimazhin, S., Bazyar, J., Chehreh, R., Daliri, S., Karamelahi, Z., Sadeghifar, J., & Vafery, Y. (2021). Effects of the COVID-19 pandemic on the intimate partner violence and sexual function: A systematic review. *Prehospital and Disaster Medicine, 36*(5), 593–598. https://doi.org/10.1017/S1049023X21000789

Akina Mama Wa Afrika. (2020). *Gendered dimensions of the economic impacts of COVID-19 in Uganda: A technical brief* https://www.akinamamawaafrika.org/wp-content/uploads/2021/11/AKINA-MAMA-WA-AFRIKA-ANNUAL-REPORT-2020.pdf

Aksunger, N., Vernot, C., Littman, R., Voors, M., Meriggi, N. F., Abajobir, A., Beber, B., Dai, K., Egger, D., Islam, A., Kelly, J., Kharel, A., Matabaro, A., Moya, A., Mwachofi, P., Nekesa, C., Ochieng, E., Rahman, T., Scacco, A., et al. (2023). COVID-19 and mental health in 8 low- and middle-income countries: A prospective cohort study. *PLoS Medicine, 20*(4), e1004081. https://doi.org/10.1371/journal.pmed.1004081

Alupo, B. (2020). *Gender and COVID-19 control measures in Uganda*. Australian Institute of International Affairs: Institute for African Women in Law. http://www.internationalaffairs.org.au/australianoutlook/gender-and-covid-19-control-measures-in-uganda/

Andreou, N., & Dayton, J. (2018). *Decent work in Uganda's informal economy*. https://balloonventures.com/wp-content/uploads/2018/09/Decent-Work-in-Ugandas-Informal-Economy.pdf

Ansah, E. W., Asamoah, A., Bimpeh, B., Anani-Adzoe, L. F., & Botha, N. N. (2023). Covid-induced intimate partner violence: Scoping review from Africa between 2020 and 2022. *Humanities and Social Sciences Communications, 10*(1), 612. https://doi.org/10.1057/s41599-023-02062-6

Asiimwe, C., Fatch, R., Cheng, D. M., Emenyonu, N. I., Ngabirano, C., Muyindike, W. R., & Hahn, J. A. (2023). Bar attendance and alcohol use before and after COVID-19 related restrictions among HIV-infected adults in South-Western Uganda. *AIDS and Behavior, 27*(6), 2005–2014. https://doi.org/10.1007/s10461-022-03934-9

Atumanya, P., Sendagire, C., Wabule, A., Mukisa, J., Ssemogerere, L., Kwizera, A., & Agaba, P. K. (2020). Assessment of the current capacity of intensive care units in Uganda; A descriptive study. *Journal of Critical Care, 55*, 95–99. https://doi.org/10.1016/j.jcrc.2019.10.019

Barrera, M., Jr., Castro, F. G., Strycker, L. A., & Toobert, D. J. (2013). Cultural adaptations of behavioral health interventions: A progress report. *Journal of Consulting and Clinical Psychology, 81*(2), 196–205. https://doi.org/10.1037/a0027085

Beesiga, B., Marson, K., Fatch, R., Emenyonu, N. I., Adong, J., Kekibiina, A., Puryear, S., Lodi, S., McDonell, M. G., Muyindike, W. R., Kamya, M. R., Hahn, J. A., & Chamie, G. (2023). Effects of a COVID-19 public health lockdown on drinking and health behavior among persons with HIV and with unhealthy alcohol use in Uganda. *AIDS and Behavior, 27*(10), 3213–3222. https://doi.org/10.1007/s10461-023-04042-y

Betthäuser, B. A., Bach-Mortensen, A. M., & Engzell, P. (2023). A systematic review and meta-analysis of the evidence on learning during the COVID-19 pandemic. *Nature Human Behaviour, 7*(3), 375–385. https://doi.org/10.1038/s41562-022-01506-4

Bogdanov, S., Augustinavicius, J., Bass, J. K., Metz, K., Skavenski, S., Singh, N. S., Moore, Q., Haroz, E. E., Kane, J., Doty, B., Murray, L., & Bolton, P. (2021). A randomized-controlled trial of community-based transdiagnostic psychotherapy for veterans and internally displaced persons in Ukraine. *Global Mental Health (Cambridge), 8*, e32. https://doi.org/10.1017/gmh.2021.27

Bolton, P., Lee, C., Haroz, E. E., Murray, L., Dorsey, S., Robinson, C., Ugueto, A. M., & Bass, J. (2014). A transdiagnostic community-based mental health treatment for comorbid disorders: Development and outcomes of a randomized controlled trial among Burmese refugees in Thailand. *PLoS Medicine, 11*(11), e1001757. https://doi.org/10.1371/journal.pmed.1001757

Boschuetz, N., Cheng, S., Mei, L., & Loy, V. M. (2020). Changes in alcohol use patterns in the United States during COVID-19 pandemic. *WMJ, 119*(3), 171–176.

Breur, C., Bloom, B., Miller, A. P., Kigozi, G., Nakyanjo, N., Ddaaki, W., Nalugoda, F., & Wagman, J. A. (2019). "The bottle is my wife": Exploring reasons why men drink alcohol in Ugandan fishing communities. *Social Work in Public Health*, 1–16. https://doi.org/10.1080/19371918.2019.1666072

Britton, P. C. (2009). The relation of coping strategies to alcohol consumption and alcohol-related consequences in a college sample. *Addiction Research & Theory, 12*(2), 103–114. https://doi.org/10.1080/16066350310001613062

Bush, K., Kivlahan, D. R., McDonell, M. B., Fihn, S. D., & Bradley, K. A. (1998). The AUDIT alcohol consumption questions (AUDIT-C): An effective brief screening test for problem drinking. Ambulatory Care Quality Improvement Project (ACQUIP). Alcohol Use Disorders Identification Test. *Archives of Internal Medicine, 158*(16), 1789–1795. https://doi.org/10.1001/archinte.158.16.1789

Center on Gender Equity and Health. (2020). *EMERGE COVID-19 and gender survey questions*. Retrieved August 15, 2020, from https://emerge.ucsd.edu/covid-19/

Cepeda, Z., Arenas, C., Vilardo, V., Hilton, E., Dico-Young, T., & Green, C. (2017). *Dominican Republic gender analysis: A study of the impact of the Zika virus on women, girls, boys and men*. http://hdl.handle.net/10546/620261

Consolata, K., & Fredrick, I. K. (2020). Assessing the relationship between gender based violence and COVID-19 pandemic in Uganda. *Kabale University Faculty of Arts and Social Sciences*. http://hdl.handle.net/20.500.12493/534

Craig, J., Kalanxhi, E., Osena, G., & Frost, I. (2020). https://doi.org/10.1101/2020.06.02.20120147

Datzberger, S., Parkes, J., Bhatia, A., Nagawa, R., Kasidi, J. R., Musenze, B. J., Naker, D., & Devries, K. (2022). Intensified inequities: Young people's experiences of Covid-19 and school closures in Uganda. *Children & Society*. https://doi.org/10.1111/chso.12627

Devereux, S. (2021). Social protection responses to COVID-19 in Africa. *Global Social Policy*. https://doi.org/10.1177/14680181211021260

Edwards, A. C., Joinson, C., Dick, D. M., Kendler, K. S., Macleod, J., Munafò, M., Hickman, M., Lewis, G., & Heron, J. (2014). The association between depressive symptoms from early to late adolescence and later use and harmful use of alcohol. *European Child & Adolescent Psychiatry, 23*(12), 1219–1230. https://doi.org/10.1007/s00787-014-0600-5

Evans-Lacko, S., Aguilar-Gaxiola, S., Al-Hamzawi, A., Alonso, J., Benjet, C., Bruffaerts, R., Chiu, W. T., Florescu, S., de Girolamo, G., Gureje, O., Haro, J. M., He, Y., Hu, C., Karam, E. G., Kawakami, N., Lee, S., Lund, C.,

Kovess-Masfety, V., Levinson, D., et al. (2018). Socio-economic variations in the mental health treatment gap for people with anxiety, mood, and substance use disorders: Results from the WHO World Mental Health (WMH) surveys. *Psychological Medicine, 48*(9), 1560–1571. https://doi.org/10.1017/S0033291717003336

Fergusson, D. M., Boden, J. M., & Horwood, L. J. (2009). Tests of causal links between alcohol abuse or dependence and major depression. *Archives of General Psychiatry, 66*(3), 260–266. https://doi.org/10.1001/archgenpsychiatry.2008.543

Foran, H. M., & O'Leary, K. D. (2008). Alcohol and intimate partner violence: A meta-analytic review. *Clinical Psychology Review, 28*(7), 1222–1234. https://doi.org/10.1016/j.cpr.2008.05.001

Gronback, L., Seekings, J., & Megannon, V. (2022). *Social protection in COVID-19 pandemic: Lessons from South Africa* (CGD Policy Paper 252, Issue).

Grossman, E. R., Benjamin-Neelon, S. E., & Sonnenschein, S. (2020). Alcohol consumption during the COVID-19 pandemic: A cross-sectional survey of US adults. *International Journal of Environmental Research and Public Health, 17*(24). https://doi.org/10.3390/ijerph17249189

Hasking, P., Lyvers, M., Carlopio, C., & Raber, A. (2011). The relationship between coping strategies, alcohol expectancies, drinking motives and drinking behaviour. *Addictive Behaviors, 36*(5), 479–487. https://doi.org/10.1016/j.addbeh.2011.01.014

Horigian, V. E., Schmidt, R. D., & Feaster, D. J. (2021). Loneliness, mental health, and substance use among US young adults during COVID-19. *The Journal of Psychoactive Drugs, 53*(1), 1–9. https://doi.org/10.1080/02791072.2020.1836435

Human Rights Watch. (2020, April 2). *Uganda: Respect rights in COVID-19 response ensure security forces refrain from violence, abuse.* Retrieved June 28, 2020, from https://www.hrw.org/news/2020/04/02/uganda-respect-rights-covid-19-response#

Hussong, A. M., Haik, A. K., & Loeb, H. M. (2023). Generation COVID: Young adult substance use. *Current Opinion in Psychology, 52*, 101640. https://doi.org/10.1016/j.copsyc.2023.101640

IHME. (2017). *Global burden of disease.* https://vizhub.healthdata.org/gbd-compare/

IHME. (n.d.). *Health research by location: Uganda*. Institute for Health Metrics and Evaluation. https://www.healthdata.org/research-analysis/health-by-location/profiles/uganda

Jalloh, M. F., Li, W., Bunnell, R. E., Ethier, K. A., O'Leary, A., Hageman, K. M., Sengeh, P., Jalloh, M. B., Morgan, O., Hersey, S., Marston, B. J., Dafae, F., & Redd, J. T. (2018). Impact of Ebola experiences and risk perceptions on mental health in Sierra Leone, July 2015. *BMJ Global Health, 3*(2), e000471. https://doi.org/10.1136/bmjgh-2017-000471

John, N. A., Bukuluki, P., Casey, S. E., Chauhan, D. B., Jagun, M. O., Mabhena, N., Mwangi, M., & McGovern, T. (2023). Government responses to COVID-19 and impact on GBV services and programmes: Comparative analysis of the situation in South Africa, Kenya, Uganda, and Nigeria. *Sex Reprod Health Matters, 31*(1), 2168399. https://doi.org/10.1080/26410397.2023.2168399

Kaggwa, M. M., Najjuka, S. M., Bongomin, F., Mamun, M. A., & Griffiths, M. D. (2022). Prevalence of depression in Uganda: A systematic review and meta-analysis. *PLoS One, 17*(10), e0276552. https://doi.org/10.1371/journal.pone.0276552

Kantor, G. K., & Straus, M. A. (1989). Substance abuse as a precipitant of wife abuse victimizations. *The American Journal of Drug and Alcohol Abuse, 15*(2), 173–189. https://doi.org/10.3109/00952998909092719

Kauhanen, L., Wan Mohd Yunus, W. M. A., Lempinen, L., Peltonen, K., Gyllenberg, D., Mishina, K., Gilbert, S., Bastola, K., Brown, J. S. L., & Sourander, A. (2023). A systematic review of the mental health changes of children and young people before and during the COVID-19 pandemic. *European Child & Adolescent Psychiatry, 32*(6), 995–1013. https://doi.org/10.1007/s00787-022-02060-0

Kgaugelo, M. (2020, April 3). Gender-based violence complaints hit 87,000 so far in lockdown, as cop arrested for allegedly raping wife. *Times Live*. https://www.timeslive.co.za/news/south-africa/2020-04-03-gender-based-violence-complaints-hit-87000-so-far-in-lockdown-as-cop-arrested-for-allegedly-raping-wife/.

Khan, K. S., Mamun, M. A., Griffiths, M. D., & Ullah, I. (2020). The mental health impact of the COVID-19 pandemic across different cohorts. *International Journal of Mental Health and Addiction*, 1–7. https://doi.org/10.1007/s11469-020-00367-0

Khantzian, E. J. (1997). The self-medication hypothesis of substance use disorders: A reconsideration and recent applications. *Harvard Review of Psychiatry, 4*(5), 231–244. https://doi.org/10.3109/10673229709030550

Kiene, S. M., Miller, A. P., Ediau, M., Tuhebwe, D., Sileo, K. M., Naigino, R. et al. (2025). A pilot randomized controlled trial of Kisoboka, a behavioral economic and motivational interviewing intervention to reduce high-risk alcohol use and improve antiretroviral therapy adherence for men in Uganda. Addiction. https://doi.org/10.1111/add.70169

Kourti, A., Stavridou, A., Panagouli, E., Psaltopoulou, T., Spiliopoulou, C., Tsolia, M., Sergentanis, T. N., & Tsitsika, A. (2021). Domestic violence during the COVID-19 pandemic: A systematic review. *Trauma, Violence & Abuse, 24*(2), 719–745. https://doi.org/10.1177/15248380211038690

Kroenke, K., Spitzer, R. L., & Williams, J. B. (2001). The PHQ-9: Validity of a brief depression severity measure. *Journal of General Internal Medicine, 16*(9), 606–613. https://doi.org/10.1046/j.1525-1497.2001.016009606.x

Lasserre, A. M., Imtiaz, S., Roerecke, M., Heilig, M., Probst, C., & Rehm, J. (2022). Socioeconomic status, alcohol use disorders, and depression: A population-based study. *Journal of Affective Disorders, 301*, 331–336. https://doi.org/10.1016/j.jad.2021.12.132

Lee, S. A. (2020). Coronavirus anxiety scale: A brief mental health screener for COVID-19 related anxiety. *Death Studies, 44*(7), 393–401. https://doi.org/10.1080/07481187.2020.1748481

Leight, J., Cullen, C., Ranganathan, M., & Yakubovich, A. (2023). Effectiveness of community mobilisation and group-based interventions for preventing intimate partner violence against women in low- and middle-income countries: A systematic review and meta-analysis. *Journal of Global Health, 13*, 04115. https://doi.org/10.7189/jogh.13.04115

Li, J., Wang, H., Li, M., Shen, Q., Li, X., Zhang, Y., Peng, J., Rong, X., & Peng, Y. (2020). Effect of alcohol use disorders and alcohol intake on the risk of subsequent depressive symptoms: A systematic review and meta-analysis of cohort studies. *Addiction, 115*(7), 1224–1243. https://doi.org/10.1111/add.14935

Lodi, S., Emenyonu, N. I., Marson, K., Kwarisiima, D., Fatch, R., McDonell, M. G., Cheng, D. M., Thirumurthy, H., Gandhi, M., Camlin, C. S., Muyindike, W. R., Hahn, J. A., & Chamie, G. (2021). The Drinkers' Intervention to Prevent Tuberculosis (DIPT) trial among heavy drinkers living with HIV in Uganda: Study protocol of a 2x2 factorial trial. *Trials, 22*(1), 355. https://doi.org/10.1186/s13063-021-05304-7

Lundberg, P., Rukundo, G., Ashaba, S., Thorson, A., Allebeck, P., Ostergren, P. O., & Cantor-Graae, E. (2011). Poor mental health and sexual risk behaviours in Uganda: A cross-sectional population-based study. *BMC Public Health, 11*, 125. https://doi.org/10.1186/1471-2458-11-125

Luo, Y., Chua, C. R., Xiong, Z., Ho, R. C., & Ho, C. S. H. (2020). A systematic review of the impact of viral respiratory epidemics on mental health: An implication on the coronavirus disease 2019 pandemic. *Frontiers in Psychiatry, 11*, 565098. https://doi.org/10.3389/fpsyt.2020.565098

Magidson, J. F., Fatch, R., Orrell, C., Amanyire, G., Haberer, J. E., Hahn, J. A., & team, M. (2019). Biomarker-measured unhealthy alcohol use in relation to CD4 count among individuals starting ART in sub-Saharan Africa. *AIDS and Behavior, 23*(6), 1656–1667. https://doi.org/10.1007/s10461-018-2364-2

Mahmud, M., & Riley, E. (2021). Household response to an extreme shock: Evidence on the immediate impact of the Covid-19 lockdown on economic outcomes and well-being in rural Uganda. *World Development, 140*, 105318. https://doi.org/10.1016/j.worlddev.2020.105318

McKinney, C. M., Caetano, R., Rodriguez, L. A., & Okoro, N. (2010). Does alcohol involvement increase the severity of intimate partner violence? *Alcoholism, Clinical and Experimental Research, 34*(4), 655–658. https://doi.org/10.1111/j.1530-0277.2009.01134.x

McNabb, K., Kaidu, T., & Kavuma, S. (2023). *The dynamics of formal employment during and after the COVID-19 pandemic in Uganda.*

Miller, A. P., Ddaaki, W. G., Bloom, B. E., Wirtz, A. L., Nakyanjo, N., Kigozi, G., & Wagman, J. A. (2021a). Perspectives of women living with HIV on addressing violence and use of alcohol during HIV services: Qualitative findings from fishing communities in Uganda. *Violence Against Women*. https://doi.org/10.1177/10778012211019054

Miller, A. P., Pitpitan, E. V., Kiene, S. M., Raj, A., Jain, S., Zúñiga, M. L., Nabulaku, D., Nalugoda, F., Ssekubugu, R., Nantume, B., Kigozi, G., Sewankambo, N. K., Kagaayi, J., Reynolds, S. J., Grabowski, K., Wawer, M., Wagman, A., & J. (2021b). Alcohol use and alcohol-related consequences are associated with not being virally suppressed among persons living with HIV in the Rakai region of Uganda. *Drug and Alcohol Dependence*. https://doi.org/10.1016/j.drugalcdep.2021.109005

Miller, A. P., Ziegel, L., Mugamba, S., Kyasanku, E., Wagman, J. A., Nkwanzi-Lubega, V., Nakigozi, G., Kigozi, G., Nalugoda, F., Kigozi, G., Nkale, J., Watya, S., & Ddaaki, W. (2021c). Not enough money and too many thoughts: Exploring perceptions of mental health in two Ugandan districts through the mental health literacy framework. *Qualitative Health Research.* https://doi.org/10.1177/1049732320986164

Miller, A. P., Mugamba, S., Bulamba, R. M., Kyasanku, E., Nkale, J., Nalugoda, F., Nakigozi, G., Kigozi, G., Nalwoga, G. K., Kagaayi, J., Watya, S., & Wagman, J. A. (2022). Exploring the impact of COVID-19 on women's alcohol use, mental health, and experiences of intimate partner violence in Wakiso, Uganda. *PLoS One, 17*(2). https://doi.org/10.1371/journal.pone.0263827

Miller, A. P., Appa, A., Muyindike, W., Fatch, R., Kekibiina, A., Beesiga, B., Adong, J., Emenyonu, N., Marson, K., Getahun, M., Kamya, M., Chamie, G., Camlin, C., & Hahn, J. A. (2024). Experiences of intimate partner violence among HIV/TB coinfected persons with unhealthy alcohol use in Uganda: Qualitative study of an incentive-based alcohol/medication adherence intervention. *Violence Against Women.* https://doi.org/10.1177/10778012231225229

Molodynski, A., Cusack, C., & Nixon, J. (2017). Mental healthcare in Uganda: Desperate challenges but real opportunities. *BJPsych International, 14*(4), 98–100. https://doi.org/10.1192/s2056474000002129

Mugamba, S., Ziegel, L., Bulamba, R. M., Kyasanku, E., Johansson Arhem, K., Sjoland, C. F., Miller, A. P., Nakigozi, G., Nalwoga, G. K., Watya, S., Kiwanuka, N., Kagaayi, J., Kiwanuka, D., Ddaaki, W., Wagman, J. A., Kigozi, G., Ekstrom, A. M., & Nalugoda, F. (2022). Cohort profile: The Africa Medical and Behavioral Sciences Organization (AMBSO) Population Health Surveillance (APHS) in rural, semi-urban and urban Uganda. *International Journal of Epidemiology.* https://doi.org/10.1093/ije/dyac164

Muller, A. E., Hafstad, E. V., Himmels, J. P. W., Smedslund, G., Flottorp, S., Stensland, S. O., Stroobants, S., Van de Velde, S., & Vist, G. E. (2020). The mental health impact of the Covid-19 pandemic on healthcare workers, and interventions to help them: A rapid systematic review. *Psychiatry Research, 293*, 113441. https://doi.org/10.1016/j.psychres.2020.113441

Murray, L. K., Dorsey, S., Haroz, E., Lee, C., Alsiary, M. M., Haydary, A., Weiss, W. M., & Bolton, P. (2014). A common elements treatment approach for adult mental health problems in low- and middle-income countries. *Cognitive and Behavioral Practice, 21*(2), 111–123. https://doi.org/10.1016/j.cbpra.2013.06.005

Murray, L. K., Hall, B. J., Dorsey, S., Ugueto, A. M., Puffer, E. S., Sim, A., Ismael, A., Bass, J., Akiba, C., Lucid, L., Harrison, J., Erikson, A., & Bolton,

P. A. (2018). An evaluation of a common elements treatment approach for youth in Somali refugee camps. *Global Mental Health (Cambridge), 5*, e16. https://doi.org/10.1017/gmh.2018.7

Murray, L. K., Kane, J. C., Glass, N., Skavenski van Wyk, S., Melendez, F., Paul, R., Kmett Danielson, C., Murray, S. M., Mayeya, J., Simenda, F., & Bolton, P. (2020). Effectiveness of the Common Elements Treatment Approach (CETA) in reducing intimate partner violence and hazardous alcohol use in Zambia (VATU): A randomized controlled trial. *PLoS Medicine, 17*(4), e1003056. https://doi.org/10.1371/journal.pmed.1003056

Najjuka, S. M., Checkwech, G., Olum, R., Ashaba, S., & Kaggwa, M. M. (2021). Depression, anxiety, and stress among Ugandan university students during the COVID-19 lockdown: An online survey. *African Health Sciences, 21*(4), 1533–1543. https://doi.org/10.4314/ahs.v21i4.6

Najmul, H., Abdinasir Yusuf, O., Audrey, G., George, O. A., Danny, A., Rashid, A., Richard John, L., Palwasha, K., & Muzamil Mahdi Abdel, H., Dorothy, Y.-M., Leonard, M., Elizabeth Henry, S., Blandina, T. M., Mark, U., David, M., Nathan, K., Rashida Abbas, F., Pascalina-Chanda, K., Florian, S., … David, M. (2020). Lockdown measures in response to COVID-19 in nine sub-Saharan African countries. *BMJ Global Health, 5*(10), e003319. https://doi.org/10.1136/bmjgh-2020-003319

Nnyombi, A., Bukuluki, P., Besigwa, S., Ocaya-Irama, J., Namara, C., & Cislaghi, B. (2022). How social norms contribute to physical violence among ever-partnered women in Uganda: A qualitative study. *Frontiers in Sociology, 7*, 867024. https://doi.org/10.3389/fsoc.2022.867024

O'Brien, M., & Tolosa, M. X. (2016). The effect of the 2014 West Africa Ebola virus disease epidemic on multi-level violence against women. *International Journal of Human Rights in Healthcare, 9*(3), 151–160. https://doi.org/10.1108/ijhrh-09-2015-0027

Ojeahere, M. I., Kumswa, S. K., Adiukwu, F., Plang, J. P., & Taiwo, Y. F. (2022). Intimate partner violence and its mental health implications amid COVID-19 lockdown: Findings among Nigerian couples. *Journal of Interpersonal Violence, 37*(17–18), NP15434-NP15454. https://doi.org/10.1177/08862605211015213

Øverup, C. S., DiBello, A. M., Brunson, J. A., Acitelli, L. K., & Neighbors, C. (2015). Drowning the pain: Intimate partner violence and drinking to cope prospectively predict problem drinking. *Addictive Behaviors, 41*, 152–161. https://doi.org/10.1016/j.addbeh.2014.10.006

Pacek, L. R., Martins, S. S., & Crum, R. M. (2013). The bidirectional relationships between alcohol, cannabis, co-occurring alcohol and cannabis use disorders with major depressive disorder: Results from a national sample. *Journal of Affective Disorders, 148*(2-3), 188–195. https://doi.org/10.1016/j.jad.2012.11.059

Pedrelli, P., Shapero, B., Archibald, A., & Dale, C. (2016). Alcohol use and depression during adolescence and young adulthood: A summary and interpretation of mixed findings. *Current Addiction Reports, 3*(1), 91–97. https://doi.org/10.1007/s40429-016-0084-0

Pfefferbaum, B., & North, C. S. (2020). Mental health and the Covid-19 pandemic. *The New England Journal of Medicine, 383*(6), 510–512. https://doi.org/10.1056/NEJMp2008017

Rehm, J., Probst, C., Shield, K. D., & Shuper, P. A. (2017). Does alcohol use have a causal effect on HIV incidence and disease progression? A review of the literature and a modeling strategy for quantifying the effect. *Population Health Metrics, 15*(1), 4. https://doi.org/10.1186/s12963-017-0121-9

Rehm, J., Kilian, C., Ferreira-Borges, C., Jernigan, D., Monteiro, M., Parry, C. D. H., Sanchez, Z. M., & Manthey, J. (2020). Alcohol use in times of the COVID 19: Implications for monitoring and policy. *Drug and Alcohol Review, 39*(4), 301–304. https://doi.org/10.1111/dar.13074

Roy, C. M., Bukuluki, P., Casey, S. E., Jagun, M. O., John, N. A., Mabhena, N., Mwangi, M., & McGovern, T. (2021). Impact of COVID-19 on gender-based violence prevention and response services in Kenya, Uganda, Nigeria, and South Africa: A cross-sectional survey. *Frontiers in Global Women's Health, 2*, 780771. https://doi.org/10.3389/fgwh.2021.780771

Ryerson, N. C., Wilson, O. W. A., Pena, A., Duffy, M., & Bopp, M. (2021). What happens when the party moves home? The effect of the COVID-19 pandemic on U.S. college student alcohol consumption as a function of legal drinking status using longitudinal data. *Translational Behavioral Medicine, 11*(3), 772–774. https://doi.org/10.1093/tbm/ibab006

Sallie, S. N., Ritou, V., Bowden-Jones, H., & Voon, V. (2020). Assessing international alcohol consumption patterns during isolation from the COVID-19 pandemic using an online survey: Highlighting negative emotionality mechanisms. *BMJ Open, 10*(11), e044276. https://doi.org/10.1136/bmjopen-2020-044276

Schwarzer, R., & Jerusalem, M. (1995). Generalized self-efficacy scale. In J. Weinman, S. Wright, & M. Johnston (Eds.), *Measures in health psychology: A user's portfolio. Causal and control beliefs* (pp. 35–37). NFER-NELSON.

Semakula, E. (2020). *Gender, police brutality, and public health in Uganda during the COVID-19 pandemic*. Institute for African Women in Law. Retrieved June 28, 2020, from https://www.africanwomeninlaw.com/post/gender-police-brutality-and-public-health-in-uganda-during-the-covid-19-pandemic

Sharma, A., & Borah, S. B. (2020). Covid-19 and domestic violence: An indirect path to social and economic crisis. *Journal of Family Violence, 1-7*. https://doi.org/10.1007/s10896-020-00188-8

Sileo, K. M., Muhumuza, C., Helal, T., Olfers, A., Lule, H., Sekamatte, S., Kershaw, T. S., Wanyenze, R. K., & Kiene, S. M. (2023). Exploring the effects of COVID-19 on family planning: Results from a qualitative study in rural Uganda following COVID-19 lockdown. *Reproductive Health, 20*(1), 31. https://doi.org/10.1186/s12978-023-01566-3

Sinclair, V. G., & Wallston, K. A. (2004). The development and psychometric evaluation of the Brief Resilient Coping Scale. *Assessment, 11*(1), 94–101. https://doi.org/10.1177/1073191103258144

Sohi, I., Chrystoja, B. R., Rehm, J., Wells, S., Monteiro, M., Ali, S., & Shield, K. D. (2022). Changes in alcohol use during the COVID-19 pandemic and previous pandemics: A systematic review. *Alcoholism, Clinical and Experimental Research, 46*(4), 498–513. https://doi.org/10.1111/acer.14792

Sokolovsky, A. W., Hertel, A. W., Micalizzi, L., White, H. R., Hayes, K. L., & Jackson, K. M. (2021). Preliminary impact of the COVID-19 pandemic on smoking and vaping in college students. *Addictive Behaviors, 115*, 106783. https://doi.org/10.1016/j.addbeh.2020.106783

Sun, Y., Wu, Y., Fan, S., Dal Santo, T., Li, L., Jiang, X., Li, K., Wang, Y., Tasleem, A., Krishnan, A., He, C., Bonardi, O., Boruff, J. T., Rice, D. B., Markham, S., Levis, B., Azar, M., Thombs-Vite, I., Neupane, D., et al. (2023). Comparison of mental health symptoms before and during the covid-19 pandemic: Evidence from a systematic review and meta-analysis of 134 cohorts. *BMJ, 380*, e074224. https://doi.org/10.1136/bmj-2022-074224

Suubi, K., Yegon E., Ajema, C., Wandera, N., Afifu, C., & Mugyenyi, C. (2022). *Impact of COVID-19 on women workers in the urban informal economy in Uganda and Kenya: Secondary data review*.

The World Bank. (2022). *Total fertility rate—Uganda (2021)*. https://data.worldbank.org/indicator/SP.DYN.TFRT.IN?locations=UG-XL

Uganda MOH. (2020). *Coronavirus (pandemic): COVID 19*. Government of Uganda. Retrieved June 28, 2020, from https://www.health.go.ug/covid/

Uganda MOH. (2022). *Uganda demographic and health survey 2021 (UDHS-7)*. Uganda Bureau of Statistics.

UN DESA. (2022). World Population Prospects 2022. https://population.un.org/wpp/

UN WOMEN. (2022). *UN women reveals concerning regression in attitudes towards gender roles during pandemic in new study*. https://www.unwomen.org/en/news-stories/press-release/2022/06/un-women-reveals-concerning-regression-in-attitudes-towards-gender-roles-during-pandemic-in-new-study

UNICEF. (2021). *COVID-19: Education replaced by shuttered schools, violence, teenage pregnancy*. United Nations.

Wagman, J. A., Gray, R. H., Campbell, J. C., Thoma, M., Ndyanabo, A., Ssekasanvu, J., Nalugoda, F., Kagaayi, J., Nakigozi, G., Serwadda, D., & Brahmbhatt, H. (2015). Effectiveness of an integrated intimate partner violence and HIV prevention intervention in Rakai, Uganda: Analysis of an intervention in an existing cluster randomised cohort. *The Lancet Global Health, 3*(1), e23–e33. https://doi.org/10.1016/S2214-109X(14)70344-4

Wandera, N., Suubi, K., Afifu, C., Emily, S., Connor, R., & Izugbara, C. (2023). *The social and economic impact of the COVID-19 policy responses on women working in the urban informal sector in Uganda*. Kampala, Uganda. International Center for Research on Women (ICRW), Kampala.

Weerakoon, S. M., Jetelina, K. K., & Knell, G. (2021). Longer time spent at home during COVID-19 pandemic is associated with binge drinking among US adults. *The American Journal of Drug and Alcohol Abuse, 47*(1), 98–106. https://doi.org/10.1080/00952990.2020.1832508

Weiss, W. M., Murray, L. K., Zangana, G. A., Mahmooth, Z., Kaysen, D., Dorsey, S., Lindgren, K., Gross, A., Murray, S. M., Bass, J. K., & Bolton, P. (2015). Community-based mental health treatments for survivors of torture and militant attacks in Southern Iraq: A randomized control trial. *BMC Psychiatry, 15*, 249. https://doi.org/10.1186/s12888-015-0622-7

WHO. (2004). *Intimate partner violence and HIV/AIDS* (Violence Against Women and HIV/AIDS: Critical Intersections Information Bulletin Series, Issue). http://www.who.int/hac/techguidance/pht/InfoBulletinIntimatePartnerViolenceFinal.pdf

WHO. (2015). *Mental Health Atlas*. http://www.who.int/mentalhealth/evidence/atlas/executive_summary_en.pdf?ua=1Geneva

WHO. (2018a). *Global status report on alcohol and health 2018*. http://www.who.int/substance_abuse/publications/global_alcohol_report/msb_gsr_2014_2.pdf?ua=1

WHO. (2018b). *Global status report on alcohol and health 2018.*

WHO. (2020). *Strengthening the health system response to violence against women in Uganda: Lessons learned from adapting and implementing WHO guidelines and tools.*

WHO. (2021). *WHO global lists of high burden countries for tuberculosis (TB), TB/HIV and multidrug/rifampicin-resistant TB (MDR/RR-TB), 2021–2025.* https://cdn.who.int/media/docs/default-source/hq-tuberculosis/who_globalhbcliststb_2021-2025_backgrounddocument.pdf?sfvrsn=f6b854c2_9

WHO. (2022). *Policy, system and practice response to alcohol consumption during the COVID-19 pandemic in seven countries of the WHO African Region. Brief 9, October 2022* (Policy Brief, Issue). https://www.who.int/publications/i/item/9789240061903

WHO. (2023). *World health statistics 2023: Monitoring health for the SDGs, sustainable development goals.*

Williams, E. C., Hahn, J. A., Saitz, R., Bryant, K., Lira, M. C., & Samet, J. H. (2016). Alcohol use and human immunodeficiency virus (HIV) infection: Current knowledge, implications, and future directions. *Alcoholism, Clinical and Experimental Research, 40*(10), 2056–2072. https://doi.org/10.1111/acer.13204

World Bank. (2023). *Poverty & equity brief: Uganda.* https://databankfiles.worldbank.org/public/ddpext_download/poverty/987B9C90-CB9F-4D93-AE8C-750588BF00QA/current/Global_POVEQ_UGA.pdf

Wu, T., Jia, X., Shi, H., Niu, J., Yin, X., Xie, J., & Wang, X. (2021). Prevalence of mental health problems during the COVID-19 pandemic: A systematic review and meta-analysis. *Journal of Affective Disorders, 281*, 91–98. https://doi.org/10.1016/j.jad.2020.11.117

Wyckoff, K. G., Narasimhan, S., Stephenson, K., Zeidan, A. J., Smith, R. N., & Evans, D. P. (2023). "COVID gave him an opportunity to tighten the reins around my throat": Perceptions of COVID-19 movement restrictions among survivors of intimate partner violence. *BMC Public Health, 23*(1), 199. https://doi.org/10.1186/s12889-023-15137-5

Zablotska, I. B., Gray, R. H., Koenig, M. A., Serwadda, D., Nalugoda, F., Kigozi, G., Sewankambo, N., Lutalo, T., Wabwire Mangen, F., & Wawer, M. (2009). Alcohol use, intimate partner violence, sexual coercion and HIV among women aged 15–24 in Rakai, Uganda. *AIDS and Behavior, 13*(2), 225–233. https://doi.org/10.1007/s10461-007-9333-5

# Part III

## Young Adults Who Drink Little or No Alcohol

# 8

# Non-drinkers and Non-drinking: A Review, a Critique, and Pathways to Policy

Emma Banister, Dom Conroy, and Maria Piacentini

**Abstract** Non-drinkers make up a growing proportion of young adults in many countries. Perhaps mirroring this, academic research focused on non-drinkers is an emerging field of work across disciplinary boundaries. In this chapter, we first provide an overview of qualitative research which has tended to focus on non-drinking as a lifestyle choice for young people, entailing issues relating to motivation, identity, and self-management; and quantitative research which have typically explored how 'views of

E. Banister
Work and Equalities Institute, University of Manchester, Manchester, UK
e-mail: emma.banister@manchester.ac.uk

D. Conroy (✉)
Faculty of Arts and Social Science, The Open University, London, UK
e-mail: d.conroy@open.ac.uk

M. Piacentini
University of Lancaster, Lancaster University Management School, Lancaster, UK
e-mail: m.piacentini@lancaster.ac.uk



D. Conroy, F. Measham (eds.), *Young Adult Drinking Styles*, Sustainable Development Goals Series, https://doi.org/10.1007/978-3-031-98528-7_8

non-drinkers' might predict drinking behaviour among young adults and young people. We then problematise understandings of 'non-drinkers' and 'non-drinking' as straightforward terms drawing on contemporary sociological theory and critical research. The chapter concludes with an exploration of how these emergent themes of the 'non-drinking literature' might be used to inform policy and practice to promote moderate alcohol consumption among young adults. We also explore a future research agenda for academics planning research concerning non-drinking and non-drinkers.

Non-drinkers and non-drinking, whether as something temporary or as a lifestyle choice, have been the focus of growing cultural and scholarly interest. This is also evident in work on Temporary Abstinence Challenges (TACs, e.g., 'Dry January' in the UK and 'Hello Sunday Morning' in Australia) and 'dry dating', explored in Chaps. 9 and 10 of this book, respectively. While many young adults drink alcohol on a regular basis, there has been an internationally recognised decline in the volume and frequency(?) of alcohol consumption among young people in high income countries over the last 20 years, particularly among adolescents (Holmes et al., 2024). The most recent data from the Drinkaware Monitor Report (2023) shows that young adults are increasingly moving towards responsible drinking, with a rise in non-drinkers (21% in 2023, compared to 14% in 2017) and a decline in frequent and high-risk drinking.

The growth of interest in non-drinking lifestyles has led to UK media speculation around Generation Z individuals (born between 1997 and 2012) who appear to be 'growing up sober curious' (BBC, 2022). The increasing use of the term 'sober curious' allows for fluidity 'encouraging an ongoing "questioning" of drinking alcohol', emphasising reflection and moderation and potentially, yet not inevitably, longer term sobriety (Lunnay et al., 2022, p. 3). The movement and its momentum suggest a wider questioning of, firstly, binary positions on drinking and not drinking, and, secondly, the necessity for individuals to identify themselves in terms of consumption. Sober curious implies a discursive engagement with societal pressures and expectations, inviting exploration of alternative lifestyle choices without necessarily fully committing to abstinence, and thereby resisting categorisation into either camp of drinker or non-drinker. Interest in 'sobriety', 'sober curiosity', or 'positive sobriety' communities has substantially grown since the first edition of this book. Although there is overlap with personal reasons for not drinking, a wider discussion of contemporary sobriety movements is beyond this chapter's scope. For more on sobriety communities, refer to Chaps. 9 and 10 in this volume, academic research (e.g., Atkinson et al., 2023; Nicholls, 2022), and popular writings on sobriety (e.g., Gray, 2017; Warrington, 2019).

This chapter is designed to collate research relating to non-drinkers and non-drinking, draw on relevant sociological theory to problematise the notion of binary 'drinker' identities, and to consider chapter implications for health promotion and the future research agenda in this area. The chapter is organised as follows: section one summarises key themes from research on non-drinkers and non-drinking. Section two problematises traditional drinker/non-drinker identities, viewing them as fluid rather than fixed, and contextualises this within omission/commission debates and the sociology of nothing (Scott, 2018). Section three discusses how this evidence base can help refresh alcohol-related health promotion policy and future research agendas. Our approach integrates a plurality of ideas, methods, and paradigms, incorporating different disciplinary perspectives.

## Non-drinking and Non-drinkers: Key Research Themes

This section summarises studies that unproblematically view non-drinkers and non-drinking as a relatively homogeneous and undifferentiated group. These studies often identify non-drinkers as an 'outgroup' defined by their lack of drinking, contrasted with the dominant 'regular drinkers'. Accordingly, this section includes post-positivist research using psychometric measures on views of non-drinkers and qualitative research on young adult non-drinkers' experiences.

Psychometric research has shown links between variability on different attitudes towards non-drinker scales and individual drinking patterns among young adults. For instance, Prototype Willingness Model studies indicate that negative evaluations of 'the prototypical non-drinker' predict increased alcohol consumption among students (e.g., Gerrard et al., 2002). Similarly, unfavourable attitudes towards non-drinkers correlate with higher levels of harmful drinking among young people (Regan & Morrison, 2013, 2017). Recent psychometric studies also suggest that non-drinkers may present threats to social activities (Cheers et al., 2024). These studies provide a framework for understanding how views about non-drinkers influence drinking behaviours, though they often reduce non-drinkers to a homogenous 'type' of person, and tend to conflate views towards non-drinkers (group or individual) with views on non-drinking (the behaviour or position).

Qualitative research shows that young adults who regularly drink often hold negative perceptions of non-drinkers, viewing them as 'boring' or judgmental (Black & Monrouxe, 2014; Jacobs et al., 2018; Emslie et al., 2012). For example, focus group studies suggest non-drinkers at student parties have little influence on their peers' drinking behaviour and are generally accepted in drinking environments (Brown et al., 2010). However, non-drinkers, particularly males, can face scrutiny, as not drinking is seen as incongruent with attributes of hegemonic masculine identities (Conroy & de Visser, 2013).

There is now fairly extensive research exploring the social/relational experiences of young adult non-drinkers (Banister et al., 2019; Conroy & de Visser, 2014, 2015; Pavlidis et al., 2019; Piacentini & Banister, 2009; Rahman, 2023). A systematic review of UK-based qualitative studies reports that young adults who consume little or no alcohol may face significant and overt forms of alcohol-related peer pressure (Morris et al., 2020). Challenges for non-drinkers include being denigrated as 'cowards' or 'weirdos' (Robertson & Tustin, 2018). The Finnish Drinking Habits Survey shows that while adult non-drinkers experience positive social environments at family events, other social occasions remain challenging, especially for younger individuals and former drinkers (Katainen et al., 2022).

Research explores how young adults strategically manage non-drinking in social situations where peers consume alcohol (Conroy & de Visser, 2014; Piacentini & Banister, 2009; Seaman & Ikegwuonu, 2010).

Interviews with young adults in Finland and Australia revealed strategies to avoid potential stigma and isolation, such as choosing certain social groups, engaging with the non-drinking 'scene', acknowledging personal choices not to drink, and asserting moral superiority over binge drinking peers (Pavlidis et al., 2019). Other strategies include 'passing as a drinker' by pretending to drink alcohol to avoid peer scrutiny (Conroy & de Visser, 2015; Jacobs et al., 2018; Romo et al., 2015) and resisting or reframing negative labels associated with being a 'type' of drinker (Piacentini et al., 2012).

Research has also examined the motivations behind non-drinking among lifelong non-drinkers and former drinkers, revealing complex and sometimes contradictory reasons. For example, de Visser and Smith's (2007) interviews with demographically diverse young men showed that light/non-drinkers often had reasons both for and against drinking. Other studies indicate that motivations for non-drinking are multi-faceted and may need reaffirmation in different situations (Conroy & de Visser, 2014, 2015; Herman-Kinney & Kinney, 2013). Some research highlights how non-drinkers manage scrutiny by rhetorically invoking their reasons. For example, a US study found that college abstainers initially used concealment strategies (e.g., claiming medical reasons) and later adopted preventive disclosure strategies (e.g., sharing genuine reasons with trusted individuals) with varying success in terms of diverting peer scrutiny (Herman-Kinney & Kinney, 2013). Mixed methods research with undergraduates who drink alcohol identified benefits of non-drinking, such as enhanced self-esteem and productivity, but also concerns about social inclusion (Conroy & de Visser, 2018).

In the next section, we critique the non-drinking literature and explore a nuanced understanding of drinking styles. This includes recognising that personal drinking styles are shaped by individual choice but understood by other people, and how categories such as 'non-drinker' are invoked, deployed, and negotiated in discussions about drinking practices.

## Problematising 'Non-drinking'

The previous section highlighted how attitudes and approaches towards non-drinking have evolved in recent years. In this section, we first contextualise traditional approaches to non-drinking in academic literature. Drawing on Emma and Maria's sociological perspective of 'nothingness' in relation to non-drinking (Banister et al., 2019), we address existing tensions and complexities in understandings and terminology. Finally, we explore Dom's collaborative research with Charlotte Morton and Christine Griffin (Bath University) on 'drinker types' as rhetorical tools in drinking practices. This section aims to emphasise the importance of generating accounts of non-drinking which permit greater agency for non-drinkers and frame the practice of non-drinking as a deliberate lifestyle choice.

The majority of non-drinking research is conducted in Western countries, primarily the UK (Burgess et al., 2022; Nicholls, 2022; Banister et al., 2019; Piacentini et al., 2012; Conroy & de Visser, 2013, 2014, 2015, 2018), Australia (Caluzzi et al., 2020; Jaensch et al., 2018), New Zealand (Ball et al., 2020; Nairn et al., 2006; Niland et al., 2017), and the United States (Goings et al., 2019; Ross et al., 2015), contexts where drinking alcohol is a predominant cultural norm and excess is normalised (Measham, 2004; Szmigin et al., 2011). This focus informs the way in which non-drinking behaviours are understood and described—generally in relation to these predominant alcohol consumption norms. Terminology in the context of researching non-drinkers is notoriously messy. The operational meaning of researchers' preferred term—'non-drinker'—is open to interpretation producing a range of difficulties and ambiguities. In the work of both Nairn et al. (2006) and Piacentini and Banister (2009), this is manifest through light-drinking individuals perceiving their self-definition as non-drinkers 'in comparative terms relative to the dominant norms within the student culture' (Piacentini & Banister, 2009, p. 281). In other words, some very light drinkers may define as non-drinkers, while others may move between drinking and non-drinking positions, practices, and identities.

Conroy and de Visser (2014, 2015) distinguish between culturally sanctioned reasons for not drinking (e.g., religion, health, athleticism) and culturally unsanctioned reasons (e.g., discomfort around drunk people, dislike of alcohol's effects or taste), framing non-drinking practices around legitimacy and acceptability (Piacentini et al., 2012). This separation highlights heterogeneity within the non-drinking population, providing a basis for choosing to reject alcohol without inviting scrutiny (Romo, 2012). While those abstaining for religious or cultural reasons constitute a significant portion of non-drinkers (Measham, 2008), they are often overlooked in academic research, possibly due to assumptions that their behaviour is easily understood or managed by others, potentially denying these individuals agency and representation in broader non-drinking discussions.

In addition to reasons for non-drinking, there is a temporal dimension to abstention. Herring et al. (2014) distinguish between different temporal orientations towards non-drinking, linked to broader narrative history: ongoing lifestyle choices ('consistent'), transitions away from drinking ('transitional'), and responses to specific life events ('turning point'). Lifelong non-drinkers are differentiated from former drinkers, termed abstainers and desistors, respectively (Herman-Kinney & Kinney, 2013). The literature lacks a comprehensive framework to fully encompass the diverse experiences within the non-drinking population and the cultural variations influencing drinking practices, including in contexts where alcohol consumption is the norm and where abstention challenges societal norms, both globally and locally.

The sociology of nothing as recently developed by Scott (2018) helps account for elements of (non-) consumption that are unseen. She positions nothing as 'not just a passively endured condition, but a reflexively managed mode of experience' and alludes to the non-drinker as an exemplar of 'commission', under which a conscious decision is made to not drink (pp. 4–5). While this may be the case for many non-drinkers (e.g., the culturally sanctioned reformed alcoholic in Banister et al., 2019), it does not fully capture the range of non-drinking positions. More specifically, it fails to capture those who are classified as non-drinkers by omission, where the decision not to drink may not be as consciously, or actively, enacted. In an earlier study (Piacentini & Banister, 2006), we reported the case of Lena whose religion prohibits alcohol. Living within her own culture, her non-consumption of alcohol would be considered an act of omission (it is just something that she happens to not do), but now she lives within a new culture (studying in the UK) her non-drinking becomes understood by others, and experienced by Lena, as an act of commission, a more conscious act, something to work at. This gives a flavour of the complexity of what it means to be a non-drinker, demonstrating how people move in and out of omission/commission depending on the cultural context within which their behaviours are enacted.

Scott (2018) uses commission to understand the active accomplishment of doing or being a non-something; it involves conscious disengagement or disidentification—demonstrably doing nothing. Applied to the alcohol context, it implies an absolute position around not drinking, with an accompanying committed effort to not drink. This emphasis links with culturally sanctioned or legitimate non-drinking positions, illustrated where non-drinking individuals actively account for their choices (Supski & Lindsay, 2017), navigate peer scrutiny (Graber et al., 2016), or reveal active appeals to alternative subject positions, which can bring sporting and academic activities to the forefront (Nairn et al., 2006). For Muslim and certain faith communities, abstention aligns with Mullaney's concept of 'never identities' (Scott, 2018). However, alcohol also maintains an 'absent presence'—it exists but is not openly discussed (Valentine et al., 2010). This highlights the importance of nuanced considerations when categorising reasons as culturally (un)sanctioned and understanding relative positions in terms of what are considered culturally sanctioned reasons for not drinking (Conroy & de Visser, 2014).

These issues are also evoked in Temporary Abstention Challenges, such as Dry January in the UK, which provide culturally sanctioned opportunities for temporary abstinence from alcohol. These temporary initiatives, noted for their positive regulative techniques (Yeomans, 2018) and widespread sponsorship (e.g., supporting alcohol and cancer charities), allow participants to demonstrably do nothing (not drink), without the potential stigma associated with long-term sober identities. Within this context, Cherrier and Gurrieri (2013) argue that temporary abstainers are still constituted by others as drinkers, mitigating the stigma reserved for the more permanent or committed abstainer.

Under active commission, non-drinkers can be actively positioned in opposition to drinkers. In contrast, not drinking can be considered as performance of omission, a more passive act of happening to not do something. Omission involves non-identification rather than disidentification; it operates below conscious awareness, not significant enough to be consciously rejected. This includes people who just do not identify as a drinker rather than explicitly identifying as a non-drinker. This disengagement with the collective identity of the non-drinker is explored in detail in Banister et al. (2019), but also hinted at in Conroy and de Visser (2014) in their discussion of a participant, Michelle, who resists being defined by her alcohol practices; 'I don't want to be labelled by what I do and don't do' (p. 7). Michelle challenges the restrictive definitions and regulations imposed by the social category of 'non-drinking' (p. 7).

Omission, as described by Scott, is a passive act with less emphasis on identity management, contrasting with previous research on non-drinking that explores the challenges of coping with being a non-drinker (Piacentini & Banister, 2009; Caluzzi et al., 2020). However, Banister et al. (2019) demonstrate how within the context of alcohol consumption, even under omission, not drinking ('not being') can be more planful than Scott (2018) envisaged. They identify two main identity refusal strategies: distancing through resistance (contesting the existence of a non-drinker as a something) and distancing through othering (accepting the existence of non-drinkers yet denying similarities to them personally). These differing positions influence how omission is enacted, including variations in identity talk, aiming to reduce the significance of alcohol consumption or non-consumption in shaping identity (p. 14).

The complexity of terminology drives home the need for deeper insights into the relational dynamics influencing consumption choices. A framework that accounts for the possibility of non-drinking as being both commission and omission allows more heterogeneous considerations of drinking behaviours, for example, potentially including light/occasional drinkers under omission and recognising that similar non-drinking positions may be dealt with very differently by different (non) consumers and in different settings (e.g., varying identity talk and construction). Such an approach offers sensitivity for understanding how non-drinking practices vary across cultural and situational contexts, depending on the audience as well as the individual (Cocker et al., 2018). Drawing on Scott's sociology of nothing permits scholars to more fully appreciate the range of (non)drinking positions adopted and the range of responses, both from the individuals themselves and their peers/audiences.

The above discussion establishes the importance of recognising the agency involved in non-drinking positions, towards producing a more balanced and sensitive account of non-drinking which more effectively reflects its diverse forms and presentations. We will now suggest how this agency can be understood in another way by drawing on work that has revealed evidence of mismatches between lay/self-identified and formal definitions of two drinker categories (e.g., 'light drinkers' and 'binge drinkers') among university students who self-identified as light- or non-drinkers (Conroy et al., 2022). As far as we are aware, no formal definition of 'non-drinking' is available in the academic literature or in policy documents. To define light drinkers, we used a definition from Herring et al. (2014) who define them as individuals who drink one/two UK units a week or less depending on whether they are female/male and report not being drunk in the previous two months.

This work suggests how students, faced with concrete definitions, were rhetorically creative in accounting for how someone might 'earn' a non-drinker category when contextual information was taken into account. This is illustrated with reference to interview talk from an 18-year-old who self-identified as a non-drinker yet could be categorised as a light drinker using formal criteria. In this interview, participant definitions for non-drinkers, in relation to historical drunken behaviour, revealed shifts in footing from absolutes (i.e., participant talk emphasising tight definitional requirements for qualifying as a light drinker) to a more permissive formulation that could accommodate drunkenness without closing off the possibility of meaningfully self-identifying as a non-drinker. Another interview with a participant who self-identified as a light drinker illustrated how if an individual decides that they are a light drinker (evident where a participant indicates that they view themselves as a light drinker) then they are, almost regardless of what and how much that individual drinks. Evidence here sharply contrasts with the underpinning assumptions of formal definitions and enables individuals to socialise within a heavy-drinking culture while still identifying as a non or light drinker.

From these studies we can see that these rhetorical devices reveal the multiple possible dimensions involved in how drinker categories such as 'non-drinking' could or should be defined. Illustrative examples drew on the amount of alcohol consumed; the frequency of drinking and the frequency of getting drunk; and contrasting motivations underlying drinking behaviour. The effect of this might be two-fold: it provides a framework for justifying limited drinking behaviour to self and others, but it also means that drinking behaviour itself (which would contradict a more credible 'non-drinker' identity) can remain congruent given the heavy-drinking culture typically experienced by university students. Here, notions of objectively recognisable 'non-drinkers' seem to evaporate, and drinker categories become utilised as rhetorical devices for managing identity within university culture, as a distinct cultural setting.

All of the above should feed into health promotion practice and policy developments in the alcohol-related market, as well as future research on non-drinking; we now turn to consider these in more detail.

## Using Non-drinking Research to Inform Policy and Practice

Non-drinking has rarely featured in health promotion policy and strategy designed to promote healthier alcohol consumption in the general population. Efforts to promote more moderate drinking traditionally focus on education about 'sensible drinking' (e.g., Department of Health, 2016). Non-drinking is, however, intermittently included in alcohol policy. For example, the Change4Life campaign encouraged participants to take two 'dry days' without alcohol consumption per week (Charles, 2012) and the Dry January initiative continues to be supported (Alcohol Change, 2024) (although such initiatives ultimately continue to emphasise alcohol consumption norms through encouraging small windows of conscious abstinence followed by a 'return' to drinking).

Health promotion strategy might usefully problematise and challenge the dominant, negative views of non-drinkers and non-drinking. Such strategic activity could point, credibly, to how numerically non-drinkers represent a large and growing group of individuals, and therefore, this is no longer a marginalised or minority position. Similarly, a dedicated social marketing campaign might challenge the suggestion that non-drinking is typically met with negative responses, instead highlighting how non-drinking may attract social praise and admiration and provide a wider variety of social and lifestyle opportunities than might otherwise be possible.

Applying non-drinking research to a broader alcohol health promotion agenda might involve appealing to the varied potential advantages of 'dry days', drawing on Conroy and de Visser's (2018) work which highlighted potential benefits of social non-drinking (e.g., experiencing 'more natural', substance-free social confidence) as identified by individuals who routinely consume alcohol. In light of our earlier discussion about omission, increased uptake of 'dry days' could potentially normalise non-drinking within mainstream social contexts by enhancing its visibility during social gatherings. Consequently, this could mitigate the tendency to crudely pigeon-hole people as 'non-drinkers' or indeed 'drinkers', encouraging people to move more fluidity between these two positions in different social settings, for example. Non-drinking research highlighting social challenges faced by non-drinkers has informed an understanding of how individuals who seek to drink alcohol in moderation can strategically manage alcohol intake (e.g., by joining social events a bit later) and approaches for successfully refusing offers of alcoholic drinks (e.g., providing innocuous reasons for non-drinking to avoid attention and peer pressure to consume more alcohol) (Conroy & de Visser, 2021).

A related policy approach might be to problematise simplistic definitions of drinking behaviour and, particularly, specific 'drinker categories', including 'non-drinker' and 'binge drinker'. This approach, again, chimes with the theoretical emphases of commission and omission described in section two of this chapter. Softening the hard boundaries between 'drinker categories' (e.g., 'non-drinkers' vs 'social drinkers') might permit young adults to reflect on non-drinking as something they can practise flexibly and freely during social occasions. Appreciating the distinctions between active and passive approaches to non-drinking may equip non-drinkers with strategies and approaches for how they present themselves in varying social settings, to ameliorate the negative impacts of their positioning on their identity, and to help them fully engage in their social worlds as a positively managed mode of experience (Scott, 2018).

There is also potential to consider how the idea of non-drinking may be incorporated into interventions aimed at reducing alcohol consumption in other settings, such as GP practices and health clinics. While we know that encouraging university students to consider the benefits of social non-drinking and how it can be strategically managed in social situations has been linked to decreased alcohol consumption (Conroy et al., 2015), little is known about how non-drinking could be approached from a more general health promotion standpoint. Furthermore, using 'dry days' as a strategy to advocate for moderate drinking poses risks, including the potential for compensatory binge drinking following dry days, as might be predicted from an 'abstinence violation effect' perspective (Curry et al., 1987). Health promotion strategies could leverage non-drinking to encourage moderate alcohol consumption among young adults. However, given the uncertainties and ambiguities surrounding non-drinking as a categorical activity, it is unclear how dry days could straightforwardly promote moderate drinking without this risk of compensatory (alcohol) consumption.

While these means of promoting moderate alcohol consumption may draw on encouraging *individual* non-drinking, a key emergent theme from the non-drinking evidence base suggests the importance of reimagining, planning, and reconfiguring *social* environments so that alcohol consumption is de-emphasised as a central feature. We note the particular responsibilities held by institutions, such as universities and higher education colleges, in this respect.

In the UK, the National Union of Students (NUS) has set up the Drug and Alcohol Impact project (https://www.drugandalcoholimpact.uk), which runs in partnership with universities and students' unions. This scheme aims to promote and generate whole campus shifts in alcohol and drug cultures. There are also rankings available of 'sober friendly universities', which show the kinds of approaches and societies in place to promote a less alcohol-oriented student experience (Fresh, 2023). Initiatives to expand opportunities for drinks-free socialising are growing, partly in response to the growing national, racial, and cultural diversity of UK student populations. For example, Leeds Students Union has introduced pottery and coffee making classes and now 'tags' relevant events as 'alcohol free' in line with increasing demands for alcohol-free social events (Leeds University Union, 2021). A more imaginative and inclusive approach to social environments for young people will help to recognise the (growing) variation in drinking habits and include non-drinkers within this vision. This kind of approach may help to normalise lighter drinking habits and to inculcate an understanding of 'drinking styles' rather than 'drinker types' in social spaces.

Industry trends indicate that the market itself also plays a pivotal role in normalising alternative consumption patterns. In recent years, major drinks companies have started to produce a variety of non-alcoholic or very low alcohol options. The emerging no/lo drinks market has reached £221m in 2021 representing around 1% of sales (Holmes et al., 2024). The rise in alternative beverages supports the coping mechanisms employed by non-drinkers in drinking environments, as discussed earlier in this chapter, including tactics for concealing abstinence. Progress in this area also holds potential to enhance 'choice' and provide viable and desirable alternative product options for non-drinkers to consume in social settings. There is also potential to normalise non-drinking, thereby challenging binary notions of socialising that strictly delineate drinking and non-drinking environments (although others have also cautioned that the rising trend in no/lo drinks could have the opposite effect, effectively further normalising *drinking,* given the expectation that consumers must drink something that strongly resembles alcohol in smell, taste, and appearance in social settings).

There are further challenges; given it is mainly alcohol companies producing these no/lo options, it informs an uneasy alliance for any associated social marketing or policy activity. Furthermore, despite the absence of duty taxes, the production complexities and potentially lower sales volumes result in no/lo prices often exceeding those of equivalent alcoholic beverages. This raises affordability issues and underscores the tendency for these socially acceptable options for moderating alcohol consumption to be more accessible to higher-income, middle-class consumers (Anderson et al., 2021) paralleling patterns observed in movements such as sober curious and positive sobriety (Lunnay et al., 2022).

Another issue concerns the use of shared branding by major drinks companies (e.g., Heineken 0.0), and the issue of surrogate marketing which allows producers to promote their alcoholic offerings by stealth (Nicholls, 2022), with Holmes et al. (2024) asking whether it is a 'necessary compromise' that public health benefits are secured in this way. This reflects debates elsewhere, including in relation to smoking, tobacco, and electronic cigarettes (vapes) (de Andrade et al., 2014).

What implications does this hold for drinking spaces and pub culture? On one hand, it could foster the evolution of pubs into more inclusive spaces where both drinking and non-drinking can coexist, emphasising socialisation, community, and connections. The development of no/lo options seems crucial for pubs to adapt to changing drinking habits and ensure their viability. Additionally, distinct non-drinking spaces are emerging, for example, 'Love From' in Kampus (situated in a 'bustling new neighbourhood' in central Manchester) and Torstig in London's trendy Hoxton, suggesting a young, affluent market segment. Interestingly, while these bars position themselves as alcohol-free (AF), their menus feature 'lo' options, which may not align with the preferences of individuals abstaining from alcohol for cultural or medical reasons. Are we moving towards a scenario where the distinction of being a non-drinker, whether temporarily or permanently, becomes less relevant and less pronounced? But do these spaces also risk only catering to 'sometimes', 'once', or 'could be' drinkers? For some, the idea of visiting a bar and consuming alcohol-mimicking beverages may not align with cultural norms; this warrants further research. Though not within the scope of this chapter, it is also worth considering alongside the rise of other non-drinking venues in the UK nightlife economy, such as dessert cafes, which offer a diverse clientele and a different approach to late-night socialising independent of alcohol consumption.

## Future Research

Considering the implications of non-drinking evidence for alcohol policy prompts reflections on fruitful future directions for research. Maintaining the profile of research on non-drinking remains crucial for several reasons. An emphasis on 'binge drinking' among young adults often oversimplifies their drinking habits, neglecting evidence of new and creative responses and widespread resilience to heavy-drinking cultures. With the growing number of young non-drinkers, their presence in diverse social settings may influence the alcohol behaviours of others within their social circles, both drinkers and non-drinkers. Exploring this impact on drinking behaviours could involve studying both drinkers and non-drinkers within the same social groups to understand how their coexistence affects group dynamics, consumption levels, identity associations, social connectedness, and overall well-being. While much research has focused on young people, it may also be valuable to investigate the lived experiences of non-drinkers in older age categories to understand how not drinking influences their mode of being.

## References

Alcohol Change. (2024). Try Dry®: The app for the Dry January® challenge and beyond. Retrieved April 12, 2024, from https://alcoholchange.org.uk/help-and-support/managing-your-drinking/dry-january/get-involved/the-dry-january-app

Anderson, P., O'Donnell, A., Kokole, D., Jane Llopis, E., & Kaner, E. (2021). Is buying and drinking zero and low alcohol beer a higher socio-economic phenomenon? Analysis of British survey data, 2015–2018 and household purchase data 2015–2020. *International Journal of Environmental Research and Public Health, 18*(19), 10347.

Atkinson, A. M., Matthews, B. R., Nicholls, E., & Sumnall, H. (2023). 'Some days I am a lunatic that thinks I can moderate': Amalgamating recovery and neo-liberal discourses within accounts of non-drinking among women active in the 'positive sobriety' community on Instagram in the UK. *International Journal of Drug Policy, 112*, 103937.

Ball, J., Edwards, R., Sim, D., Cook, H., & Denny, S. (2020). What explains the decline in adolescent binge-drinking in New Zealand? *International Journal of Drug Policy, 84*, 102826.

Banister, E., Piacentini, M. G., & Grimes, G. (2019). Identity refusal: Distancing from non-drinking in a drinking culture. *Sociology, 53*, 744–761.

BBC (2022). Why Gen Zers are growing up sober curious. Available: https://www.bbc.co.uk/worklife/article/20220920-why-gen-zers-are-growing-up-sober-curious

Black, L. F., & Monrouxe, L. V. (2014). 'Being sick a lot, often on each other': Students' alcohol-related provocation. *Medical Education, 48*(3), 268–279.

Brown, A. L., Koelsch, L., & Yufik, T. (2010). The exception to the rule: Nondrinkers at college student parties: 834. *Alcoholism: Clinical & Experimental Research, 34*(6), 219A.

Burgess, A., Yeomans, H., & Fenton, L. (2022). 'More options... less time' in the 'hustle culture' of 'generation sensible': Individualization and drinking decline among twenty-first century young adults. *The British Journal of Sociology, 73*(4), 903–918.

Caluzzi, G., MacLean, S., & Pennay, A. (2020). Re-configured pleasures: How young people feel good through abstaining or moderating their drinking. *International Journal of Drug Policy, 77*, 102709.

Charles, G. (2012). Change4Life tackles sensible drinking mission. Campaign. Retrieved October 3, 2019, from https://www.campaignlive.co.uk/article/change4life-tackles-sensible-drinking-mission/1115582

Cheers, C., Pennay, A., de la Piedad Garcia, X., & Callinan, S. (2024). Development and validation of the Cheers Attitudes towards Non-drinkers Scale (CANS). *Journal of Health Psychology, 29*(10), 1101–1114.

Cherrier, H., & Gurrieri, L. (2013). Anti-consumption choices performed in a drinking culture: Normative struggles and repairs. *Journal of Macromarketing, 33*(3), 232–244.

Cocker, H., Piacentini, M., & Banister, E. (2018). Managing dramaturgica dilemmas: Youth drinking and multiple identities. *European Journal of Marketing, 52*(5/6), 1305–1328.

Conroy, D., & de Visser, R. (2013). 'Man up!': Discursive constructions of nondrinkers among UK undergraduates. *Journal of Health Psychology, 18*(11), 1432–1444.

Conroy, D., & de Visser, R. (2014). Being a non-drinking student: An interpretative phenomenological analysis. *Psychology & Health, 29*(5), 536–551.

Conroy, D., & de Visser, R. (2015). The importance of authenticity for student non-drinkers: An interpretative phenomenological analysis. *Journal of Health Psychology, 20*(11), 1483–1493.

Conroy, D., & de Visser, R. O. (2018). Benefits and drawbacks of social non-drinking identified by British university students. *Drug & Alcohol Review, 37*, S89–S97.

Conroy, D., Sparks, P., & de Visser, R. (2015). Efficacy of a non-drinking mental simulation intervention for reducing student alcohol consumption. *British Journal of Health Psychology, 20*(4), 688–707.

Conroy, D., & de Visser, R. O. (2021). Strategies for managing alcohol intake and refusing offers of alcoholic drinks. In The Palgrave Handbook of Psychological Perspectives on Alcohol Consumption (pp. 325–348). Cham: Springer International Publishing.

Conroy, D., Griffin, C., & Morton, C. (2022). Defending, contesting and rejecting formal drinker categories: how UK university students identify as 'light-drinkers' or 'non-drinkers'. Drugs: Education, *Prevention and Policy, 29*(5), 509-518.

Curry, S., Marlatt, G. A., & Gordon, J. R. (1987). Abstinence violation effect: Validation of an attributional construct with smoking cessation. *Journal of Consulting and Clinical Psychology, 55*(2), 145–149.

de Andrade, M., Hastings, G., & Angus, K. (2014). Promotion of electronic cigarettes: Tobacco marketing reinvented? *BMJ, 348*(7939), 15–17.

de Visser, R. O., & Smith, J. A. (2007). Alcohol consumption and masculine identity among young men. *Psychology and Health, 22*(5), 595–614.

Department of Health. (2016). *Alcohol guidelines review*. Report from the Guidelines Development Group to the UK Chief Medical Officers. Retrieved October 3, 2019, from https://assets.publishing.service.gov.uk/government/uploads/system/uploads/attachment_data/file/545739/GDG_report-Jan2016.pdf

Drinkaware (2023). Monitor 2023 Hub. Available: https://www.drinkaware.co.uk/research/drinkaware-monitors/monitor-2023-hub?gad_source=1&gad_campaignid=22298792539&gbraid=0AAAAAD6s1rBDPcM9b-B86GK0LYvnZlyXa&gclid=Cj0KCQjw8p7GBhCjARIsAEh-ghZ0SL_cVtAxrXSEcb-eC09RKmNV0-260EHVprdTqbV8nA0G4jj2IZP-saAjNAEALw_wcB

Emslie, C., Hunt, K., & Lyons, A. (2012). Older and wiser? Men's and women's accounts of drinking in early mid-life. *Sociology of Health & Illness, 34*(4), 481–496.

Fresh. (2023). Top 10 universities for sober students Retrieved April 12, 2024, from https://www.thisisfresh.com/blog/2023/12/18/top-10-universities-for-sober-students/

Gerrard, M., Gibbons, F. X., Reis-Bergan, M., Trudeau, L., Vande Lune, L. S., & Buunk, B. (2002). Inhibitory effects of drinker and nondrinker prototypes on adolescent alcohol consumption. *Health Psychology, 21*(6), 601–609.

Goings, T. C., Salas-Wright, C. P., Belgrave, F. Z., Nelson, E. J., Harezlak, J., & Vaughn, M. G. (2019). Trends in binge drinking and alcohol abstention among adolescents in the US, 2002–2016. *Drug and Alcohol Dependence, 200*, 115–123.

Graber, R., de Visser, R., & Abraham, C. (2016). Staying in the 'sweet spot': A resilience-based analysis of the lived experience of low-risk drinking and abstention among British youth. *Psychology & Health, 31*(1), 79–99.

Gray, C. (2017). The Unexpected Joy of Being Sober. Octopus Publishing Group.

Herman-Kinney, N. J., & Kinney, D. A. (2013). Sober as deviant: The stigma of sobriety and how some college students "stay dry" on a "wet" campus. *Journal of Contemporary Ethnography, 42*(1), 64–103.

Herring, R., Bayley, M., & Hurcombe, R. (2014). 'But no one told me it's okay to not drink': A qualitative study of young people who drink little or no alcohol. *Journal of Substance Use, 19*(1/2), 95–102.

Holmes, J., Angus, C., Kersbergen, I., Pryce, R., Stevely, A., & Wilson, L. (2024). *No- and low-alcohol drinks in Great Britain: Monitoring report*, Sheffield, University of Sheffield. Retrieved April 12, 2024, from https://sarg-sheffield.ac.uk/wp-content/uploads/2024/01/SARGNoLoMonitoringReportJan24Revised.pdf

Jacobs, L., Conroy, D., & Parke, A. (2018). Negative experiences of non-drinking college students in Great Britain: An interpretative phenomenological analysis. *International Journal of Mental Health & Addiction, 16*(3), 737–750.

Jaensch, J., Whitehead, D., Prichard, I., & Hutton, A. (2018). Exploring young peoples' use of alcohol at outdoor music festivals in Australia. *Journal of Applied Youth Studies, 2*(3), 32–42.

Katainen, A., Härkönen, J., & Mäkelä, P. (2022). Non-drinkers' experiences of drinking occasions: A populationbased study of social consequences of abstaining from alcohol. *Substance Use & Misuse, 57*(1), 57–66.

Leeds University Union. (2021). Freshers' fun without the drinking: Alcohol-free Welcome events at LUU. Retrieved April 12, 2024, from https://www.luu.org.uk/news/2021/09/16/freshers-fun-without-the-drinking-alcohol-free-welcome-events-at-luu/

Lunnay, B., Nicholls, E., Pennay, A., MacLean, S., Wilson, C., Meyer, S. B., Foley, K., Warin, M., Olver, I., & Ward, P. R. (2022). Sober curiosity: A qualitative study exploring women's preparedness to reduce alcohol by social class. *International Journal of Environmental Research and Public Health, 19*(22), 14788.

Measham, F. (2004). The decline of ecstasy, the rise of 'binge' drinking and the persistence of pleasure. *Probation Journal, 51*(4), 309–326.

Measham, F. (2008). The turning tides of intoxication: Young people's drinking in Britain in the 2000s. *Health Education, 108*(3), 207–222.

Morris, H., Larsen, J., Catterall, E., Moss, A. C., & Dombrowski, S. U. (2020). Peer pressure and alcohol consumption in adults living in the UK: A systematic qualitative review. *BMC Public Health, 20*, 1–13.

Nairn, K., Higgins, J., Thompson, B., Anderson, M., & Fu, N. (2006). "It's just like the teenage stereotype, you go out and drink and stuff": Hearing from young people who don't drink. *Journal of Youth Studies, 9*(3), 287–304.

Nicholls, E. (2022). Help or harm? Exploring the expanding 'No and Low' alcohol market in the UK. *IAS Blog*. Retrieved April 12, 2024, from https://www.ias.org.uk/2022/03/22/help-or-harm-exploring-the-expanding-no-and-low-alcohol-market-in-the-uk/

Niland, P., McCreanor, T., Lyons, A. C., & Griffin, C. (2017). Alcohol marketing on social media: Young adults engage with alcohol marketing on Facebook. *Addiction Research & Theory, 25*(4), 273–284.

Pavlidis, A., Ojajarvi, A., & Bennett, A. (2019). Young people and alcohol abstention: Youth cultural practices and being a non-drinker in Finland and Australia. *Journal of Youth Studies, 22*(8), 1101–1116.

Piacentini, M. G., & Banister, E. N. (2006). Getting hammered? Students coping with alcohol. *Journal of Consumer Behaviour: An International Research Review, 5*(2), 145–156.

Piacentini, M. G., & Banister, E. N. (2009). Managing anti-consumption in an excessive drinking culture. *Journal of Business Research, 62*(2), 279–288.

Piacentini, M. P., Chatzidakis, A., & Banister, E. N. (2012). Making sense of drinking: The role of techniques of neutralisation and counter-neutralisation in negotiating alcohol consumption. *Sociology of Health & Illness, 34*(6), 841–857.

Rahman, N., Sofija, E., & Sebar, B. (2023). 'I Just Don't Drink': Examining the Experiences of Young Adult Abstainers in Australia's Changing Drinking Trends. *YOUNG, 31*(1), 38–56.

Regan, D., & Morrison, T. G. (2013). Adolescents' negative attitudes towards non-drinkers: A novel predictor of risky drinking. *Journal of Health Psychology, 18*(11), 1465–1477.

Regan, D., & Morrison, T. G. (2017). Temporal stability and predictive validity of the Regan attitudes toward non-drinkers scale. *SAGE Open, 7*(2).

Robertson, K., & Tustin, K. (2018). Students who limit their drinking, as recommended by national guidelines, are stigmatized, ostracized, or the subject of peer pressure: Limiting consumption is all but prohibited in a culture of intoxication. *Substance Abuse: Research and Treatment, 12*, 1178221818792414.

Romo, L. K. (2012). "Above the influence": How college students communicate about the healthy deviance of alcohol abstinence. *Health Communication, 27*(7), 672–681.

Romo, L. K., Dinsmore, D. R., Connolly, T. L., & Davis, C. N. (2015). An examination of how professionals who abstain from alcohol communicatively negotiate their non-drinking identity. *Journal of Applied Communication Research, 43*(1), 91–111.

Ross, C. S., Maple, E., Siegel, M., DeJong, W., Naimi, T. S., Padon, A. A., et al. (2015). The relationship between population-level exposure to alcohol advertising on television and brand-specific consumption among underage youth in the US. *Alcohol and Alcoholism, 50*(3), 358–364.

Scott, S. (2018). A sociology of nothing: Understanding the unmarked. *Sociology, 52*(1), 3–19.

Seaman, P., & Ikegwuonu, T. (2010). *Drinking to belong*. Joseph Rowntree Foundation. Retrieved November 1, 2019, from https://www.jrf.org.uk/sites/default/files/jrf/migrated/files/alcohol-young-adults-full.pdf

Supski, S., & Lindsay, J. (2017). 'There's something wrong with you' how young people choose abstinence in a heavy drinking culture. *Young, 25*(4), 323–338.

Szmigin, I., Bengry-Howell, A., Griffin, C., Hackley, C., & Mistral, W. (2011). Social marketing, individual responsibility and the "culture of intoxication". *European Journal of Marketing, 45*(5), 759–779.

Valentine, G., Holloway, S. L., & Jayne, M. (2010). Contemporary cultures of abstinence and the nighttime economy: Muslim attitudes towards alcohol and the implications for social cohesion. *Environment and Planning, 42*(1), 8–22.

Warrington, R. (2019). Sober Curious. HarperOne.

Yeomans, H. (2018). New Year, new you: A qualitative study of dry January, self formation and positive regulation. *Drugs: Education, Prevention and Policy, 26*(6), 460–468.

# 9

# 'It Seems Like Even More of a Reason to Drink': A Literature Review of Temporary Abstinence Challenges (TAC) and Evidence Concerning Immediate Post-Challenge Drinking Plans Among Young Adults

**Ashlea Bartram and Dom Conroy**

**Abstract** Temporary Abstinence Challenges (TAC), that is, taking breaks from consuming any alcohol for defined periods (e.g. one month) have grown in popularity, internationally, over the last two decades (e.g. Dry January, Sober October in the UK; Dry July in Australia). TACs are of interest to social scientists and health promotion practitioners and policy makers because evidence has provided some support for their role in reducing alcohol use, enhancing skills at refusing alcoholic drinks and other benefits including increased quality of life. Questions have been

---

A. Bartram (✉)
National Centre for Education and Training on Addiction, Flinders University, Adelaide, SA, Australia
e-mail: ashlea.bartram@flinders.edu.au

D. Conroy
Faculty of Arts and Social Science, The Open University, London, UK
e-mail: d.conroy@open.ac.uk



D. Conroy, F. Measham (eds.), *Young Adult Drinking Styles*, Sustainable Development Goals Series, https://doi.org/10.1007/978-3-031-98528-7_9

raised and developed around the extent to which TACs may foster longer-term changes in alcohol consumption, over the risks of potential 'backfire' effects (e.g. compensatory 'binging' post-TAC participation). In this chapter, we first outline the current evidence base and field discussion linked to TACs, outlining findings from key studies, and draw attention to key debates relating to TAC participation among young adults. In the second section we explore material from a longitudinal study of TAC participation involving increasing/higher risk young adult drinkers. We explore data that concerned these individuals' immediate plans relating to alcohol consumption post-TAC participation. The chapter concludes with suggestions for future research priorities in the TAC literature.

## Introduction

Temporary abstinence challenges (TACs)—where people abstain from alcohol for a limited period of time, often a month—have skyrocketed in popularity over the past fifteen years. Although people can and do undertake these challenges informally (Siconolfi et al., 2023), the increase in popularity has largely been driven by a number of high profile organised TACs, which typically involve communications campaigns, registration systems, and support materials, and sometimes include fundraising elements. These include Dry July (https://www.dryjuly.com) and febfast (https://febfast.org.au) in Australia, Dry January (https://dryjanuary.org.uk) in the UK, the Buddhist Lent Dry Campaign in Thailand (Jirarattanasopha et al., 2019), IkPas (https://ikpas.nl) in the Netherlands, and Tournée Minérale (https://www.tourneeminerale.be/) in Belgium. Many of these campaigns are very popular. Dry January in particular has achieved very high awareness and engagement among drinkers, with 78% of drinkers reporting that they knew about Dry January 2016 (De Visser et al., 2017). The 2023 Dry January campaign had 175,000 registrants—more than a forty-fold increase since it started in 2013 (Alcohol Change, 2023). Many more people take part informally without registering, with an estimated 6.5 million English adults trying to abstain in January without registering in 2021 (Alcohol Change, 2020). Outside of the official campaign, the term 'Dry January' appears to have entered the public lexicon in the UK, with British media outlets such as the Mirror dedicating regular articles and even webpages to the topic (Mirror, 2024).

Empirical research on TACs has gathered pace and they have also received attention in broader alcohol-related health promotion discussion and debate. Work designed to bring together and critically articulate the newfound prominence of TACs within both research and everyday discussion is therefore timely. In this chapter, we first outline the current evidence base and field discussion linked to TACs and draw attention to key debates relating to TAC participation among young adults. In the second section, we focus on one discrete area of TAC participation—evidence concerning immediate post-TAC drinking plans as apparent from a sample of young adults. The chapter concludes with an agenda for TAC-related research designed to understand adjacent drinking practices among young adults in the future and policy/practice implications.

## Exploring Temporary Abstinence Challenges

TACs are of interest to health promoters for their potential to reduce harms from alcohol consumption, particularly if they prompt people to make changes to their drinking beyond the period of abstinence. TACs have been shown to attract relatively heavy drinkers who might benefit from reducing their alcohol consumption (de Visser et al., 2016; de Visser & Piper, 2020; de Ternay, 2022). Participants are also more likely to be female, which is a demographic that is underrepresented in traditional alcohol treatment settings (Davey, 2021). Young people typically comprise a minority of TAC participants. For example, early data from Australian TACs showed that 14% of Dry July 2013 participants and just 5% of febfast participants were aged 18–24 years—despite the latter being a fundraiser for youth support services (Dry July, 2014; Hillgrove & Thomson, 2012). Similarly, in the UK, just 6% of people who participated in Dry January 2016 and completed baseline and follow-up surveys were aged 18–25 (de Visser, 2020). More broadly, increasing numbers of young people are abstaining from drinking in many countries, including those where TACs are most prominent (see Caluzzi & Pennay Chap. 3). However, young people, like older adults, face expectations that alcohol consumption is normative, and may find TACs helpful in that they provide socially sanctioned reasons not to drink (Bartram et al., 2017; Conroy & de Visser, 2014; Cheers et al., 2020; Frank et al., 2020). At the other end of the consumption spectrum, Siconolfi et al. (2023) note that younger people are underrepresented in the alcohol treatment-seeking population, with TACs potentially providing a low-stigma entry path to support to reduce harms from alcohol consumption.

Robert (2016, 2018, 2022) has characterised TACs as a form of public pedagogy that supports participants to learn about 'responsible drinking' through 'exemplary' abstinence. Robert means 'exemplary' not just in its common usage of being praiseworthy (although participants can be positioned this way (Bartram et al., 2018)), but as something that provides an example that helps to facilitate learning, by making a subject more comprehensible and by inspiring imitation (Robert, 2022). TACs, Robert (2016, 2022) argues, do this by providing an embodied experience for participants. Campaign messaging prompts participants to attend to the embodied aspects of the TACs and guides participants to interpret and evaluate their experiences as physically and psychologically beneficial (Robert, 2016). TACs, by providing a socially sanctioned reason to avoid drinking, can support participants to develop skills and self-efficacy in drink refusal (Bartram et al., 2017; Conroy & de Visser, 2014; Conroy & de Visser, 2018; de Visser et al., 2016). Yeomans (2019) points out that TACs, in contrast to many state-led attempts to change drinking behaviour, are presented as fundamentally positive experiences, serving to reveal that you can 'enjoy' abstinence rather than just having to regulate your consumption in the interests of your long-term health.

Although TACs share a common element of temporary abstinence, other elements such as seasonality, fundraising, and participant supports vary from TAC to TAC. In terms of seasonality, Dry January occurs in winter at the beginning of a new year. It draws on associations with new year's resolutions and plans to 'detox' (and reduce spending) following a period of excess to promote positive self-formation (Yeomans, 2019; Taylor, 2019). It also capitalises on the idea that people go out less in the middle of winter, potentially making abstention easier. Australia's febfast follows a similar 'new year' logic but delays the start of the TAC by a month in recognition of the extended summer holidays many Australians take, while Dry July, like Dry January, is timed for winter. In Thailand, where 94% of the population identify as Buddhist, the Buddhist Lent Dry Campaign is set during Buddhist Lent, a three-month period in the monsoon season during which Buddhist lay people pledge to do charitable deeds and refrain from 'bad' deeds, similar to Christian Lent or Muslim Ramadan (Jirarattanasopha et al., 2019). Some TACs, such as Dry July, are primarily oriented towards fundraising, while others such as Dry January and the Buddhist Lent Dry Campaign have explicit public health objectives (although Dry January still provides the option to fundraise) (Robert, 2022). Many TACs offer support materials via e-mail and on their website for registered participants, although the nature of these supports and how they characterise participation may vary from campaign to campaign (Bartram et al., 2018). In contrast, the Buddhist Lent Dry Campaign has not historically had a registration system, although in some communities, local events are held at the beginning of the campaign to enable people to make a public pledge to abstain (Saengow, 2019). Collectively, these different elements may render each TAC attractive to different types of participants with differing motives, although it is not yet clear whether or how each element affects the outcomes of TACs, as outcomes have not been systematically studied across campaigns (Butters et al., 2023).

## Outcomes from TAC Participation

The principal outcome of interest from TAC participation is, arguably, reduced typical alcohol intake and/or reduced subsequent occurrence of episodic 'binge drinking' (or, more formally, Heavy Episodic Drinking defined as consumption of 60g pure alcohol in a single occasion, World Health Organisation, 2024). However, health and well-being outcomes have also been studied in association with TAC participation. Outcomes from TAC participation have been most extensively studied for Dry January and the Buddhist Lent Dry Campaign. Studies of Dry January have shown that participation in Dry January is associated with a range of benefits, including changes in self-rated physical health, psychological well-being, drink refusal self-efficacy (DRSE), and alcohol intake at both one and six months after participation (de Visser & Nicholls, 2020; de Visser & Piper, 2020; de Visser et al., 2016). Similar improvements to health and well-being outcomes have been reported in other TAC evaluation studies. For example, recent evaluation of post-challenge survey responses from 49,022 Tournée Minérale campaign participants (requiring 1 month of alcohol abstinence) indicated that alcohol abstinence contained both benefits (e.g. improved sleep) and disadvantages (e.g. increased soft drink consumption) (Thienpondt et al., 2024).

Improvements were larger among participants who successfully remained abstinent during the TAC, but there were also modest changes for participants who did not remain abstinent (de Visser & Nicholls, 2020; de Visser & Piper, 2020; de Visser et al., 2016). These changes were not observed among a control group of adult drinkers who did not attempt to abstain from alcohol in January (de Visser & Piper, 2020). A small minority of Dry January participants reported increases in drinking days per week, drinks per day, and frequency of drunkenness six months after participation, but these 'rebound effects' were not common (e.g. only 11% had an increased frequency of drunkenness at 6-month follow-up) (de Visser et al., 2016). Nonetheless, there may be value in establishing for whom or in what circumstances these negative consequences may occur (Butters et al., 2023).

Successfully remaining abstinent during Dry January was predicted by identifying as male rather than female, having a lower AUDIT score, having greater DRSE for emotion regulation, and reading supportive e-mails from the organisers (de Visser & Nicholls, 2020). A comparison with the general population of adult drinkers found that TAC participants who officially registered for Dry January were more likely to successfully remain abstinent (70%) than those who did not register but reported trying to have a Dry January (36%) (de Visser & Piper, 2020). Collectively, this suggests that facilitating higher levels of engagement with a TAC by encouraging registration and use of support e-mails is of value. However, fundraising or completing Dry January with a companion was not associated with success (de Visser et al., 2016).

Outcomes for the Buddhist Lent Dry Campaign have been similarly positive. Drawing on a nationally representative survey conducted in

2016, Saengow (2019) found that during Buddhist Lent, a third of current drinkers abstained from alcohol completely, 16% abstained for a certain period, and 19% decreased the quantity of alcohol that they consumed. Although Buddhist Lent Dry Campaign has no registration system akin to Dry January, drinkers were more likely to abstain if they reported exposure to the campaign media or made a public commitment to abstain (Jirarattanasopha et al., 2019; Saengow, 2019; Witvorapong & Watanapongvanich, 2020). The effects of the national campaign were significantly enhanced when a tailored community intervention was also available, with effects on alcohol abstinence evident during and three months after the campaign, but not at six months post-campaign (nine months after its start) (Jirarattanasopha et al., 2019).

Concluding discussion above of outcomes associated with TAC participation we note that TAC participation cannot reliably be understood as a standalone event that individuals engage with in isolation but as part of a broader journey and drinking biography of attempts to reduce. By young adulthood, many individuals will have a varied and complex history and relationship with alcohol which will inevitably intersect with TAC participation in nuanced ways. We will focus in more detail on young adult's participation in TACs in the next section.

## Young Adult's Participation in TACs

So far in this chapter we have described outcomes and experiences of TAC participation in general. We turn now to consider specific characteristics of young people and young adult's participation in TACs. Young adults typically drink less frequently than older adults (NHS Digital, 2022). As such, young TAC participants may have fewer social occasions to navigate during their TAC month than older participants (de Visser, 2020).

Despite the potential value of TACs for young people, to date there has been limited investigation of young people's engagement with and experiences of TACs. The most detail comes from de Visser's (2020) exploration of the characteristics and motivations of Dry January 2016 participants aged 18–25 years, drawing on baseline and end-of-TAC surveys. de Visser (2020) found that, prior to participation, younger participants were heavier drinkers, had significantly lower DRSE in social settings, but significantly greater emotional and opportunistic DRSE than older participants—suggesting that younger participants were qualitatively different in their drinking patterns than older participants. The three most important reasons young people reported for taking part were to give their body a break from booze, to save money, and for health reasons. Compared to older participants, younger people were more likely to take part to save money, and less likely to take part for health reasons or to lose weight. While charity was the least important reason for both young and older participants to take part in Dry January, it was more important for younger participants, with 17% of young people fundraising compared to 10% of older participants (de Visser, 2020). Despite these differences in motives, younger and older participants held similar plans for after Dry January, with 8.5% of young people planning to stop drinking and 76% planning to drink less—however, the study did not include a longer-term follow-up so it was not possible to assess the extent to which these plans were realised (de Visser, 2020).

Two-thirds (67%) of younger Dry January participants completed the challenge without drinking, which was significantly greater than the 61% of older participants who completed the challenge (de Visser, 2020). de Visser notes that young adults typically drink less frequently than older adults (NHS Digital, 2022). As such, young TAC participants may have fewer social occasions to navigate during their TAC month than older participants (de Visser, 2020). For both younger and older participants, reading all of the support e-mails was predictive of completing the challenge, but younger participants were less likely to have made use of these e-mails and generally rated their content as less helpful—suggesting a need to ensure promotional material and support are relevant to this age group. Other predictors of completing the challenge differed between younger and older participants, with a lower frequency of drunkenness pre-challenge predicting challenge completion for younger participants while lower AUDIT, greater emotional DRSE, and fundraising predicted challenge completion for older participants (de Visser, 2020).

Siconolfi et al. (2023) explored TAC participation among a cohort of young adults aged 18–19 years primarily living in California in the

USA. While there are no large-scale formal TACs with registration programs akin to Dry January in the USA, market-led TACs exist (e.g. https://www.theluckiestclub.com/courses/the-sober-90, https://thisnakedmind.com/programs-training/), and anecdotal reports suggest many people embark on their own personal TACs. Siconolfi et al. (2023) found that 7% of the cohort reported participating in a TAC in the past year, with 85% of these abstaining for the entire period. Following their participation about 15% did not resume drinking and another 52% reported drinking less; less than 1% reported a subsequent increase in drinking. Motives for participation most commonly related to general health, rather than specifically to drinking, although participants had a greater readiness to quit drinking alcohol than non-participants. Compared to non-participants, participants were more likely to have engaged in past-month heavy drinking, had higher past-year AUDIT scores, a greater number of alcohol-related consequences, and a greater prevalence of past-year substance use treatment—suggesting that young TAC participants in the USA were at comparatively higher risk of alcohol-related harms.

Collectively, these two studies provide some indication that TAC participation could support young people to reduce their alcohol consumption, but that their experiences may qualitatively differ from older participants, reflecting their different drinking patterns, drinking contexts, and motives for TAC participation. However, each study has some limitations. The US study by Siconolfi et al. (2023) assessed participation and outcomes retrospectively so may have been subject to recall bias, with young people more likely to report participation if successful. It also made no comparison with older people. In addition, it took place in a setting in which there were no formal campaign registration or supportive communications, both of which have been shown to increase challenge success for TAC participants more broadly (de Visser & Nicholls, 2020; de Visser & Piper, 2020; Jirarattanasopha et al., 2019; Saengow, 2019; Witvorapong & Watanapongvanich, 2020). The UK study by de Visser (2020) lacked a longer-term follow-up to assess outcomes of participation. It also could not assess if differences between younger and older participants were related to campaign participation or reflected differences between younger and older drinkers per se (as de Visser (2020) noted, young people may drink less to spend less money in January in general). Future studies may benefit from including control groups of both non-participants and older participants, a prospective design, and longer-term follow-up.

There is a need to investigate whether young people's experiences differ across different campaigns that vary in terms of seasonality (e.g. Autumn vs Summer), educational timings (e.g. fresher's week/month vs exam periods), and the extent to which the TAC in question contains an emphasis on fundraising or not (e.g. from a UK perspective, Dry January vs Sober October). For example, concerns about saving money may be more prevalent among post-Christmas campaign participants, while campaigns that emphasise fundraising (along with general health benefits) may offer a socially acceptable, low stigma framing for younger people's participation. Given differences in young people's drinking patterns and motivations for participation, and the different drinking contexts in which they are likely to be embedded, there is also a need for a more qualitative, in-depth exploration of young people's experiences of TAC participation—the focus of the next section of this chapter.

## Understanding Immediate Post-Challenge Plans

As discussed in the previous section, speculation has surrounded whether and how TACs instil new behaviour plans, modify psychological mechanisms associated with behaviour change, and catalyse a new relationship with alcohol. Pinning down the timescale of this new relationship with alcohol is clearly important; TAC participation that results in reduced drinking for a few weeks is useful but less valuable if it is not sustained into the medium to longer term. In addition, TAC participation might lead to compensatory drinking or even 'backfire effects' where participants consume potentially even higher levels of alcohol than before participation and justify this in compensatory terms through having engaged in (partially or fully) TAC participation.

In the current section, we explore individuals' immediate plans relating to alcohol consumption post-TAC participation regardless of whether this was successful or not. Identifying and understanding these initial plans is important if TACs are to be effectively appraised in terms of (1) evidence of their shorter-term successes in reducing drinking plans and inculcating a new relationship with alcohol, and (2) evidence of backfire effects as described above.

We explore individuals' immediate plans relating to alcohol consumption post-TAC participation by drawing on illustrative interview data from a broader UK-based longitudinal study (ethically approved by University of East London, ETH1920-0124). This study had originally been designed to focus on experiences of participation in two different types of TAC (Sober October and Dry January). For this illustration, we draw exclusively on semi-structured interview data extracts taken from a 'post TAC participation time point' in the study which occurred 2–3 days before or after the final date of the TAC challenge (e.g. 31 October for Sober October participants). We will focus on interview extracts taken from interviews with six participants who were identified as all either 'increasing risk drinkers' or drinkers whose self-report drinking responses indicated greater likelihood of higher risk episodic drinking (see Table 9.1). Participants were aged 24–31; four were lifelong UK residents, while Angela and Ryan had been UK residents for 12–14 months preceding their interviews.

Participants were interviewed between December 2019 and February 2021. Project data was collected during the period of the COVID-19

**Table 9.1** Empirical illustration sample details

| Pseudonym | Sex | Age (years) | Ethnicity | Units[a], HED[b] | TAC type | TAC days completed (% overall challenge) |
|---|---|---|---|---|---|---|
| Marion | Female | 24 | White British | 25, 2 | Dry January | 31 (100) |
| Rachel | Female | 24 | White British | 24, 1 | Dry January | 31 (100) |
| Angela | Female | 24 | French | 10, 1 | Sober October | 10 (32) |
| Ryan | Male | 21 | Black Somalian | 10, 1 | Sober October | 31 (100) |
| Naomi | Female | 31 | Black British | 8, 1 | Dry January | 31 (100) |
| Tanya | Female | 25 | Black British | 8, 1 | Dry January | 31 (100) |

[a] Alcohol consumption in week prior to TAC participation
[b] HED = heavy episodic drinking

pandemic and associated societal lockdowns. While the pandemic clearly influenced many alcohol-relevant parts of life including social contact and socialising, our dataset overall produced minimal evidence implicating a major role of the pandemic/pandemic restrictions on alcohol consumption/non-consumption. Most participants completed the entire TAC successfully (i.e. without drinking any alcohol); Angela was the exception and completed 10 days (32%) of her TAC. All participants are identified by pseudonyms.

The post-TAC participation time point data included below were collated and subjected to Reflective Thematic Analysis involving data immersion, data coding, and generating an initial set of theme titles (Braun & Clarke, 2019). Three themes in total are presented: Theme 1—Recognising accomplishments and looking ahead; Theme 2—Compensation vs restraint post-challenge; and Theme 3—The bearing of seasonal characteristics on drinking plans immediately following TAC participation. These themes are discussed below with illustrations from relevant textual data.

## Theme 1: Recognising Accomplishments and Looking Ahead

Whether participants planned restraint and caution or noted the possibility for compensatory indulgence with alcohol in the weeks following TAC participation, and whether abstinence during TAC participation had been mainly heeded, most participants had developed a reflective relationship with alcohol looking into the immediate future. Angela, who only completed 10 days of Dry January, said:

> (TAC participation) has made me a lot more reflective on my alcohol consumption… I've noticed that I can drink quite quickly. It might be quite hard to say no as well… what I did find difficult… I didn't find it difficult at all... but when I found it difficult at times that I did drink was when I thought to myself in the balance is it really worth having a drink right now during Sober October? There were like 2–3 times where I did drink because I did actually think 'yes it is (worth it)' … so, in that sense, even though I,

> not failed, even though I drank during Sober October I felt like it made me really just really, really look at… like who I'm drinking with and how I'm drinking uhm… yeah, I guess I just kind of understood then… yeah, just how I like to… I understood how I like to drink. Angela (Sober October)

For someone whose TAC participation might have been judged a 'failed attempt', the breadth, level, and intricacies of reflection here are striking. Temporary abstinence provided feedback on how quickly Angela consumed alcohol, the relative ease of refusing alcoholic drinks, choices around drinking companions, personal drinking styles ('how I'm drinking') possibly relating to consumption intensity, and fundamental questions around decisional balance linked to the choice about whether to break the period of abstinence itself as part of participation. Interesting in this extract are two occasions where there is movement towards and then away from self-implication in talk about personal drinking practices ('difficult' to 'not difficult'; 'failed' to 'not failed'). This speaks to the role of different types of TAC participation and raises questions around the core purpose of participation and how it may be drawn on in different ways for challenge participants. Elsewhere in her interview, Angela had also noted the social changes that had happened, possibly coincidentally but notably, during the early period of TAC participation that involved making key changes to friendships and social networks in her life.

In her interview, Tanya also struck a reflective tone when considering how forward-looking drinking plans might work in the immediate period following TAC participation:

> Having (been abstinent) for so long I don't necessarily feel inclined to break it so to speak… if I was to have alcohol in this month, it would be just like something that came up naturally as opposed to feeling 'Oh, now January is done, I need to celebrate the end by having alcohol'. Tanya (Dry January)

Unlike Angela, Tanya had completed the entire period of Dry January. However, it is worth noting that Angela typically drank more alcohol on a regular basis than Tanya and evidently had a different set of challenges and objectives around drinking practices to engage with during and following TAC participation. Interesting in Tanya's extract is how one month of abstinence is understood and approached—Tanya seems interested in keeping this going for as long as possible on one level at least, leaving the resumption of drinking practices to chance, ultimately. Phrasing here is difficult to follow entirely with 'inclined' suggesting reluctance or at least considered deliberation on Tanya's part about how she navigates her relationship with alcohol immediately post-TAC participation.

## Theme 2: Compensation Vs Restraint Post-Challenge

All participants except Angela had abstained for the full duration of the TAC. For many participants, TAC completion, celebrated though it frequently was, presented individuals with decisions around when and how they might resume alcohol consumption following a month of abstinence (whether full or partial).

> I feel like people finish January and it's almost like 'Oh, I can finally go out and drink again' you see people on social media people congratulating themselves by going out and getting drunk after doing Dry January [laughing]... it's not really changing your drinking habits, is it? If that's what Dry January has set out to do in the long-term, it's not, if everyone's going out to celebrate that they've done it, they've done this month achievement... it seems like even more of a reason to drink... they're like, ah, I can go out and drink for the rest of the month because I've done it for one month [laughing]. Rachel (Dry January)

> I probably am going to drink in November... surprisingly I haven't touched anything since the end ... I mean, it's Nov 2nd, so it's not that bad... I'm not that person that would jump for joy, crack open the new brandy... I like the idea of setting aside the weekend (for drinking), that seems more sustainable long term... and for people who find (TACs) more difficult I wonder if the temptation would be, once (the next month) hits, to overindulge maybe so I can imagine it would be more sustainable to not quit altogether. Ryan (Sober October)

Rachel's interview extract illustrates a pattern in the data concerning previous reactions she had witnessed from individuals who, having completed TAC challenges, immediately consumed alcohol in large volumes for potentially prolonged periods ('rest of the month'). This behaviour appeared directly in relation and seemingly proportionately to TAC participation almost like a currency; with a stock of abstinence acquired, a 'pass-card' had been acquired for resuming alcohol consumption in a relatively excessive way. The choice of words here was important—'I *can* finally go out and drink… *because* I've done it for one month'—and conveyed a sense that this would be heavier drinking with justification and therefore relatively liberated from feelings of guilt or normative judgement.

Ryan was one of several participants who spoke about a new challenge following on from TAC participation—how to successfully resume drinking and incorporate alcohol consumption back into life. Ryan's extract suggested a cautious, tentative re-entry to consuming alcohol post-TAC participation. However, the closing parts of the extract hit on some of the inherent tensions involved in this re-entry and the range of choices available, to him or anyone post-TAC, around the type of drinking practice ('more sustainable'), choices around enduring abstinence practices ('quit altogether'), the possibility of compensatory behaviour ('crack open the brandy'), and how these factors might vary on perceived difficulty of TAC participation.

## Theme 3: The Bearing of Seasonal Characteristics on Drinking Plans Immediately Following TAC Participation

Ryan's extract in the previous theme suggested how resuming alcohol consumption might be treated with caution and even hesitation following TAC participation. A final selection of material suggested how seasonal differences between two of the most culturally prominent UK TACs (Dry January and Sober October) might also influence immediate post-TAC drinking plans but also broader drinking practices leading up to TAC participation. Interview extracts from Rachel and Naomi illustrate this:

> If TAC participation is about trying to help people in the long-term then I think Dry January's very good at that short-term maybe whereas I feel like with Sober October there's more temptation, people are going out more, and it's quite a busy month, I guess... maybe because not as many people do it in October (whereas) in January, everyone's doing it and no-one's really going out. Rachel (Dry January)

> I did drink a lot the week before because I knew that I wasn't going to be asking for a while... I definitely indulged like clearing out your fridge before you started out... I drank a lot from Christmas to New Year's. Naomi. (Dry January)

In her extract, Rachel expressed the viewpoint that TACs may help individuals achieve different objectives linked to their drinking practices depending on which season the TAC is undertaken in. Rachel appears to suggest that, relative to Sober October participation, Dry January might have shorter-term effects (possibly carrying over into longer-term consumption changes), might involve less temptation to drink, and might be more straightforward to accomplish given the relatively fewer opportunities to socialise/drink at the start of the year and the increased likelihood that other people might be participating in the TAC ('everyone's doing it').

Relatedly, Naomi spoke in her interview about alcohol consumption rituals linked to Dry January participation that involved excessive drinking during the period immediately before the TAC that occurred partly because of seasonal festivities but also linked to (or rationalised by) the desire to 'clear out/clear up' remaining alcoholic drinks. Naomi's extract is interesting because it suggests a certain type of compensatory style of drinking that may occur immediately prior to TAC participation, in contrast to the post-TAC compensatory drinking discussed above.

## Conclusion

In this chapter, we have reviewed the literature regarding TACs and young people and presented findings from a qualitative study of young TAC participants regarding their immediate post-TAC plans. There is good evidence that participation in TACs may lead to longer-term reductions in alcohol consumption among participants in general. Evidence is also positive, but more limited, for younger participants. There is a need for more studies with longer-term follow-up of young adult participants, to investigate the extent to which changes in alcohol consumption are sustained. The qualitative findings presented here showed that young adult participants were prompted by the TAC to reflect on their alcohol consumption and keen to consider their plans for the future. However, they were sensitive to the potential for rebound effects, particularly through compensatory drinking post-TAC (and, in Naomi's case, pre-TAC). Participants also noted that seasonal aspects of TACs might shape their post-TAC plans—a potential difference between TACs that has not yet been systematically studied. Future research, both qualitative and quantitative, is needed to understand the longer-term effects of TAC participation for young people, as well as how these may vary between campaigns with different timing and that emphasise different motives for participation.

## References

Alcohol Change. (2020). Press release: 6.5 million people plan to do Dry January 2021, up from 3.9 million in 2020. https://alcoholchange.org.uk/blog/press-release-6-5-million-people-plan-to-do-dry-january-2021-up-from-3-9-million-in-2020

Alcohol Change. (2023). The Dry January story. https://alcoholchange.org.uk/help-and-support/managing-your-drinking/dry-january/about-dry-january/the-dry-january-story

Bartram, A., Eliott, J., & Crabb, S. (2017). 'Why can't I just not drink?' A qualitative study of adults' social experiences of stopping or reducing alcohol consumption. *Drug and Alcohol Review, 36*(4), 449–455.

Bartram, A., Hanson-Easey, S., & Eliott, J. (2018). Heroic journeys through sobriety: How temporary alcohol abstinence campaigns portray participant experiences. *The International Journal of Drug Policy, 55*, 80–87.

Braun, V., & Clarke, V. (2019). Reflecting on reflexive thematic analysis. *Qualitative Research in Sport, Exercise and Health, 11*(4), 589–597.

Butters, A., Kersbergen, I., Holmes, J., & Field, M. (2023). Temporary abstinence challenges: What do we need to know? *Drug and Alcohol Review, 42*(5), 1087–1091.

Cheers, C., Callinan, S., & Pennay, A. (2020). The 'sober eye': Examining attitudes towards non-drinkers in Australia. *Psychology & Health, 36*(4), 385–404.

Conroy, D., & de Visser, R. (2014). Being a non-drinking student: An interpretative phenomenological analysis. *Psychology & Health, 29*(5), 536–551.

Conroy, D., & de Visser, R. O. (2018). Benefits and drawbacks of social non-drinking identified by British university students. *Drug and Alcohol Review, 37*, S89–S97.

Davey, C. (2021). Online sobriety communities for women's problematic alcohol use: A mini review of existing qualitative and quantitative research. *Frontiers in Global Women's Health, 2*, 773921.

de Ternay, J., Leblanc, P., Michel, P., Benyamina, A., Naassila, M., & Rolland, B. (2022). One-month alcohol abstinence national campaigns: a scoping review of the harm reduction benefits. *Harm Reduction Journal, 19*(1), 24.

de Visser, R. O. (2020). Young people and temporary alcohol abstinence during Dry January. In I. D. Conroy & F. Measham (Eds.), *Young adult drinking styles: Current perspectives on research, policy and practice* (pp. 253–272). Palgrave Macmillan.

de Visser, R. O., & Nicholls, J. (2020). Temporary abstinence during Dry January: Predictors of success; impact on well-being and self-efficacy. *Psychology & Health, 35*(11), 1293–1305.

de Visser, R. O., & Piper, R. (2020). Short- and longer-term benefits of temporary alcohol abstinence during 'Dry January' are not also observed among adult drinkers in the general population: Prospective cohort study. *Alcohol and Alcoholism, 55*(4), 433–438.

de Visser, R. O., Robinson, E., & Bond, R. (2016). Voluntary temporary abstinence from alcohol during "Dry January" and subsequent alcohol use. *Health Psychology, 35*(3), 281–289.

de Visser, R. O., Robinson, E., Smith, T., Cass, G., & Walmsley, M. (2017). The growth of 'Dry January': Promoting participation and the benefits of participation. *European Journal of Public Health, 27*(5), 929–931.

Dry July. (2014). Annual Report 2013-14 Australia. https://www.dryjuly.com/about/impact-reports

Frank, V. A., Herold, M. D., Schroder, S., Bjonness, J., & Hunt, G. (2020). Legitimizing and negotiating abstinence: Young adults' narratives about practicing situational and long term abstinence in Denmark. *International Journal of Drug Policy, 81*, 102655.

Hillgrove, T., & Thomson, L. (2012). Evaluation of the impact of febfast participation. Final report. Victorian Health Promotion Foundation (VicHealth), Carlton, Australia.

Jirarattanasopha, V., Witvorapong, N., & Hanvoravongchai, P. (2019). Impact of Buddhist Lent Dry Campaign on alcohol consumption behaviour: A community level study. *Health & Social Care in the Community, 27*(4), 863–870.

Mirror. (2024). *Dry January*. Retrieved 13 May 2024, from https://www.mirror.co.uk/all-about/dry-january

NHS Digital. (2022). *Health Survey for England, 2021 part 1. Part 3: Drinking alcohol.* Retrieved 6 May 2024, from https://digital.nhs.uk/data-and-information/publications/statistical/health-survey-for-england/2021/part-3-drinking-alcohol#frequency-of-drinking-in-the-last-12-months-by-age-and-sex

Robert, J. (2016). Temporary sobriety initiatives as public pedagogy: Windows of opportunity for embodied learning. *Health, 20*(4), 413–429.

Robert, J. (2018). Meeting the sober self, recognizing the drinking self: Back to baseline experimentation in temporary sobriety initiatives. *Contemporary Drug Problems, 45*(3), 283–302.

Robert, J. (2022). *Alcohol, binge sobriety and exemplary abstinence.* Bloomsbury Academic.

Saengow, U. (2019). Drinking abstinence during a 3-month abstinence campaign in Thailand: Weighted analysis of a national representative survey. *BMC Public Health, 19*(1), 1688.

Siconolfi, D., Tucker, J. S., Pedersen, E. R., Perez, L. G., Dunbar, M. S., Davis, J. P., Rodriguez, A., Seelam, R., & D'Amico, E. J. (2023). Sober curiosity and participation in temporary alcohol abstinence challenges in a cohort of U.S. emerging adults. *Journal of Studies on Alcohol and Drugs, 85*(2), 201–209.

Taylor, C. (2019). Your money: How Dry January is changing finances. *Reuters*, 14 January. Retrieved 19 November 2023, from https://www.reuters.com/article/us-money-savings-dryjanuary-idUSKCN1P80ZI/

Thienpondt, A., Van Cauwenberg, J., Van Damme, J., & Deforche, B. (2024). Process evaluation of the Belgian one-month-without alcohol campaign

'Tournée Minérale': A mixed method approach. *BMC Public Health, 24*(1), 383.

Witvorapong, N., & Watanapongvanich, S. (2020). Using pre-commitment to reduce alcohol consumption: Lessons from a quasi-experiment in Thailand. *Socio-economic Planning Sciences, 70*, 100723.

World Health Organisation. (2024). Alcohol, heavy episodic drinking (drinkers only) past 30 days. https://www.who.int/data/gho/indicator-metadata-registry/imr-details/458#:~:text=Definition%3A,to%206%20standard%20alcoholic%20drinks

Yeomans, H. (2019). New year, new you: A qualitative study of Dry January, self-formation and positive regulation. *Drugs: Education, Prevention & Policy, 26*(6), 460–468.

# 10

# "I Always Joke that I Became a Bit of a Prude": Exploring Young Women's Lived Experiences of Sober Dating in the UK Using Sociological (Auto-) Ethnographic, Insider Research

Claire Davey and Millie Gooch

**Abstract** 'Sober dating' is the act of spending time with other people to pursue a romantic or sexual connection whilst not consuming alcohol. Sober dating has emerged as a constituent part of a broader trend of declining alcohol consumption—particularly among young adults—across high-income countries, including the UK, and a rise in popular engagement with Temporary Abstinence Challenges, online sobriety communities and 'sober curiosity'. Emerging research seeks to understand why young people are drinking less or not at all, yet there is limited research that explores how young people 'do' sobriety—how they navigate daily activities and life stages without alcohol—including leisure and

---

C. Davey (✉)
Faculty of Arts, Humanities and Education, Canterbury Christ Church University, Canterbury, UK

M. Gooch
Sober Girl Society, London, UK
e-mail: millie@sobergirlsociety.com



D. Conroy, F. Measham (eds.), *Young Adult Drinking Styles*, Sustainable Development Goals Series, https://doi.org/10.1007/978-3-031-98528-7_10

pleasure. This chapter offers an (auto-)ethnographic exploration that draws on the authors' positionalities as intimate insider researchers, to understand how young women, who no longer consume alcohol, navigate dating practices: 'sober dating'. First, we outline the contemporary context within which the phenomenon of sober dating has occurred and unpack a range of initial themes and questions regarding the practice. We consider the role of online dating applications, online sobriety communities, and no- and low-alcohol drinks in the emergence of sober dating. We subsequently explore interview data and auto-ethnographic reflections to understand women's lived experiences of sober dating. The chapter concludes by discussing these experiences within current debates around neoliberal feminism and highlights some implications and considerations for future research and sobriety support initiatives.

## Introduction: Exploring the Contemporary Context of Sober Dating

'Sober dating' can be described as the act of spending time with other people to pursue a romantic or sexual connection whilst not consuming alcohol. According to a recent report from online dating application Tinder (www.tinder.com) (2023), 88% of 4000 surveyed singles from the United States (US), United Kingdom (UK), Canada and Australia were interested in going on a sober date, and top sober dating activities cited by participants included a picnic in the park (41%), a casual stroll with coffee or tea (39%), or an outdoor movie or concert (33%) (p. 9). The decline in usage of beer and wine emojis within Tinder profiles (40% and 25%, respectively) speaks further to this conscious uncoupling between alcohol and the dating process (ibid.).

Indeed, 52% of those surveyed in the aforementioned study were planning to drink less alcohol going forward or not at all (ibid.), which suggests that there is a strong relationship between alcohol refusal whilst dating and pursuit of a low- or no-alcohol lifestyle. Sobriety is not necessarily exclusively used as a tool to form initial connections with potential partners but may feature as part of their ongoing relationship. A preference for authenticity was identified as a key factor in driving these behaviours. The report summarised, "Today's young singles believe that working on their mental well-being can help with their dating life, and that having a partner who values self-care is critical to a happy relationship" (ibid.). Such themes regarding authenticity, wellness, and the role of technology recur throughout this chapter.

Sober dating can be identified as contemporary phenomenon within longer, cultural histories of temperance which have subsequently informed drinking cultures and attitudes towards sobriety in the UK, Australia and Canada—and most noticeably a strong abstinence-based recovery culture in the US since the Prohibition era (1920–1933) (Levine, 1993; Berridge, 2005). More recently, however, there has been a decline in alcohol consumption among young adults across high-income countries (Pape et al., 2018; Vashishtha et al., 2020), including the UK (Oldham et al., 2018). In England particularly, between 2004 and 2021, alcohol consumption has steadily declined by 14% from 11.6 litres per adult per year, to 10 litres per adult per year, with a small increase between 2014 and 2021 of 6% (9.4L to 10L) (NHS Digital, 2022).

In turn, the rate of people who do not drink alcohol at all has been steadily growing between 2005 and 2017, particularly among those under the age of 45, rising between 5 and 6% in this age group (Office for National Statistics (ONS), 2017). More current research published by NHS Digital (2022), as part of the Health Survey for England 2021, shows that 21% of adults aged 16+ had not consumed alcohol at all in the last 12 months. On average, women were more likely to not drink (24%) compared to men (18%). The youngest men and women (aged 16–24) had above average rates of long-term alcohol refusal at 34% and 42%, respectively, with lower rates across older age groups, as shown in the following excerpt from the Health Survey for England data (Table 10.1).

These trends towards non-drinking have coincided with the rise in popular engagement with Temporary Abstinence Challenges (Butters et al., 2023), online sobriety communities (Davey, 2021) and 'sober curiosity' (Kalia, 2019; Warrington, 2019). Online sobriety communities[1]

[1] Online sobriety communities first emerged in 2015 and have proliferated in number since. They are typically hosted on Social Networking Sites, such as Facebook and Instagram. They aim to help

**Table 10.1** Rates of not drinking 'at all in the last 12 months' among individuals aged 16+ years by age and sex

| | Age group | | | | | | | |
|---|---|---|---|---|---|---|---|---|
| | 16–24 | 25–34 | 35–44 | 45–54 | 55–64 | 65–74 | 75+ | Total |
| Sex | % | % | % | % | % | % | % | % |
| Men | 34 | 17 | 18 | 17 | 14 | 11 | 20 | 18 |
| Women | 42 | 25 | 22 | 20 | 17 | 18 | 25 | 24 |
| Total | 38 | 21 | 20 | 19 | 15 | 15 | 23 | 21 |

*Note*: Data adapted from NHS Digital (2022)

specifically have played an informative role in the facilitation and development of sober dating practices, including through the organisation of sober social dating events, and the growth of no- and low-alcohol drink alternatives (Davey, 2022a) often consumed at these events. These activities which, to date, have received very little attention from academia and public health, will be explored further in this chapter.

Recent research has sought to understand *why* young people are drinking less or not at all; the University of Sheffield identified eight key themes that young people used to explain the decline in youth drinking:

> The potential for alcohol-related harm; Contemporary youth cultures and places of socialisation; The affordability of alcohol; Displacement of alcohol by other substances; Access and the regulatory environment; Disputing the decline; Future Orientations; and Parenting and the home environment. (Whitaker et al., 2023, p. 1)

These broadly align with studies of Australian youth (Caluzzi et al., 2020, 2021), however Caluzzi et al. (2020) also found that Social Networking Sites (SNS) played a role in how young people presented

individuals to change their drinking behaviours through a range of services, including but not limited to: peer-to-peer support, sobriety coaching, group workshops, and social events. They also share content about alcohol-free living through mediums such as social media posts, podcasts, blogs, webinars, and in-person events. Examples include Sober Girl Society (www.sobergirlsociety.com), Sober & Social (www.soberandsocial.com) and Bee Sober (www.beesoberofficial.com). In alignment with contemporary Temporary Abstinence Challenges (Robert, 2016), online sobriety communities seem to have higher proportions of members (or members who engage) that are female; and, seem to reflect a demographic segment of being white and of higher socioeconomic means (Davey, 2021).

themselves, and thus acted as a tool of self-governance regarding drinking behaviours. In addition, a desire for agency, authenticity, and control of the self, were identified in Conroy and de Visser's (2015) study of student non-drinkers, along with the idea that sobriety is a strategy of caring for the self, both physically and mentally (Davey, 2022b).

Emerging studies of women's contemporary sobriety in the UK has shown that women's choices not to drink have also been informed by their experiences of sexual assault and male violence (Atkinson et al., 2023; Davey, 2021, 2023b). This may pose additional challenges and considerations for women who 'do' sober dating or who may be thinking about dating without alcohol.

Existing academic research has predominantly focussed on *why* young people are drinking less than previous generations, however, there is limited understanding regarding *how* they 'do' sobriety and how *not* drinking impacts daily activities or relationships—particularly for those who were former drinkers. The increasing focus on, and consumption of, no- and low-alcohol drinks has shed light on how individuals use these alternative products to 'do' friendship-making practices and celebrations without consuming alcohol (Nicholls, 2021; Davey, 2023a). Yet there is still more to be learned regarding how sober individuals 'do' leisure and pleasure and offer an alternative narrative to that provided by the wealth of drinking studies that has explored alcohol's intimate connection with these experiences (Bancroft et al., 2014; Nicholls, 2019).

This (auto-)ethnographic (McNamara, 2009; Merrill & West, 2009; Pink et al., 2016) chapter seeks to address this imbalance by providing an explorative insight into the contemporary phenomenon of sober dating through drawing on our own positionalities as intimate insider researchers (Merton, 1972; Taylor, 2011), and sociological research interviews with participants—all with lived experiences of sobriety, sober dating, and online sobriety communities as young women in the UK.

First, we draw on our insider knowledge from participating within the UK's contemporary 'positive sobriety movement' (Atkinson et al., 2023) to consider the role of online dating applications, online sobriety communities and no- and low-alcohol drinks brands in the emergence of sober dating. We then explore the lived experiences of young, sober women who embark upon sober dating by drawing on immersive interview data from a broader sociological, ethnographic study of women in sobriety (Davey, 2023b) and Millie's auto-ethnographic reflections. We weave these (auto-)ethnographic findings with wider debates around neoliberal feminism to form a discussion regarding the key implications and considerations.

## The Role of No- and Low-Alcohol Brands, Online Dating Applications and Online Sobriety Communities in the Emergence of Sober Dating

In this section, we discuss how the rise of sober dating has been facilitated, enabled, and promoted by commercial interests that seek to capitalise on contemporary sobriety trends in both the US and the UK. Specifically, we utilise our insider knowledge to explore the role of online dating applications, no- and low-alcohol drinks brands, and online sobriety communities in shaping the way in which individuals 'do' sober dating.

Tinder, the online dating application, sought to capitalise on the trends identified within their 'The Future of Dating, 2023' report, cited previously, by organising an in-person sober dating event—'Skate Dates'—at Somerset House, London. This initiative encouraged users to engage in sober, active dates by offering skate sessions at the iconic venue. It was designed to provide a fun and healthy alternative to alco-centric dating practices and showcase the benefits of alcohol-free dating activities. The campaign received positive feedback and saw high participation rates, underscoring the growing demand for sober dating experiences.

Yet Tinder is not the only online dating application to recognise and facilitate this shift towards sober dating; Thursday Dating (www.getthursday.com), a UK-based online application that focuses on in-person dates on Thursdays, partnered with Caleño (www.calenodrinks.com), a popular non-alcoholic spirit brand, for a unique social experiment. During a Thursday dating event, attendees were served a set menu of cocktails, only to discover at the end that these drinks were made with Caleño non-alcoholic spirits—that alcohol had been substituted for an alcohol-free alternative. The event sought to highlight that dating does not require alcohol and captured the surprised reactions of unsuspecting participants who realised they had been sober throughout the evening. This could be read as an attempt by a dating business to inform and re-shape mainstream dating practices for those who would ordinarily consume alcoholic beverages. These examples suggest that sober dating is becoming a constituent part of the broader contemporary movement towards sober lifestyles and social practices.

Similar collaborations have taken place between non-alcoholic spirit brand Clean Co. and online sobriety community Sober & Social, who organised a Valentine's Day sober dating event at Swingers Crazy Golf Club—once more combining both physical activity with alcohol substitution to facilitate a sober dating experience. Sober & Social was keen to ensure that sober individuals did not miss out on the traditional dating opportunities that Valentine's Day presents, due to their alcohol refusal. Indeed, the challenges faced by those who seek to sober date (further explored later in this chapter) have been identified by sobriety coaches as a commercial opportunity to provide paid support. For example, Tawny Lara, an author, speaker, and advocate for sober living positions herself as the 'The Sober Sexpert' to those who are looking for insights and advice on navigating dating without alcohol. Her book, *Dry Humping: A Guide to Dating, Relating, and Hooking Up Without the Booze* (2023) discusses the challenges and benefits of sober dating, addressing common concerns such as social anxiety and the pressure to conform to traditional social norms. She offers strategies for setting boundaries, communicating openly, and finding sober-friendly date activities. Thus, a support industry and commercial eco-system is emerging around this social practice.

Online sobriety communities and sober dating coaches may be meeting the needs of those who want to change their drinking behaviours outside of the (limited) pathways available through public health provision. It is clear that they offer assistance to women, who are currently underserved by existing modalities and healthcare provision—and arguably offer a less predatory environment than some have asserted Alcoholics Anonymous to be (Whitaker, 2020). However, this marketisation of sobriety raises concerns and considerations regarding the safeguarding and support of individuals who may be vulnerable, and for whom difficult dating experiences such as ghosting, rejection, and physical intimacy may present emotional triggers. It is evident that sober dating is another means through which contemporary sobriety culture is becoming increasingly commercialised, whereby there is a profit motive associated with helping those who are trying to change their drinking behaviours. Particularly with regard to the emergence of sober dating coaches or 'experts', individuals need to use their discernment when engaging services to ensure that such support 'professionals' have appropriate qualifications or supervision requirements until such time when the industry can be regulated more effectively (Farmer et al., 2022; Plante, 2018).

## The Challenges of Navigating Sober Dating After Giving Up Alcohol: Insights from Katie, Francesca and Tina[2]

This section draws on transcripts from individual and immersive semi-structured interviews with three young and single women—Katie, Francesca and Tina—to investigate the challenges of navigating sober dating after giving up alcohol. These interviews were conducted by Claire as part of her PhD research—an ethnography of women's experiences of sobriety and their use of online sobriety communities (Davey, 2023b). To understand participants' experiences of sober dating specifically, Claire asked open questions, similar to the below:

> I wanted to move on and talk about relationships and dating, so the physical but also romantic side of things. I wondered if you could talk to me a bit about your experiences of dating in sobriety and how you navigate that?

We weave together the empirical findings from this data sample and auto-ethnographic reflections from Millie to generate a meaningful, explorative discussion to increase understanding of the experiences of women who take part in sober dating, including: deciding whether to

[2] Not their real names—all participants have been pseudonymised.

disclose their status as a sober person, changes in navigating physical intimacy, and finding a middle-ground between two extremes of dating—drinking or hiking.

## Theme 1: "It's not something that I'll be super up-front about": Deciding Whether to Disclose Status as a Non-drinker

> It's [sobriety] not something that I…I have it on my profiles and I mean it usually does come up in the conversation pre-date but it's not like it's something I'm keeping a secret but I just, I think knowing my past self and how I think I would…I think I would have probably judged, not necessarily judged people who didn't drink, but I think I'd feel really uneasy around someone, if I knew myself and knew how much I was drinking to go on a date with someone who was just going to stay sober. I think I'd find that quite daunting and yeah so it's – it's not something I keep a secret, but it's not something that I'll be super up-front about either.
>
> Katie, 29 years old, 2 years in sobriety, single

The prominent use of dating applications, such as Tinder or Bumble (www.bumble.com), among participants led to interesting discussions regarding disclosure of sober status within dating profiles or instant message exchanges. Writing a dating profile enables users to declare whether they are drinkers or not—some have dedicated icons to show that they are a 'non-drinker' or 'sober', and Bumble even has a 'sober filter' which enables you to see only the profiles of people who are also sober. Katie suggests that she declares the status on her profile but doesn't necessarily approach the subject with prospective dates, unless necessary, through fear of judgement and stigmatisation. The fear of being pre-judged as boring led some participants to downplay their sobriety to potential dating partners, yet there was typically some degree of disclosure ahead of a first date, often to avoid an awkward moment when ordering something to drink. Indeed, Millie feels that 'being upfront about sobriety from the beginning helps to set clear expectations and weed out those who might not respect' her decision.

Whilst dating applications have helped to normalise non-drinking as a lifestyle choice, and provided some standardised terminology, research participants demonstrated that their disclosure of their sobriety status is individually negotiated. For example, some participants were quite specific about the terminology they use on apps to disclose their sobriety, that is, choosing the term 'sober' rather than 'non-drinker'. To many, 'sober' conveyed that they had past experiences of alcohol consumption but had ceased drinking, whereas 'non-drinker' gave the impression that they had never consumed alcohol (e.g., for religious reasons). 'Sober' was also felt to be a contemporary term that was worn digitally as a fashion or political label. Thus, the choice of terminology was important in expressing their identity. Further, participants conveyed how they must repeatedly renegotiate this with every new connection and dating experience, and sometimes alter or adapt their approach based on prior experiences. Thus, despite the increased normalisation and commercialisation of sober dating conveyed in the previous section, some women embark upon sober dating tentatively, agentically navigating each experience and the functionality of specific dating applications to best support their dating goals.

## Theme 2: "I became a bit of a prude": Changes in Navigating Physical Intimacy

> Yeah, oh my god, perhaps surprising, but perhaps not unsurprising but it's [dating] changed completely. I think when I was still drinking, I could go on a first date, I'd be four drinks in and suddenly they were definitely much more attractive and appealing than they were before I'd had four drinks. All those barriers come down, don't they. You just have a first kiss in the back room of a bar and you don't even notice or remember it happening, and it doesn't feel awkward…Things feel natural, and flowing and organic and in the moment, and everything seems easier… For me that was definitely a pattern – I'd hook up with people much more quickly and then when I stopped drinking, I feel like I flipped completely. I always joke that I became a bit of a prude, and I was really socially awkward at the end of the date when you say goodbye to someone…So I definitely find it harder to

> initiate intimacy, particularly around the first time. I feel a bit more self-conscious and awkward, and things flow less naturally in some ways.
>
> Francesca, 34 years old, 4 years in sobriety, single

Here, Francesca reflects on the ways in which intimacy during sober dating can feel fragmented, awkward and, to a certain extent, 'performed', particularly when initiating intimacy for the first time. When participants recounted these stories, they were often accompanied with physical displays of cringing, or embarrassment. For the majority of participants, they had come of age and experienced dating in the era of post-feminism (Banet-Weiser et al., 2020; Rivers, 2017) and the surge of the neoliberal Night Time Economy, whereby it was common (yet not always socially acceptable) for women to engage in 'hook ups' or 'one-night stands' (Niland et al., 2013; Griffin et al., 2013). Indeed, alcohol can serve as an effective tool to fast-track intimacy. In her interview, Francesca reflects on the stark change that sobriety created, whereby without alcohol, it takes her much longer—and, in some cases, many more dates—to get comfortable and familiar enough to engage in physical intimacy. Millie frames this as a positive step: the ability to determine 'whether a spark is real or merely a product of alcohol-induced euphoria'. Other participants also saw this as a process of developing more 'authentic' connections. Investing more time in getting to know someone was the only sober strategy that participants had to develop intimacy without alcohol. There were no examples of participants using alternative substances. This complexity or difficulty with sober dating is, unfortunately, something which the rise of in-person sober dating events (discussed in the prior section) is unable to address. While such challenges are acknowledged and discussed within contemporary sobriety culture (Gray, 2017; Lara, 2023), it is an area in which individuals may require more support and time prior to adjusting. Such feelings of awkwardness or embarrassment may also pose a significant barrier to those who are curious about sober dating.

## Theme 3: "I get fucked or I hike": Finding a Middle Ground Between Two Extremes of Dating Activities

> The thing that I find really hard is that people are either like go for drinks whatever, or I don't know what your dating situation is but at the minute there's very much a focus on going on hikes. I don't want to hike. I don't want to do that. There is this really big prominence in apps where people are like "I get fucked or I hike". And I can't do either of those things, or I don't want to do either of those things… I like going playing mini golf or going to Christmas markets, or going cinema, or going for tea, I don't mind any of that stuff, but no hikes.
>
> Tina, 28 years old, 5 years in sobriety, single

It was identified by many participants that dating culture in the UK is intimately linked to drinking culture. As such, this presents difficulties when planning and organising alternative activities for dates—particularly first dates. Participants reflected on the challenge of having to re-learn how to date if they were unable to drink or go to the pub on a date. Millie found that this prompts 'creative' dating ideas, which leads to finding new hobbies and interests, or the re-discovery of old ones—water sports, for example. Those in longer-term sobriety were perhaps more accepting of the idea of going to a pub and consuming a non-alcoholic drink, but some wanted to remove the possibility of alcohol from the date completely. This is the challenge that the in-person events hosted by Tinder, Thursday Dating or Sober & Social are seeking to address.

During her interview, Tina spoke of the current dating trend to go on hikes. She suggests that one extreme dating practice (of getting 'fucked') has been replaced with another extreme—hiking. Indeed, a few other participants suggested that hiking dates were enjoyable. However, Tina's reflections show how sobriety has, perhaps to too great an extent, become intrinsically linked with themes of wellness and exercise; it is assumed that people who are sober must also be invested in these—as part of a broader lifestyle of health, which Tina is not. Instead, she identified the need for a middle ground—for fun and accessible leisure activities that do not centre alcohol or extreme physical activity.

## Discussion

Common threads weave through these (auto-)ethnographic narratives of sober dating. In this section we identify and discuss them in more detail, raising key implications and considerations for those who may be embarking upon sober dating or looking to support those who are.

The lived experiences shared within this chapter strongly suggest that sober dating is informed by, and intrinsically linked to, contemporary obligations of wellness and self-care that are facilitated by a longer-term sober lifestyle (Davey, 2022b). Young(er) adults are highly cognisant of their mental, physical, and even financial health (Caluzzi et al., 2020, 2021) and, in turn, desire to meet someone who shares and supports this identity and/or lifestyle. Sober dating is posited as a way to 'do' self-care, through both the decision not to drink, but also in the choice of dating activity—with a strong tendency towards physical and outdoor activities. This may also speak to the imperative that young people face to maintain an idealised body image, particularly young women (Pruis & Janowsky, 2010). However, such sober dating practices, and sober lifestyle practices more generally, work to exclude those like Tina, or those with less socioeconomic resources, who have less time, energy or interest in engaging with such bodily discipline or may have limited access to outdoor spaces (Masterton et al., 2021). It may also provide difficulties for those who want to avoid alcohol during dates but do not want to commit to, or adhere to, a sober lifestyle altogether.

As such, sober dating could be perceived as a constituent part of a neoliberal socioeconomic model whereby investment in the individual is encouraged, to foster the "right' kinds of dispositions for surviving in neoliberal society: confidence, resilience, and positive mental attitude' (Gill, 2017, p. 606), and empowerment is gained through purchasing products or services (Banet-Weiser, 2012)—including no- and low-alcohol drinks, or the engagement of sober dating gurus. These are market-led solutions to a public health issue which the government is inadequately funding (Bulman, 2017) due to neoliberal ideologies of a minimised state (Springer et al., 2016). However, market-driven solutions for those who are seeking to drink less—and date sober—inherently privilege access to those who have the socioeconomic capital to pay—typically white, heteronormative, middle- and upper-class individuals.

We can also see here that such self-care coalesces with discourses of neoliberal feminism. By 'neoliberal feminism' we refer to a belief that women face gender inequality whilst rejecting the role that socioeconomic structures play in creating or maintaining such inequality—and that through their own choices, self-responsibility, self-care and self-empowerment, women can eradicate such inequality (Rottenberg, 2014). Women's narratives shared in this chapter suggest that 'doing' sober dating is positioned as a form of self-empowerment and self-respect—a means to prevent unwise or regrettable attachments to men—whereby more discernment regarding choice of partner is valued highly, perhaps part of the broader reframing of single-hood and single women as an empowering identity (Traister, 2016; Gray, 2018).

Sober dating is perceived as a means to be more authentic and establish authentic relationships, thus echoing Banet-Weiser's (2021) analysis that 'the appearance of authenticity remains central to how individuals organize their everyday activities and craft their very selves'—including through non-drinking and dating practices. This reflects existing research findings that demonstrate how sobriety is often perceived as a 'true' self, or a return to a truer, authentic self (Nicholls, 2021; Conroy & de Visser, 2015). However, the pressure and scrutiny of authenticity has never been so high than with the rise of SNS and online dating apps where authenticity is constructed and judged through digital representations (Peterson, 2005; van Driel & Dumitrica, 2021). The search and aspiration for authenticity, both in oneself and in others, appears to be informing contemporary engagement with sober dating practices.

It is clear, however, that while there are evidently trends in popular sober dating practices, sober dating requires a social contract to be negotiated at the start of every foray into a new connection. The experiences shared in this chapter suggest that this is individually navigated and negotiated by women dependent upon their needs, preferences and former experiences. It is also apparent that this requires additional intentional, emotional and administrative labour to set up and enter into this contract, whether in person or via an online dating application—a form of sobriety 'work'. Avoiding this initial labour can lead to miscommunication and misalignment in expectations, yet sometimes it is avoided because despite the growing popularity of sober dating, those who do so are still in the minority. The findings suggest that young sober women are attempting to walk a precarious tightrope of (non-)disclosure whereby they are seeking to balance their identity or lifestyle as a sober person with their desire to increase their chances of meeting a compatible partner.

Further, we can see how the rise in sobriety is fundamentally shifting how women 'do' dating as a form of leisure and pleasure. This includes the dating activity, but also how they approach key milestones, such as physical intimacy. This may have ushered in changing social mores regarding hook-ups and casual intimacy that have typically been a feature of the Night Time Economy and alco-centric spaces since the 'ladette' era of the late 1990s/early 2000s (Jackson & Tinkler, 2007; Measham, 2002). For some this conservatism may feel like a regression in confidence and self-assuredness—even a shift in feminist positionality away from practices of intimacy that were heralded an act of equality in the era of post-feminism (Banet-Weiser et al., 2020; Rivers, 2017), as evidenced by popular cultural icons in film and media at that time, such as Bridget Jones (Fielding, 1996), Carrie Bradshaw (Bushnell, 1996) and Ally McBeal (Ally McBeal, 1997–2002).

## Conclusion

This exploratory chapter has provided insights, from intimate insider (auto-)ethnographic research, into the contemporary phenomenon of sober dating, including the roles of online dating applications, online sobriety communities, and no- and low-alcohol drinks in its growth. This chapter has also drawn on (auto-)ethnographic reflections from young sober women to further understand lived experiences of sober dating—both its challenges and affordances.

These findings contribute to the emerging field of non-drinking studies to better understand how people 'do' sobriety and non-drinking practices. In sum, sober dating resides at the intersection of changes in contemporary (non-)drinking practices and dating practices; it is facilitated by, and significantly dependent on, technology mediums such as online sobriety communities and online dating applications, to enable individuals to 'do' sober dating. It also reflects how the increased alcohol-refusal of younger generations is informing broader, mainstream, social practices such as dating. The desire to practice sober dating is intrinsically linked to why individuals are not drinking; sober dating must be understood within the context of individuals' broader lifestyle goals of health, well-being, and authenticity. However, there are evidently more individuals who use sobriety as a tool for dating rather than as a long-term lifestyle choice.

This chapter has demonstrated how young women agentically navigate the challenges and affordances of sober dating to meet their own needs and preferences for a relationship that is most likely to support their own sobriety, relationship goals, and lifestyle. However, the challenges shared by women within their narratives allude to a potential precarity and fragility during the process of sober dating that may require increased awareness and support. Such findings raise broader questions regarding the availability, provision of, and stigma related to, sex education and relationship counselling throughout the life course. While the findings identify the prominent impact of, and commercial opportunity for, sober dating, ethical considerations have been raised regarding accessibility and exclusion, and the potential for the growing marketisation of sobriety to have a detrimental impact on vulnerable individuals.

This chapter has offered merely an introductory overview of this emerging social trend and signals multiple opportunities for further research. Moreover, it emphasises the need for academia to engage with the commercial sector—at the frontiers of enabling social change—for research purposes, to better understand contemporary leisure and non-drinking practices.

## References


*Ally McBeal*. 1997–2002. [TV series]. Fox.

Atkinson, A. M., et al. (2023). 'Some days I am a lunatic that thinks I can moderate': Amalgamating recovery and neo-liberal discourses within accounts of non-drinking among women active in the 'positive sobriety' community on Instagram in the UK. *International Journal of Drug Policy, 112*. https://doi.org/10.1016/j.drugpo.2022.103937

Bancroft, A., et al. (2014). Working at pleasure in young women's alcohol consumption: A participatory visual ethnography. *Social Research Online, 19*(3), 65–78. https://doi.org/10.5153/sro.3409

Banet-Weiser, S. (2012). Authentic: The Politics of Ambivalence in a Brand Culture. New York: New York University Press.

Banet-Weiser, S. (2021). Ruptures in authenticity and authentic ruptures: Producing white influencer vulnerability. *Kids & Technology Essay Series*. Retrieved September 19, 2023, from https://static1.squarespace.com/static/5ea874746663b45e14a384a4/t/6182cc1d7a68be7ccf6f64e2/1635961886253/Banet-Weiser_Nov21.pdf

Banet-Weiser, S., Gill, R., & Rottenberg, C. (2020). Postfeminism, popular feminism and neoliberal feminism? Sarah Banet-Weiser, Rosalind Gill and Catherine Rottenberg in conversation. *Feminist Theory, 21*(1), 3–24. https://doi.org/10.1177/1464700119842555

Berridge, V. (2005). *Temperance: Its history and impact on current and future alcohol policy.* Technical Report. Joseph Rowntree Foundation, London. Retrieved December 7, 2024, from https://researchonline.lshtm.ac.uk/id/eprint/427981/

Bulman, M. (2017). Drug and alcohol treatment funding slashed across England by 16% in four years. Independent. 25 August. Available at: https://www.independent.co.uk/news/uk/home-news/spending-on-drug-andalcohol-treatment-slashed-by-ps105m-in-four-years-a7912531.html [Accessed 4 October 2023].

Bushnell, C. (1996). *Sex and the city*. Grove Atlantic Inc.

Butters, A., et al. (2023). Temporary abstinence challenges: What do we need to know? *Drug and Alcohol Review, 42*(5), 1087–1091. https://doi.org/10.1111/dar.13625

Caluzzi, G., Pennay, A., & MacLean, S. (2020). Reflexive habitus and the new obligation of choice: Understanding young people's light drinking and alcohol abstinence. *Journal of Youth Studies, 24*, 886–900. https://doi.org/10.1080/13676261.2020.1778658

Caluzzi, G., et al. (2021). 'No one associates alcohol with being in good health': Health and wellbeing as imperatives to manage alcohol use for young people. *Sociology of Health & Illness, 43*(2), 493–509. https://doi.org/10.1111/1467-9566.13237

Conroy, D., & de Visser, R. (2015). The importance of authenticity for student non-drinkers: An interpretive phenomenological analysis. *Journal of Health Psychology, 20*(11), 1483–1493. https://doi.org/10.1177/1359105313514285

Davey, C. (2021). Online sobriety communities for women's problematic alcohol use: A mini review of existing qualitative and quantitative research. *Frontiers in Global Women's Health, 2021*, 2. https://doi.org/10.3389/fgwh.2021.773921

Davey, C. (2022a). Patterns of consumption at the UK's first 'Alcohol-Free Off-Licence': Who engaged with no- and low-alcohol drinks and why? *European Journal of Food Drink and Society, 2*(1) https://doi.org/10.21427/FGNV-SF35

Davey, C. (2022b). 'Goodbye mindless drinking and hello mindful living': A feminist analysis of women's sobriety as a practice of self-care. *Cultivate, 4*, 58–77. Retrieved December 7, 2024, from https://www.cultivatefeminist-journal.com/issue-4

Davey, C. (2023a). 'It's kind of like weaning. I had to wean myself off of wine': Navigating no- and low-alcohol drinks as potential harm reduction tools and relapse triggers by women in recovery in the UK. *Drug and Alcohol Review, 43*(1), 156–164. https://doi.org/10.1111/dar.13766

Davey, C. (2023b). The sober self, sisterhood, and non-drinking practices: A feminist ethnography of women's recovery culture within online sobriety communities. Unpublished PhD Thesis, Canterbury Christ Church University.

Farmer A. Y., et al. (2022). Knowledge of Predatory Practices within the Substance Use Disorder Treatment Industry: Development of a Measurement Instrument. *International Journal of Environmental Research and Public Health, 19*(13), 7980. https://doi.org/10.3390%2Fijerph19137980.

Gill, R. (2017). The affective, cultural and psychic life of postfeminism: A postfeminist sensibility 10 years on. *European Journal of Cultural Studies, 20*(6), 606-626. https://doi.org/10.1177/1367549417733003

Fielding, H. (1996). *Bridget Jones's diary*. Picador.

Gray, C. (2017). *The unexpected joy of being Sober*. Aster.

Gray, C. (2018). *The unexpected joy of being Single*. Aster.

Griffin, C., et al. (2013). Inhabiting the contradictions: Hypersexual femininity and the culture of intoxication among young women in the UK. *Feminism and Psychology, 23*(2), 184–206. https://doi.org/10.1177/0959353512468860

Jackson, C., & Tinkler, P. (2007). 'Ladettes' and 'Modern Girls': 'Troublesome' young femininities. *The Sociological Review, 55*(2), 251–272. https://doi.org/10.1111/j.1467-954X.2007.00704.x

Kalia, A. 2019. Five ways to be sober-curious (and make a success of not drinking). *The Guardian*, September 1. Retrieved July 27, 2024, from https://www.theguardian.com/lifeandstyle/2019/sep/01/five-ways-sober-curious-success-not-drinking?msclkid=a783a878d10511eca3e210bf253af245 [Accessed 27 July 2024].

Lara, T. (2023). *Dry humping: A guide to dating, relating, and hooking up without the booze*. Quirk Books.

Levine, H. G. (1993). Temperance cultures: Concern about alcohol problems in Nordic and English-speaking cultures. In M. Lader, G. Edwards, & D. C. Drummon (Eds.), *The nature of alcohol and drug-related problems* (pp. 16–36). Oxford University Press.

Masterton, W., Park, K., Carver, H., & Parkes, T. (2021). Greenspace programmes for mental health: A survey study to test what works, for whom and in what circumstances. *Health and Place, 72*. https://doi.org/10.1016/j.healthplace.2021.102669

McNamara, P. (2009). Feminist ethnography: Storytelling that makes a difference. *Qualitative Social Work, 8*(2), 161–177. https://doi.org/10.1177/1473325009103373

Measham, F. (2002). 'Doing gender' – 'Doing drugs': Conceptualising the gendering of drugs cultures. *Contemporary Drug Problems, 29*(2), 335–373. https://doi.org/10.1177/009145090202900206

Merrill, B., & West, L. (2009). *Using biographical methods in social research*. SAGE Publications Ltd.

Merton, R. K. (1972). Insiders and outsiders: A chapter in the sociology of knowledge. *American Journal of Sociology, 78*(1). https://doi.org/10.1086/225294

NHS Digital. (2022). *Health Survey for England, 2021 part 1. Part 3: Drinking alcohol*. Retrieved October 2, 2023, from https://digital.nhs.uk/data-and-information/publications/statistical/health-survey-for-england/2021/

part-3-drinking-alcohol#estimated-weekly-alcohol-consumption-by-sex-and-age

Nicholls, E. (2019). *Negotiating femininities in the neoliberal night-time economy: Too much of a girl? (Genders and sexualities in the social sciences)*. Macmillan.

Nicholls, E. (2021). Sober Rebels or Good Consumer-Citizens? Anti-Consumption and the 'Enterprising Self' in Early Sobriety. *Sociology, 55*(4), 768–784. https://doi.org/10.1177/0038038520981837

Niland, P., et al. (2013). 'Everyone can loosen up and get a bit of a buzz on': Young adults, alcohol and friendship practices. *International Journal of Drug Policy, 24*, 530–537. https://psycnet.apa.org/doi/10.1016/j.drugpo.2013.05.013

Office for National Statistics (ONS). (2017). Adult drinking habits in Great Britain. Retrieved May 28, 2021, from https://www.ons.gov.uk/peoplepopulationandcommunity/healthandsocialcare/drugusealcoholandsmoking/datasets/adultdrinkinghabits

Oldham, M. et al. (2018). *Youth drinking in decline*. The University of Sheffield. Retrieved September 19, 2023, from https://www.sheffield.ac.uk/news/polopoly_fs/1.806889!/file/Oldham_Holmes_Youth_drinking_in_decline_FINAL.pdf

Pape, H., Rossow, I., & Brunborg, G. (2018). Adolescents drink less: How, who and why? A review of the recent research literature. *Drug and Alcohol Review, 37*(1), 98–114. https://doi.org/10.1111/dar.12695

Peterson, R. (2005). In search of Authenticity. *Journal of Management Studies, 42*(5), 1083–1098. https://doi.org/10.1111/j.1467-6486.2005.00533.x

Pink, S., et al. (2016). *Digital ethnography: Principles and practice*. SAGE.

Plante, A. (2018). 'Buyer beware' when it comes to addiction treatment. Harvard Health Blog. 10 August. Available at: https://www.health.harvard.edu/blog/buyer-beware-when-it-comes-to-addiction-treatment-2018042514506 [Accessed 3 November 2023].

Pruis, T., & Janowsky, J. (2010). Assessment of body image in younger and older women. *The Journal of General Psychology, 137*(3), 225–238. https://doi.org/10.1080/00221309.2010.484446

Rivers, N. (2017). *Postfeminism(s) and the arrival of the fourth wave: Turning tides*. Palgrave Macmillan.

Robert, J. (2016). Temporary sobriety initiatives: emergence, possibilities and constraints. *Journal of Media & Cultural Studies, 30*(6), 646–658. https://doi.org/10.1080/10304312.2016.1231786.

Springer, S., Birch, K., and MacLeavy, J. (Eds). (2016). The Handbook of Neoliberalism. London: Routledge. Robert, J. (2016). Temporary sobriety initiatives: emergence, possibilities and constraints. *Journal of Media & Cultural Studies, 30*(6), 646–658. https://doi.org/10.1080/10304312.2016.1231786.

Taylor, J. (2011). The intimate insider: Negotiating the ethics of friendship when doing insider research. *Qualitative Research, 11*(1), 03–22. https://doi.org/10.1177/1468794110384447

Tinder. (2023). The future of dating. Report. Retrieved July 17, 2024, from https://filecache.mediaroom.com/mr5mr_tinder/179342/Copy_of_FOD_Report_2023_FINAL.pdf

Traister, R. (2016). *All the single ladies*. Simon and Schuster.

van Driel, L., & Dumitrica, D. (2021). Selling brands while staying 'Authentic': The professionalization of Instagram influencers. *Convergence: The International Journal of Research into New Media Technologies, 27*(1), 66–84. https://doi.org/10.1177/1354856520902136

Vashishtha, R., et al. (2020). Trends in adolescent drinking across 39 high-income countries: Exploring the timing and magnitude of decline. *European Journal of Public Health, 31*(2), 424–431. https://doi.org/10.1093/eurpub/ckaa193

Warrington, R. (2019). Sober Curious: The Blissful Sleep, Greater Focus, Limitless Presence, and Deep Connection Awaiting Us All on the Other Side of Alcohol. London: HarperOne.

Whitaker, H. G. (2020). *Quit like a woman: The radical choice to not drink in a culture obsessed with alcohol*. Bloomsbury.

Whitaker, V., et al. (2023). Young people's explanations for the decline in youth drinking in England. *BMC Public Health, 23*. https://doi.org/10.1186/s12889-022-14760-y

# 11

# "No Time for a Hangover": The Role of No- and Low-Alcohol Drinks in Young People's Lives

Emily Nicholls

**Abstract** Recent years have seen the growth of a rapidly expanding market of No- and Low (NoLo)-alcohol drinks in high-income countries where drinking rates are declining, particularly amongst young people. This chapter considers the current state of the field of research into NoLo consumption, drawing on original primary research in the UK to highlight examples of the ways in which these products are being used by young people and their motivations for consuming them. The chapter demonstrates how—for young drinkers—NoLos use is shaped by enduring neoliberal imperatives to drink discerningly, responsibly and in moderation, to be productive and get ahead in 'hustle culture' and to take personal responsibility for one's health and well-being.

E. Nicholls (✉)
Department of Sociology, University of York, York, UK
e-mail: emily.nicholls@york.ac.uk



D. Conroy, F. Measham (eds.), *Young Adult Drinking Styles*, Sustainable Development Goals Series, https://doi.org/10.1007/978-3-031-98528-7_11

# Introduction

Recent years have seen increased policy, public and academic interest in the expanding No- and Low (NoLo)-alcohol drinks market in the United Kingdom (UK) and other high-income countries. Whilst the definition and labelling of 'NoLos' is contested and inconsistent, these can broadly be defined as drinks designed to resemble alcohol in terms of taste, branding and appearance but with a reduced Alcohol by Volume percentage (typically between 0.0 and 1.2 ABV%) (see Department of Health and Social Care (2018) for more detail on defining 'alcohol free' products). The NoLo market is a lucrative area of rapid growth, with some UK supermarkets reporting sales more than doubling year-on-year in 2021 (Campbell, 2022). NoLo beer in particular has experienced a surge in popularity and was identified in 2019 as one of the 'fastest-growing drinks trends in the UK' (Robinson, 2019, cited in Corfe et al., 2020). Today, the range of NoLo products available spans from the mass-produced NoLo equivalents of the 'flagship' products offered by huge global players in the alcohol industry to artisanal or craft products made by small-scale breweries who exclusively produce NoLo drinks.

This growth is perhaps unsurprising in high-incomes countries where drinking rates are declining (see Chaps. 2 and 3). In these contexts, drinking has been theorised as 'in decline' since the early 2000s, particularly amongst young people (Herring et al., 2014; Pape et al., 2018; Pavlidis et al., 2019). For example, in the UK, young people are today consuming alcohol less frequently and in smaller amounts than previous cohorts and are starting to drink later (Oldham et al., 2018). These changes are mirrored across other parts of Europe and Australia, particularly amongst adolescents (Livingston et al., 2018; Ball et al., 2020; Vashishtha et al., 2021). Abstention rates have also increased; findings from Ng Fat et al. (2018) suggest that almost 30% of young people aged 16–24 in the UK abstain from alcohol consumption, whilst consumption amongst older generations such as the post-war 'Baby Boomers' has not undergone equivalent changes (Burgess et al., 2022). Decreases in youth drinking may also have been accelerated further during the COVID-19 pandemic in 2020; however, research on the impacts of the pandemic on longer-term alcohol consumption is inconclusive, with some research indicating an *increase* in consumption (Roberts et al., 2021) and a lack of consensus on the longer-term impacts. Alongside these changes in consumption practices and the increasing popularity of 'dry months' across Europe, Australia and North America (de Visser et al., 2017; Butters et al., 2023), there has been a proliferation of online communities promoting 'mindful drinking' and/or 'sober curiosity' (Davey, 2021). Whilst these are not targeted exclusively at young people, a growing number of associated 'sober socials'—such as sober raves and 'conscious clubbing' events (Hill et al., 2022)—are likely to appeal to this demographic.

Returning to NoLos, UK-based survey research suggests that those aged 18–34 are the most likely age group to have tried one (with 25% consuming one in the last 12 months), and the most likely to report that consuming NoLos has led to them reducing their alcohol consumption or stopping drinking completely (Corfe et al., 2020). Such findings suggest that young people are playing a key role in the expanding popularity of NoLo products, leading to claims that this cohort is 'spearheading' the growth of the no- and low-alcohol market (BBC, 2020). Again, similar patterns are observed in other contexts—the global NoLo beer market alone is worth almost $10 billion and is predicted to expand further (Lawton, 2022, cited in Waehning & Wells, 2024), with research starting to explore the implications of the growing market across the European Union (Kokole et al., 2022), the United States (Myles et al., 2022) and Australia (Harrison et al., 2024).

Those offering a cynical interpretation might argue that the increase in the range of NoLos represents an attempt by the alcohol industry to present young people with new ways to engage with the market through the consumption of 'alcohol-adjacent' products. Arguably, this could be a key way to maintain a consumer base in the face of declining drinking rates, particularly if these cohorts maintain their reduced or non-consumption rates into midlife and beyond. Researchers also express concern about NoLo regulation and the ways in which products are marketed/promoted to young people and more widely (Porretta & Donadini, 2008; Corfe et al., 2020), the unclear health claims and benefits associated with NoLos (de Bruijn et al., 2012) and the ways in which they might act as a 'gateway' to future alcohol consumption or encourage 'brand allegiance' amongst young people (including those under the legal drinking age) (Kaewpramkusol et al., 2019). Furthermore, if NoLos are consumed in addition to existing alcohol consumption—a strategy that has been promoted in NoLo marketing (Nicholls, 2023)—then the possibilities for NoLos to facilitate more moderate drinking practices or reductions in alcohol consumption may be limited. The presence of NoLo drinks in traditional drinking spaces may also reinforce social norms and expectations around drinking and perpetuate the notion that 'everybody drinks' because these products so strongly resemble alcohol in appearance, smell and taste (Miller et al., 2022).

On the other hand, the possibility that NoLo products could help to alleviate alcohol harm must be further considered; for example, if NoLos are used as 'substitutes' for alcohol. Miller et al. (2022) caution that substitution is unlikely to be an appealing option for those consciously seeking the embodied and intoxicating effects of alcohol, and Corfe et al. (2020) present survey findings indicating that 50% of NoLo drinkers admitted that drinking NoLos had *not* changed their overall alcohol consumption levels (with heavier drinkers more likely to say this). However, the increasing availability of NoLos might nevertheless be regarded as a progressive development, offering consumers the choice to consume viable alternatives to alcohol in settings where they might usually drink. There is also evidence to suggest that despite retaining a small share of overall alcohol sales, new NoLo and 'light' products *have* contributed to a reduction in the total number of grams of alcohol purchased by British households in recent years (Anderson et al., 2020; Kokole, 2021). Thus, the substitution model cannot be entirely disregarded, with Vasiljevic et al. (2018) suggesting that the increased availability of low/er strength alcohol products does have at least the potential to reduce overall levels of alcohol consumption and Corfe et al. (2020) acknowledging that the consumption of NoLo products could make a difference to health outcomes for individuals. For example, NoLo products may help consumers to have more alcohol-free nights, consume fewer units, stop drinking alcohol completely for the short or long term or to drink more moderately over a sustained period of time (Rehm et al., 2016).

Such goals may be important for individuals in neoliberal contexts where—even whilst drinking is normalised and expected (Cherrier & Gurrieri, 2013)—'good' consumer-citizens are compelled to 'drink responsibly' and 'moderation' is positioned as an inherently valued goal (Caluzzi et al., 2020). Consuming alcohol in particular ways may also serve as a marker of taste and status (Järvinen et al., 2014), with the 'right' products and practices facilitating the construction of the elite, discerning drinker (Nanney et al., 2020). More widely, the good citizen is also a 'productive' and 'enterprising' member of society (Rose, 1998) and Cederström and Spicer (2015) chart the rise of 'healthism', the increasing pressure to take individual responsibility for proactively managing one's mental and physical health and well-being. Binge drinking and its consequences are likely to be incompatible with these aims and goals, whilst moderation or abstinence (and—as this chapter will show—NoLo consumption) can be framed as ways of working towards them.

Further research is still required to address the question of whether/how NoLos might exacerbate or alleviate alcohol-related harm. To answer this, a greater understanding of how these products are actually being used by consumers in their everyday (non)drinking routines is required. Such research can also be situated and considered against the backdrop of neoliberalism and healthism outlined above whilst building on a currently limited understanding of consumer practices in relation to NoLos (Anderson et al., 2021). This chapter works towards addressing this gap in the existing literature, drawing on primary research to highlight the ways in which young drinkers and non-drinkers incorporate NoLos into their everyday consumption routines. The chapter draws on data from a recent research project on NoLo consumption within the UK to highlight the ways in which NoLos may be used strategically to maximise productivity, construct discerning (non)drinking identities and facilitate more moderate overall alcohol consumption to support both mental and physical health. In these ways, youth NoLo consumption practices are clearly shaped by neoliberal imperatives to drink discerningly, responsibly and in moderation, to be productive and 'get ahead' and to take personal responsibility for one's mental—and to a lesser extent physical—health and well-being.

## The 'NoLo' Project: Understanding NoLo Consumption Practices in the UK

The NoLo Project elicited the views of NoLo consumers based in the UK and explored their (non)drinking practices and routines using semi-structured, in-depth interviews (alongside analysis of marketing and social media materials for two brands). Interviews took place in 2021; despite their proximity to the recent COVID-19 pandemic there was little discussion of lockdown and social distancing measures and NoLo consumption did not appear to have been significantly affected by the pandemic. The interviews allowed for rich discussions of participants' drinking biographies and histories, including consideration of the contexts, spaces and environments in which they consumed NoLo drinks and their motivations for doing so. Fifteen UK-based drinkers and non-drinkers who had consumed NoLos at least three times in the preceding six months took part, recruited through social media platforms, online groups (including local groups and online 'mindful drinking' communities) and snowballing following institutional ethical approval. All interviews were transcribed, coded into themes and thematically analysed drawing on an inductively and deductively developed coding framework (Braun & Clarke, 2006) that was cross-referenced where relevant with the media analysis.

Seven participants identified as male and eight female, and nine identified as middle-class and three as working-class (three did not identify with a class). All resided in the UK at the time of the research and the sample was predominantly White British. Ages ranged from 22 to 68; the discussion here will focus on the experiences and narratives of the six participants aged 32 and below at the time of interview (with half in their twenties and half in their early thirties). This allows for a specific focus on the (non)drinking practices and NoLo consumption of a younger cohort, all of whom were regular—and generally enthusiastic—NoLo drinkers. One of the six young adult participants identified as a drinker who was taking a short-term break from drinking during pregnancy, two identified as former drinkers and three were 'hybrid' drinkers who regularly consumed both alcohol and NoLos.

## 'We Want to Go on a Hike Today': Productivity and Hustle Culture

One of the most significant motivators for NoLo consumption across the data was the desire to avoid feeling tired and/or hungover the day after drinking, and thus to 'maximise' one's capacity to make the most of work and leisure time:

> The reason that I started drinking alcohol-free… I wanted to have a drink of an evening, probably more a Friday or a Saturday night, to be like, "Work's finished". You know, celebrate the end of the week. So me and Nate were sharing a bottle of prosecco, and the next day, I was waking up and I was like, "You know what, I feel rough. I'm already knackered from a new job, and we want to go on a hike today or whatever, but I'm just feeling exhausted". I said to Nate, "I'm just getting tired of this," and I was only having a couple of glasses. It was actually him that then bought me a bottle of alcohol-free gin. (Emma, 31, hybrid drinker)

Emma describes how NoLos can produce some of the sense of relaxation associated with alcohol and be used to celebrate the end of the working week with her partner (Nicholls & Conroy, 2021) but without leaving her feeling 'rough', 'knackered' or 'exhausted'. Importantly, this frees her up to have a full, active weekend (e.g. 'going on a hike'). Other participants also talked about the ways in which NoLos still 'hit the spot' (Liam, 26, hybrid) as they resemble alcohol in taste and produce associated feelings of relaxation or celebration, but without the risk of an unjustifiable 'write-off day' (Alice, 32, short-term non-drinker) afterwards. Much like Emma, Hannah (30, non-drinker) described how drinking NoLos meant she could get up early on a weekend morning to exercise (specifically noting how the morning after consuming alcohol this would not be possible). Framings of mornings as a particularly important period for productivity were echoed by others:

> I literally work every weekend with the business. So, I know that I do not have time to have a hangover. I need to be up at 6:30, like get up and go. (Georgie, 22, hybrid)

As the youngest participant in the sample, Georgie highlighted both the pleasures and the necessity of 'waking up on a Saturday morning hangover free'. She embodies the position of the entrepreneurial and enthusiastic member of what Burgess et al. (2022) call 'hustle culture' (where young people faced with increasingly uncertain and anxious futures are forced to use their leisure time creatively for self-development and/or income generation). After working full-time during the week, the weekend demands of her 'side hustle' (an independent cake business) mean she 'does not have time to have a hangover' if she is to successfully grow her small business and embody the notion of the 'enterprising' and future-focused self (Rose, 1998).

As these examples show, across the data there was a sense that even one's leisure time must be used productively, with hangovers to be avoided primarily because they limit one's capacity to make the most of one's day (rather than due to the associated physically unpleasant sensations, which were rarely mentioned). This facilitates a 'blurring' between work and leisure where even one's supposed 'down-time' must be used in productive and future-focused ways (Caluzzi et al., 2021) that centre exercise, CV-building and/or self-development. In such framings, the hangover shifts from a bonding experience (Fjær, 2012) and extension of supposedly 'carefree' leisure activities characterised by binge drinking and calculated hedonism (Szmigin et al., 2008) to an unjustifiable waste of time. NoLos in these contexts offer an opportunity for young people to enjoy some of the perceived benefits of alcohol consumption (taste, relaxing, transition to leisure time) but without the risk of a hangover and the associated consequences.

## 'Not Your Standard Supermarket Beer': Choice, Craft and the Discerning (Non)Drinker

Younger participants were also particularly likely to celebrate the 'choice' that they felt the expanding NoLo market offers, positioning themselves as 'active consumers' (Georgie, 22, hybrid) who felt NoLos supported them to make an 'informed choice' (Liam, 26, hybrid) about their drinking practices. Half of the younger participants positioned themselves as knowledgeable 'craft' consumers who were particularly invested in sampling a range of artisanal NoLo products typically produced by small-scale, independent brewers (including ales, porters, stouts and sour beers). For example, Liam described 'ticking off new NoLo drinks' as a 'hobby', mirroring the practices of alcohol consumers who track or display consumption using apps or guides to 'tick off' and rank beers (Chorley et al., 2016). Those who appreciated craft products talked at length about discovering and purchasing new, specialist and niche drinks, showcasing their knowledge about how to serve drinks and/or pair them with food and stressing the importance of taste, aesthetic and/or the 'local' origins of products. Whilst in general the relatively recent (at the time of research) COVID-19 pandemic did not appear to shape young people's NoLo consumption significantly, some participants did describe 'lockdowns' as opportunities to research online and purchase new NoLo products (including from specialist websites). In this way, the expanding NoLo market increasingly presents young people with the means to embody particular types of (non)drinking identities as discerning and 'sophisticated' consumers (Chapman et al., 2018; Ikäheimo, 2020). This was perhaps particularly important for former drinkers such as Hannah and Luke, who positioned themselves as discerning consumers with sophisticated tastes and extensive knowledge acquired through their years as drinkers. As Hannah (30, non-drinker) noted, the expanding NoLo market allowed her to better 'replicate' her previous consumption practices and ensure she was 'not missing out' by having to drink 'standard or boring [NoLo] beer' in sobriety. Others echoed this language:

> A lot of people will say, "What is the point of drinking alcohol-free beer if there is no alcohol in it?". I would assume that those people would be happy with your standard supermarket beer and don't have too much of an interest in the craft scene, but I do. I really like unique local sellers of beer or wine and things like that and exploring it as more than just a vehicle for getting drunk. (Luke, 29, non-drinker)

Here, Luke positions himself as a sophisticated consumer (and indeed elsewhere in the interview as a 'total snob') who can appreciate the 'uniqueness' and flavour of craft NoLos, in contrast to 'standard supermarket beer'. As observed here, notions of taste and/or the idea of using NoLos to explore a craft 'scene' or even as part of an 'alternate lifestyle' (Liam, 26, hybrid) could also be used to justify NoLo consumption in the face of possible accusations that drinking alcohol-adjacent products (but without the intoxication effects) is 'pointless'. Young people who drink craft NoLos are increasingly able to rationalise their consumption choices by drawing on processes of—implicitly classed-based—othering. This allows them to align with the discerning (and middle-class) consumer and establish distance from the (implicitly working-class) consumer of 'standard', cheap, mass-produced lager (Thurnell-Read, 2016). This type of drinker is depicted as merely using alcohol as 'a vehicle for getting drunk' and lacks any appreciation of the 'sophisticated' pleasures of consumption (Wallace, 2019) available to young people who consume craft NoLos.

## 'A Level I'm Comfortable With': Hybridity and Drinking in Moderation

For the young (and indeed older) drinkers in the sample, NoLo consumption could also be incorporated into one's drinking regimes as a substitute for alcohol in particular contexts. Such findings contribute to ongoing debates around 'addition' versus 'substitution' in relation to NoLo usage (Miller et al., 2022), suggesting that—amongst a small sample at least—NoLos may be consumed instead of rather than on top of alcohol in some settings. According to survey research, one-third of NoLo consumers aged 18–34 cited a desire to cut down on alcohol consumption as a reason they drank NoLos (Corfe et al., 2020), and this was evidenced across the sample, where the substitution approach aided directly in the construction of moderate and responsible drinking identities amongst young people (and/or in the construction of their imagined *future* or long-term relationships with alcohol). For example, Hannah (30, non-drinker) explained that—prior to stopping drinking completely—she adopted a conscious strategy to 'cut back on alcohol midweek' by switching to NoLos in the evening. Now sober for one month, Hannah envisaged a longer-term period of abstinence, but also speculated about a possible 'hybrid' future where she mostly consumes NoLos but has the occasional and infrequent alcoholic drink. Similarly, whilst not drinking at the time of interview due to pregnancy, Alice also reflected on how the expanding range of NoLos and what she perceived to be a decreasing stigma towards non-drinking was helping her to envision a more balanced future relationship with alcohol for both herself and her partner:

> You can mix it up. It doesn't have to be that you are entirely booze-free or you drink all of the time. It can be a mixture of both. You can do the two together. (Alice, 32, short-term non-drinker)

Such strategies represent one way to try to maintain a more 'balanced' or moderate relationship with alcohol in contexts where 'moderation' is encouraged but remains a slippery and contested concept (Yeomans, 2013). Other participants were already active hybrid drinkers; whilst co-consumption of NoLos and alcohol in a single drinking session was rare, common strategies including switching to NoLos at particular times (NoLos during the week, alcohol at weekends) or in certain spaces (NoLos at home, alcohol when out in bars, pubs or restaurants):

> I think, what I'll probably maintain for quite a while is not drinking [alcohol] at home, just when I go out. I mean I'll have one beer, and then go home, or have one beer with a meal. I just like having the options... I know I'm drinking at a level I'm comfortable with, because it's, literally, one or two a week at most. (Liam, 26, hybrid)

Here, Liam describes what he views as a 'comfortable' and sustainable level of consumption (limiting alcohol consumption to public space) whilst positioning himself as a low-level and 'responsible' drinker (even when he goes out he will just drink 'one beer' or 'one or two a week at most'). Others also talked about switching to NoLo consumption at home and/or during the week, or reserving alcohol consumption for 'occasions', whilst noting that the stigma around not drinking (either long-term or just on a particular occasion) had significantly reduced, making it much more acceptable to choose a NoLo alternative in social contexts. Linking back to earlier discussions, there was an emphasis on being an 'active consumer' (Georgie, 22, hybrid); thus taking responsibility for one's (non)drinking practices, whilst wider structural issues impacting on substance use were downplayed (Atkinson & Sumnall, 2020). These kinds of practices also of course sit within wider discourses around 'responsible consumption' (Caluzzi et al., 2020), expectations around 'disciplining' the body (Beck, 1992) and framings of moderation and self-control as both a personal responsibility and a moral obligation (Room, 2011).

## 'It Doesn't Affect My Mood At All': Supporting Mental Health and Well-Being

Finally, NoLo consumption was bound up with notions of health and well-being. Whilst physical health was discussed as a key motivator for consuming NoLos (with a particular focus on stopping or reducing alcohol consumption to support 'healthy futures' (Nicholls, 2023) and avoid future health conditions), this was much more common amongst older participants. Younger participants were much more likely to associate alcohol with risks to mental—rather than physical—health, and to use NoLo consumption as a means to enjoy some of the pleasure of alcohol (as discussed above) but without the negative effects on mood and well-being, particularly in relation to stress, anxiety and depression. Again, these kinds of findings may be unsurprising as younger cohorts come of age in a society where more open discussion of mental health and well-being is encouraged (Bradbury, 2020):

> The main benefit for me [of a NoLo] is it doesn't have the side-effects of the drug aspect of alcohol. It doesn't affect my mood at all. (Liam, 26, hybrid)

For Liam, the primary benefit of NoLo consumption is the lack of the mood-altering side effects that can be associated with alcohol, particularly the day after drinking. As a young man experiencing depression and low mood, elsewhere in the interview Liam describes strategically using NoLo consumption to be more 'proactive' about managing his mental health, recognising alcohol as a depressant and subjecting every decision to drink it to a 'cost–benefit analysis' where he must consider the implications for his mental well-being (whilst admitting he sees considerations of physical health as a less significant factor). Other young participants agreed that physical health was not a huge motivator for NoLo consumption—suggesting a potential lack of knowledge regarding the physical health risks associated with alcohol (Sanderson et al., 2009)—instead indicating that mental health (particularly in relation to anxiety) had been a much more significant factor in decisions to switch to consuming NoLos and/or to stop drinking alcohol completely.

This is not to say that discussions of physical health were *completely* absent amongst the younger participants as reasons for drinking NoLos, stopping drinking or reducing alcohol consumption (see also Pavlidis et al., 2019). However, any presumed physical health benefits of NoLo consumption tended to be described as 'added bonuses' rather than as a primary motivator for drinking NoLos. For example, Luke (29, non-drinker) described a recent 'spiral' into other more positive health choices (such as stopping smoking and weight loss[1]), whilst others indicated that NoLo consumption helped them break out of unhealthy 'cycles' of sleeping poorly, binging unhealthy food or missing exercise after drinking alcohol. In this sense, NoLos were not necessarily positioned as a 'healthier' choice in and of themselves (and where they were, this was primarily in relation to reduced calorie count rather than the reduction of risks associated with alcohol consumption such as cancer or hypertension), but rather as a tool that supported participants to adopt other 'health-promoting' behaviours demanded under neoliberalism (Crawford, 1980). Wider discourses of healthism are also threaded through these discussions of NoLo consumption, echoing earlier research findings suggesting young people experience increasing pressure to be 'healthy' and may frame drinking (particularly excessively) as incompatible with good mental and physical health (Caluzzi et al., 2021) or even a 'destructive force' in relation to health and well-being (Törrönen et al., 2021).

[1] Whilst 'health' and 'weight loss' are distinct, they were discussed interchangeably by some participants, for example in a tendency to associate the reduced calories in NoLos (compared to alcohol) with 'healthy' choices and to discuss weight loss when asked about physical health.

## Conclusion

For young people, NoLos may be regarded as useful tools that, on the one hand, provide many of the benefits and advantages of alcohol consumption, for example in relation to relaxation, taste, marking periods of transition and celebration and/or providing comparatively new ways to embody the identity of the discerning and tasteful consumer. At the same time, NoLos are felt to lack the more negative perceived effects of drinking (including hangovers, tiredness and/or negative implications for mental and physical health) and—amongst drinkers—to support 'hybrid' consumption practices where NoLos function as a substitute for alcohol.

NoLo consumption can also be explicitly framed as a mechanism to support young people in constructing identities as productive, discerning, moderate and health-conscious consumers in contemporary neoliberal contexts. For example, the lack of hangovers facilitates a more 'productive' use of both work and leisure time and supports young people to navigate 'hustle culture' and work on health, income generation and/or self-improvement during a period of unprecedented anxiety and uncertainty for youth in relation to their futures (Burgess et al., 2022). Associations of NoLos with increased productivity mirror the marketing strategies used to promote 'energy drinks' (products containing caffeine or other stimulants which are targeted predominantly at young people) as boosting mental and/or physical 'performance' (Buchanan et al., 2018). Against a backdrop of healthism where individuals experience increasing pressure to proactively manage health as an individualised and moral obligation, NoLo consumption may also be associated with directly supporting mental health and with enabling wider 'health-promoting' behaviours. The conscious consumption of 'craft' and artisanal NoLos products also facilitates the construction of the discerning, sophisticated and tasteful consumer, potentially aiding in the construction of specific class and gendered identities such as the young 'hipster' (Spracklen et al., 2013).

For drinkers specifically, NoLos may also facilitate more moderate or reduced alcohol consumption, through the proactive and calculated adoption of hybrid consumption models where NoLos can function as a 'substitute' for alcohol at particular times or in particular contexts. In this way, NoLos directly support processes of what Burgess et al. (2022) term 'conscious moderation' and facilitate the construction of particular types of 'responsible' and restrained (non)drinking identities amongst young people. Dominant drinking cultures that normalise binge drinking and 'living in the moment' (Griffin et al., 2009) sit at odds with such values, yet these tensions can be navigated through 'responsible' consumption, whereby consumers can continue to buy into dominant drinking cultures yet show restraint by drinking in moderation and/or participating in periods of abstinence. In this sense, NoLos can be strategically deployed as a way to manage what Lupton (2018) terms the 'neoliberal paradox', that is, the expectation or even pressure to consume (particularly in 'cultures of intoxication' where drinking is normalised as a form of 'empowerment') versus the need to simultaneously maintain control and avoid unhealthy 'excess'. NoLo consumption is thus a distinct practice that might support young adult consumers to embody particular (non)drinking identities of moderation or abstinence, allowing them to show 'responsible' and future-focused behaviour without disengaging completely from the dominant drinking cultures in which young people are often entangled.

These findings expand a limited evidence base around how NoLos are being used by different groups of consumers, contributing to a more detailed and nuanced understanding of the ways in which NoLos are used by both young adult drinkers and non-drinkers. Whilst focusing on a UK context, such findings will likely have resonance in other global contexts where drinking is 'in decline' and NoLo markets are expanding. An enhanced grasp of these practices can ultimately help inform wider discussions about the potentialities of NoLos to alleviate or exacerbate alcohol-related harm. There *was* evidence across the data of substitution (i.e. both younger and older participants replacing alcohol with NoLos in particular contexts and settings) and little to suggest that NoLos were simply being consumed in addition to existing alcohol consumption. Switching to NoLo products and/or abstaining from alcohol in particular contexts and scenarios may contribute to reduced individual alcohol consumption and, more widely, help to normalise socialising without alcohol and function as 'a spring board for more moderate future consumption'

(Conroy & de Visser, 2018, p. 593). Having said this, there is still no strong evidence base to indicate that an expansion of the NoLo market would reduce alcohol-related harm at a societal level; further research into NoLo consumption practices amongst different cohorts/demographics and the resulting implications for public health is imperative.

## References

Anderson, P., Jané-Llopis, E., O'Donnell, A., Manthey, J., & Rehm, J. (2020). Impact of low and no alcohol beers on purchases of alcohol: Interrupted time series analysis of British household shopping data, 2015–2018. *BMJ Open, 10*(10), e036371.

Anderson, P., Kokole, D., & Llopis, E. J. (2021). Production, consumption, and potential public health impact of low-and no-alcohol products: Results of a scoping review. *Nutrients, 13*(9), 3153.

Atkinson, A. M., & Sumnall, H. (2020). Neo-liberal discourse of substance use in the UK reality TV show, The Jeremy Kyle Show. *Drugs: Education, Prevention and Policy, 27*(1), 15–26.

Ball, J., Edwards, R., Sim, D., Cook, H., & Denny, S. (2020). What explains the decline in adolescent binge-drinking in New Zealand? *International Journal of Drug Policy, 84*, 102826.

BBC. (2020). *'Nolo beer' sales rocket thanks to young teetotallers*. https://www.bbc.co.uk/news/business-51833135

Beck, U. (1992). *Risk society: Towards a new modernity*. SAGE.

Bradbury, A. (2020). Mental health stigma: The impact of age and gender on attitudes. *Community Mental Health Journal, 56*(5), 933–938.

Braun, V., & Clarke, V. (2006). Using thematic analysis in psychology. *Qualitative Research in Psychology, 3*(2), 77.

Buchanan, L., Yeatman, H., Kelly, B., & Kariippanon, K. (2018). A thematic content analysis of how marketers promote energy drinks on digital platforms to young Australians. *Australian and New Zealand Journal of Public Health, 42*(6), 530–531.

Burgess, A., Yeomans, H., & Fenton, L. (2022). 'More options… less time' in the 'hustle culture' of 'generation sensible': Individualization and drinking decline among twenty-first century young adults. *The British Journal of Sociology, 73*(4), 903–918.

Butters, A., Kersbergen, I., Holmes, J., & Field, M. (2023). Temporary abstinence challenges: What do we need to know? *Drug and Alcohol Review, 42*(5), 1087–1091.

Caluzzi, G., MacLean, S., Livingston, M., & Pennay, A. (2021). 'No one associates alcohol with being in good health': Health and wellbeing as imperatives to manage alcohol use for young people. *Sociology of Health and Illness, 43*(2), 493–509.

Caluzzi, G., MacLean, S., & Pennay, A. (2020). Re-configured pleasures: How young people feel good through abstaining or moderating their drinking. *International Journal of Drug Policy, 77*, 102709.

Campbell, P. (2022). Viewpoint: *The Rise of NoLo*. Talking Retail. https://www.talkingretail.com/opinion/talking-points/viewpoint-the-rise-of-nolo-02-12-2022/#:~:text=The%20NoLo%20market&text=This%20unexplored%20territory%20highlighted%20a,200%20million%20in%20supermarkets%20alone.

Cederström, C., & Spicer, A. (2015). *The wellness syndrome*. Polity Press.

Chapman, N. G., Nanney, M., Lellock, J. S., & Mikles-Schluterman, J. (2018). Bottling gender: Accomplishing gender through craft beer consumption. *Food, Culture & Society, 21*(3), 296–313.

Cherrier, H., & Gurrieri, L. (2013). Anti-consumption choices performed in a drinking culture: Normative struggles and repairs. *Journal of Macromarketing, 33*(3), 232–244.

Chorley, M., Rossi, L., Tyson, G., & Williams, M. (2016). Pub crawling at scale: Tapping untappd to explore social drinking. *Proceedings of the International AAAI Conference on Web and Social Media, 10*(1), 62–71.

Conroy, D., & de Visser, R. O. (2018). Benefits and drawbacks of social non-drinking identified by British university students. *Drug and Alcohol Review, 37*, 589–597.

Corfe, S., Hyde, R., & Shepherd, J. (2020). *Alcohol-free and low-strength drinks: Understanding their role in reducing alcohol-related harms*. Social Market Foundation / Alcohol Change. https://www.smf.co.uk/publications/no-low-alcohol-harms/

Crawford, R. (1980). Healthism and the medicalization of everyday life. *International Journal of Health Services, 10*(3), 365–388.

Davey, C. (2021). Online sobriety communities for women's problematic alcohol use: a mini review of existing qualitative and quantitative research. *Frontiers in Global Women's Health, 2*, 773921.

de Bruijn, A., van den Wildenberg, E., & van den Broeck, A. (2012). *Commercial promotion of drinking in Europe: Key findings of independent monitoring of alcohol marketing in five European countries. Dutch Institute for Alcohol Policy.* https://eucam.info/wp-content/uploads/2014/04/ammie-eu-rapport_final.pdf

de Visser, R. O., Robinson, E., Smith, T., Cass, G., & Walmsley, M. (2017). The growth of 'Dry January': Promoting participation and the benefits of participation. *European Journal of Public Health, 27*(5), 929–931.

Department of Health & Social Care. (2018). *Low Alcohol Descriptors Guidance.* https://assets.publishing.service.gov.uk/government/uploads/system/uploads/attachment_data/file/763840/low-alcohol-descriptors-guidance.pdf

Fjær, E. G. (2012). The day after drinking: Interaction during hangovers among young Norwegian adults. *Journal of Youth Studies, 15*(8), 995–1010.

Griffin, C., Bengry-Howell, A., Hackley, C., Mistral, W., & Szmigin, I. (2009). Every time I do it I absolutely annihilate myself': Loss of (self-) consciousness and loss of memory in young people's drinking narratives. *Sociology, 43*(3), 457–476.

Harrison, N. J., Norris, C. A., Bartram, A., Murphy, M., Pettigrew, S., Dell, A. O., et al. (2024). "They start on the zero-alcohol and they wanna try the real thing": Parents' views on zero-alcohol beverages and their use by adolescents. *Australian and New Zealand Journal of Public Health, 100119.*

Herring, R., Bayley, M., & Hurcombe, R. (2014). "But no one told me it's okay to not drink": A qualitative study of young people who drink little or no alcohol. *Journal of Substance Use*, 19(1-2), 95-102.

Hill, K. M., Johansson, M., Smith, J., Brown, K., & Davies, E. L. (2022). Connecting through dance: Understanding conscious clubbing event experiences. *Qualitative Health Research, 32*(11), 1721–1731.

Ikäheimo, J. (2020). Exclusive craft beer events: Liminoid spaces of performative craft consumption. *Food, Culture & Society, 23*(3), 296–314.

Järvinen, M., Ellergaard, C. H., & Larsen, A. G. (2014). Drinking successfully: Alcohol consumption, taste and social status. *Journal of Consumer Culture, 14*(3), 384–405.

Kaewpramkusol, R., Senior, K., Nanthamongkolchai, S., & Chenhall, R. (2019). Brand advertising and brand sharing of alcoholic and non-alcoholic products, and the effects on young Thai people's attitudes towards alcohol use: A qualitative focus group study. *Drug and Alcohol Review, 38*(3), 284–293.

Kokole, D. (2021). *Who drinks zero and low alcohol beer in Great Britain?* Institute of Alcohol Studies. https://www.ias.org.uk/2021/12/08/who-drinks-zero-and-low-alcohol-beer-in-great-britain/

Kokole, D., Jané Llopis, E., & Anderson, P. (2022). Non-alcoholic beer in the European Union and UK: Availability and apparent consumption. *Drug and Alcohol Review, 41*(3), 550–560.

Livingston, M., Callinan, S., Raninen, J., Pennay, A., & Dietze, P. M. (2018). Alcohol consumption trends in Australia: Comparing surveys and sales-based measures. *Drug and Alcohol Review, 37*, S9–S14.

Lupton, D. (2018). *Fat* (2nd ed.). Routledge.

Miller, M., Pettigrew, S., & Wright, C. J. (2022). Zero-alcohol beverages: Harm-minimisation tool or gateway drink? *Drug and Alcohol Review, 41*(3), 546–549.

Myles, C. C., Weil, B. V., Wiley, D., & Watson, B. (2022). Representations of low (er) alcohol (craft) beer in the United States. *Nutrients, 14*(23), 4952.

Nanney, M., Chapman, N. G., Lellock, J. S., & Mikles-Schluterman, J. (2020). Gendered expectations, gatekeeping, and consumption in craft beer spaces. *Humanity & Society, 44*(4), 449–468.

Ng Fat, L., Shelton, N., & Cable, N. (2018). Investigating the growing trend of non-drinking among young people; Analysis of repeated cross-sectional surveys in England 2005–2015. *BMC Public Health, 18*, 1090.

Nicholls, E. (2023). 'Not Just Living in the Moment': Constructing the 'Enterprising' and future-oriented self through the consumption of no-and-low-alcohol drinks. *Sociological Research Online, 13607804231191063.*

Nicholls, E., & Conroy, D. (2021). Possibilities and pitfalls? Moderate drinking and alcohol abstinence at home since the COVID-19 lockdown. *International Journal of Drug Policy, 88*, 103025.

Oldham, M., Holmes, J., Whitaker, V., Fairbrother, H., & Curtis, P. (2018). *Youth drinking in decline*. Sheffield.

Pape, H., Rossow, I., & Brunborg, G. S. (2018). Adolescents drink less: How, who and why? A review of the recent research literature. *Drug and Alcohol Review, 37*, S98–S114.

Pavlidis, A., Ojajarvi, A., & Bennett, A. (2019). Young people and alcohol abstention: Youth cultural practices and being a non-drinker in Finland and Australia. *Journal of Youth Studies, 22*(8), 1101–1116.

Porretta, S., & Donadini, G. (2008). A preference study for no alcohol beer in Italy using quantitative concept analysis. *Journal of the Institute of Brewing, 114*(4), 315–321.

Rehm, J., Lachenmeier, D. W., Llopis, E. J., Imtiaz, S., & Anderson, P. (2016). Evidence of reducing ethanol content in beverages to reduce harmful use of alcohol. *The Lancet Gastroenterology & Hepatology, 1*(1), 78–83.

Roberts, A., Rogers, J., Mason, R., Siriwardena, A. N., Hogue, T., Whitley, G. A., & Law, G. R. (2021). Alcohol and other substance use during the COVID-19 pandemic: A systematic review. *Drug and Alcohol Dependence, 229*, 109150.

Room, R. (2011). Addiction and personal responsibility as solutions to the contradictions of neoliberal consumerism. In K. Bell, A. Salmon, & D. McNaughton (Eds.), *Alcohol, Tobacco, Obesity and The New Public Health* (pp. 47–58). Routledge.

Rose, N. (1998). *Inventing our selves: Psychology, power and personhood.* Cambridge University Press.

Sanderson, S. C., Waller, J., Jarvis, M. J., Humphries, S. E., & Wardle, J. (2009). Awareness of lifestyle risk factors for cancer and heart disease among adults in the UK. *Patient Education and Counseling, 74*(2), 221–227.

Spracklen, K., Laurencic, J., & Kenyon, A. (2013). 'Mine's a Pint of Bitter': Performativity, gender, class and representations of authenticity in real-ale tourism. *Tourist Studies, 13*(3), 304–321.

Szmigin, I., Griffin, C., Mistral, W., Bengry-Howell, A., Weale, L., & Hackley, C. (2008). Re-framing 'binge drinking' as calculated hedonism: Empirical evidence from the UK. *International Journal of Drug Policy, 19*(5), 359–366.

Thurnell-Read, T. (2016). 'Real ale' enthusiasts, serious leisure and the costs of getting 'too serious' about beer. *Leisure Sciences, 38*(1), 68–84.

Törrönen, J., Samuelsson, E., Roumeliotis, F., Room, R., & Kraus, L. (2021). 'Social health', 'physical health', and wellbeing: Analysing with bourdieusian concepts the interplay between the practices of heavy drinking and exercise among young people. *International Journal of Drug Policy, 91*, 102825.

Vashishtha, R., Pennay, A., Dietze, P., Marzan, M. B., Room, R., & Livingston, M. (2021). Trends in adolescent drinking across 39 high-income countries: Exploring the timing and magnitude of decline. *European Journal of Public Health, 31*(2), 424–431.

Vasiljevic, M., Coulter, L., Petticrew, M., & Marteau, T. M. (2018). Marketing messages accompanying online selling of low/er and regular strength wine and beer products in the UK: A content analysis. *BMC Public Health, 18*(1), 147.

Waehning, N., & Wells, V. K. (2024). Product, individual and environmental factors impacting the consumption of no and low alcoholic drinks: A systematic review and future research agenda. *Food Quality and Preference*, 105163.

Wallace, A. (2019). 'Brewing the truth': Craft beer, class and place in contemporary London. *Sociology, 53*(5), 951–966.

Yeomans, H. (2013). Blurred visions: Experts, evidence and the promotion of moderate drinking. In T. T. Smith & J. Holmwood (Eds.), *Sociologies of moderation: Problems of democracy, expertise and the media*. Wiley Blackwell.

# Part IV

## Young Adult Drinking Spaces: Staying Inside; Going Outside; Digital Spaces

# 12

# Social Media, Alcohol Marketing, and Young Adults' Drinking Cultures

Ian Goodwin and Antonia Lyons

**Abstract** Young people are heavy users of social media, and social media play a central role in young adults' drinking cultures and practices. Social media are replete with positive references to alcohol, which are positively associated with alcohol use. Yet social media have also been linked to recent declines in youth drinking seen in high-income countries. Alcohol marketing on these platforms is interactive, engaging, and dynamic. This chapter briefly overviews some key developments in research on social media and drinking cultures in young adults, and considers three contemporary technological developments: (1) the rapid growth of a mobile social media ecology with diverse and differentiated platforms; (2)

I. Goodwin (✉)
School of Cultures, Languages and Linguistics, University of Auckland, Auckland, New Zealand
e-mail: ian.goodwin@auckland.ac.nz

A. Lyons
Department of Social and Community Health, Centre for Addiction Research, University of Auckland, Auckland, New Zealand
e-mail: antonia.lyons@auckland.ac.nz



D. Conroy, F. Measham (eds.), *Young Adult Drinking Styles*, Sustainable Development Goals Series, https://doi.org/10.1007/978-3-031-98528-7_12

alcohol marketing on data-driven and algorithmic platforms; and (3) evolving media automation, which means that users generate data that continually intersects with recursive, automatic algorithmic decision making. We conclude by considering what these shifts mean for alcohol researchers and those working in health promotion and alcohol policy, and the unique challenges they pose.

Social media are now pivotal to the traditional concerns of alcohol researchers, as well as to those interested in youth culture, leisure practices, and the life experiences of young adults more generally. The study of social media and drinking cultures is a dynamic field in which technologies, commercial activities, and young people's practices have changed rapidly. In this chapter, we provide a brief overview of some of the key developments in the research on social media and drinking cultures in young adults, and then focus on three conceptual issues that are relevant for researchers seeking to gain insight into young adults' contemporary drinking cultures and practices.

Social media are "networked database platforms that combine public with personal communication" (Meikle, 2016, p. 6). Early research exploring young adults, drinking, and social media focused overwhelmingly on Facebook (Boyle et al., 2017), which made sense when Facebook dominated online sociality. With over 3.03 billion monthly active users as of October 2023 (Statistica, 2023), Facebook remains the largest social media platform in the world and retains a central role in many Internet users' lives, one that we still need to understand (Sujon et al., 2018). Yet there has been a notable proliferation of social media characterised by intensive engagement across numerous, differentiated, and always-on platforms, leading to a more dynamic form of 'cybernetic' sociality associated with multiple information flows and real-time feedback. Young adults have been particularly enthusiastic adopters of platforms like Instagram, Snapchat, and TikTok (Auxier and Anderson, 2021). Moreover, use of both Snapchat and Instagram is associated with an exceptionally steep 'age gradient', with their popularity dropping much faster with age than older platforms like Facebook (Ortiz-Ospina, 2019).

Research has consistently demonstrated links between alcohol content on social media platforms and the health and well-being of young people. This work demonstrates the pervasiveness of positive references to alcohol on young people's social media profiles (e.g. Beullens & Schepers, 2013; Vanherle et al., 2023), and its positive association with intentions to drink in ways that may pose a health risk (Mesman et al., 2020). For example, being exposed to alcohol content on social media has been found to be directly and indirectly related to alcohol consumption in emerging adults, but this was not the case for alcohol content seen in traditional media (Geusens & Beullens, 2023). A range of theories are drawn on to explain these associations, including social identity (Pegg et al., 2018), drinking identities, and possible and future selves (e.g. Geusens & Beullens, 2023). The research in this field has primarily used observational designs, and these consistently demonstrate associations between online alcohol content and drinking behaviours. This raises concerns that social media create "intoxigenic digital spaces" (Griffiths & Casswell, 2010, p. 525) or in other words, online alcohol-promoting environments, that are potentially damaging to public health (McCreanor et al., 2013).

Simultaneously, social media and changes in communication technology have been identified as one factor (of many) that contributes to the overall decline in young people's drinking evidenced in recent years in high-income countries (Room et al., 2020). Increasingly young people have used social media to socialise with peers, connect with others, and start romantic relationships, meaning there are fewer opportunities to drink alcohol (Luomanen & Alasuutari, 2022). Research also suggests that young people in high-income countries have increasing concerns about their futures and economic security, and see drinking alcohol as a risky practice that needs moderating due to health and well-being factors, as well as managing their time in responsible ways (Goodwin & Griffin, 2017; Pennay et al., 2024). Evidence also indicates that heavy drinking does not function as a way to rebel, or form identities, for young people in the same way it did in previous generations (Livingston et al., 2024). Social media can heighten the risks of heavy drinking, with behaviours while intoxicated captured in photos and videos on mobile devices and potentially shared widely through platforms. Such records of drinking activities can be permanent and may jeopardise job-seeking, education, and future success (Pennay et al., 2024).

Researchers have also sought to gain understanding of young adults' drinking-related social media activities as a form of online drinking *culture*. Here the emphasis has been on investigating how drinking displays online relate to the forging of young adults' identities (e.g. Lindsay & Supski, 2017; Goodwin & Griffin, 2017; Niland et al., 2014), and examining the close links between alcohol consumption, social media use, and the maintenance of young adults' intimate social ties and broader social worlds (e.g. Niland et al., 2015). Focusing on drinking as a leisure practice imbued with power relations, some of this work has usefully documented how class, gender, and ethnicity structures young adults' engagement with online drinking displays (e.g. Atkinson & Sumnall, 2016; Hutton et al., 2016; Moewaka Barnes et al., 2016, 2017). These studies highlight that drinking and its online display are recognised as a means for young adults to exercise considerable autonomy and agency as they engage in leisure practices, narrate their own sense of identity, forge and maintain friendships, and develop sociality. Simultaneously however, such practices are subject to, and potentially reproductive of, broader power relations that can limit, constrain, or shape young adults' lives in problematic or even disempowering ways.

Scholars in this field have also developed a growing critical awareness of the ways in which the software architectures and affordances of platforms (i.e. their functionalities and the online actions they both enable and constrain) influence the social interactions and user activities that occur on them, including drinking-related displays and behaviours. While platforms do not simplistically determine what users do, they are far from neutral facilitators of user activities (Bucher, 2018). The particular form and functionality of the virtual environments made available through specific platforms has "wide-ranging consequences (whether intentional or not) for the types of public interaction and participation made possible" (Wahl-Jorgensen, 2018, p. 78). More broadly, social media platforms are routinely designed to create powerful imperatives to share personal and social information with others in the network (Wahl-Jorgensen, 2018; van Dijck, 2013). One of the key aspects of such 'architectural' influences on social media platforms is the data-driven and algorithmic nature of their interfaces, which are designed to hone in on the data the user provides to shape the user experience (Bucher, 2018).

This includes popular user-generated content such as drinking photos (Goodwin et al., 2016). It also encompasses any demographic information supplied, users' professed interests, their specific social network, and their geographic location. By using algorithmic code to examine such data, the system comprehensively learns a wide range of "individual preferences that determine the unique feed of content that the user will see" (Carah & Meurk, 2017, p. 370). This process is tied to novel platform business models that "exploit the possibilities of networked digital media" (Meikle, 2016, p. 6) for profit, and this includes the involvement of alcohol corporations that now use algorithmic sorting of content to maximise marketing opportunities, as we describe in more detail later.

Overall, much of the research in this area is exploratory, cross-sectional, and observational. There is much less experimental research, and studies that have been conducted have tended to focus on the effects of exposure to digital alcohol marketing content (see Noel et al., 2020, for a review). Evidence at this point highlights a proliferation of social media platforms that young adults routinely engage with, a pervasiveness of both user-generated and commercial alcohol content within their online cultures, and an increasing awareness of the architectures and underlying commercial imperatives of social media platforms by both users and researchers.

In the following sections, we concentrate on three conceptual issues that provide insight into these contemporary technological developments, including (1) the rapid growth of a mobile social media ecology with diverse and differentiated social media platforms engaged within real-time; (2) the novel characteristics of alcohol marketing on data-driven and algorithmic social media platforms that are increasingly integrated with the lived experiences of young people within drinking cultures; (3) how this data-driven and participatory process has culminated in user experiences and alcohol marketing on social media being increasingly bound up with media automation, whereby user agency generates data that intersects with recursive, automatic algorithmic decision making within novel marketing strategies.

## A Social Media Ecology That Is Mobile, Always-On and Involves Multiple Different Platforms

Smartphones now host social media, and they have become more powerful, cheaper, smaller, and increasingly part of everyday life (Mackey, 2016). Contemporary social media are therefore 'mobile first'. Even Facebook, originally accessed through the desktop PC, has evolved into a mobile platform that has enabled it to play a more central role in young people's sociality and the last-minute micro-coordination of social events (Bertel & Ling, 2016). A range of studies have demonstrated the increasingly central role of mobile social media in enhancing young adults' sense of pervasive and perpetual virtual contact with physically absent friends (e.g. Thulin, 2017; Thulan et al., 2020). These developments have important spatial and temporal effects on young adults' sociality. The ability to sustain perpetual contact with peer networks, alongside a continual ambient background awareness of absent others, produces an increasingly 'always-on' social media culture. Early studies on smartphones, social media, and drinking have highlighted that novel 'real-time' influences on young adults' drinking experiences are emerging as central to nightlife experiences, enabling an intensified synchronisation of young adults' sociality while linking disparate drinking spaces (e.g. see Truong, 2018; Hebden, 2023). This suggests social media have become a much more integral part of the drinking experience, continuously involved in drinking practices, event planning, deciding where and what to drink, and with whom.

An always-on social media culture has also provided a much firmer basis for the proliferation of numerous and differentiated social media platforms that increasingly fill different social niches and serve different purposes in young adults' social lives, nightlife experiences, and leisure practices. A *social media ecology* perspective captures the complex ways in which users now negotiate multiple platforms to meet their social and communicative needs (Zhao et al., 2016). Young adults select which platform to use based on the audience and the nature of the content they wish to share, sometimes preserving strict boundaries between platforms while at other times deliberately sharing content across platforms (Zhao et al., 2016). As a result, young adults now routinely engage with a multifaceted social media ecology, and their drinking cultures therefore increasingly interrelate to the varying social norms and practices that are emerging across a multiplicity of social media. For example, research has highlighted the unique technological affordances of micro-blogging on Twitter as a means for widely sharing drinking content that may promote alcohol consumption (Alhabash et al., 2018; Cavazos-Rehg et al., 2015). Other research has demonstrated that alcohol posts are positively framed on both Facebook and Instagram (Hendriks et al., 2018), suggesting the online practices prevalent on both may allow for the entrenchment and promotion of drinking in young adults' everyday lives. In an attempt to tease out differences that may exist across social media platforms, Boyle et al. (2017) used hypothetical, photographic vignettes of glamorised or negative portrayals of alcohol consumption, asking young adults where they would likely come across this content. Results showed that Instagram (now X) was viewed as most likely destination for photos depicting alcohol use as attractive and glamorous, while Snapchat was the most likely for sharing negative portrayals. Other research shows that TikTok has emerged with its own distinctive form of drinking displays associated with popular short form videos that that minimise the negative effects of drinking while demonstrating "a propensity to promote rapid consumption of multiple drinks and to juxtapose alcohol use with positive associations such as humor and camaraderie" (Russell et al., 2021, p. 615). BeReal is a more recent social media platform that emphasises authenticity and sharing 'in the moment', encouraging spontaneity, fun, and close relationships, and removing the need for polished self-presentations (Reddy & Kumar, 2024). Research has yet to explore how BeReal is used in drinking practices and cultures, although it may be appealing for friends who regularly drink together.

The concept of 'social media repertoires' was introduced by Boczkowski et al. (2018) to help make sense of users' now routine and frequent engagement with a range of different platforms. Repertoires point to shared constellations of meanings that help young adult users stabilise, understand, and navigate what is acceptable and desirable on each platform. Repertoires are always dynamic, and particularly subject to change as new platforms are introduced. However, there are key recognisable differences across different social media: WhatsApp is a multifaceted communication space; Facebook is a space for the display of a carefully crafted and socially acceptable self; Instagram is an environment for more stylised forms of self-presentation; Twitter (now X) is valued for information and informality; and Snapchat is a platform for more spontaneous and ludic forms of connection (Boczkowski et al., 2018). In this way there is a certain relational *calculus* involving the entire social media ecology here, one that shapes an understanding of matters such as what to post where, what comments are appropriate, what one should share and what one should not (Boczkowski et al., 2018). This calculus involves both relational and emotional dynamics across a variety of social domains. Most young adults now undertake their sociality, work, cultural lives, and leisure practices within this social media ecology, in a variegated, dynamic, and complex fashion that alcohol researchers need to understand. Young people construct their identities across multiple social media platforms in ongoing, dynamic, and differentiated ways, and these processes may play a role in relationships between exposure to alcohol content on social media and alcohol use (e.g. see Pegg et al., 2018; Geusens & Beullens, 2023).

Different platform repertoires produce divergent online cultures that provide increasing agency for young adult users whilst also limiting what can be achieved and what is considered normative and acceptable (Buehler, 2017). Differences in the technological affordances offered by social media matter to this meaning-laden process. For example, Snapchat's key technological innovation when it was introduced in 2011 may well have been the ephemeral nature of the content posted to the platform: rather than archiving content, it is displayed for a limited time before disappearing. This results in the platform offering less social support than other platforms, but it also leads to users experiencing Snapchat as more lightweight, enjoyable, and fun than other platforms, and it tends to reduce "self-presentational concerns" (Bayer et al., 2016). It is easy to see why Snapchat was subsequently appropriated by young adults as a key part of their drinking cultures, given they view drinking with close friends as pleasurable, involving having fun and being sociable (Lyons & Willot, 2008). The perceived appropriateness of Snapchat vis-à-vis sites like Facebook as a destination for 'negative' drinking events (Boyle et al., 2017) also makes sense considering its emphasis on ephemerality, and the success of Snapchat's ephemeral affordances helps explain why other platforms subsequently incorporated their own options for posting temporary content into their interfaces (e.g. the 'stories' feature on Instagram). Similarly, TikTok's emphasis on short-form vertical video has proven highly popular with users, allowing for new forms of ludic sociality that have quickly become associated with positively framed drinking displays (Russell et al., 2021). Following TikTok's success with short-form vertical video it has also recently been incorporated into the interfaces of other platforms (e.g. YouTube).

Better understanding of young people's drinking practices requires insight into such dynamic interconnections between the social and the technological. Detailed analyses of the specific technological affordances offered by divergent social media are required: both singularly in terms of the unique cultures they facilitate *and* in terms of their *relative* place within the whole. Affordances affect the particular repertoires young adults associate with specific platforms, the subsequent comparative position the platform holds within the social media ecology, and its subsequent role in facilitating specific aspects of young people's drinking practices and displays.

## Social Media and Novel Alcohol Marketing Strategies: User Experiences, Data, and Algorithms

Research has demonstrated that commercial alcohol interests moved quickly to take advantage of young adults' enthusiasm for alcohol-related content on social media (Nicholls, 2012; Niland et al., 2017). Various studies of the wide range of marketing activities by alcohol corporations on social media have become a focus of analysis (McCreanor et al., 2013; Room & O'Brien, 2021). In a systematic review of 47 studies in this growing field, Lobstein et al. (2017) concluded that branded marketing messages were highly appealing to young adults, violated alcohol advertising codes, and showed a positive association between exposure to digital marketing and higher levels of drinking. Studies were cross-sectional and did not use controlled interventions or experimental designs, so cannot determine causality. Some scholars argue there is evidence for causal relationships between traditional forms of alcohol advertising exposure and consumption in young people (Sargent & Babor, 2020). This is likely to be a particularly pressing issue for social media given this is where the marketing spend of alcohol corporations is increasingly concentrated (Room & O'Brien, 2021), and where there are vast numbers of young users. Reviews have demonstrated that among young people, being exposed to digital marketing is related to higher levels of alcohol consumption (Lobstein et al., 2017) while engaging with this marketing is related to increased drinking (Noel et al., 2020). This has raised a series of public policy concerns about the difficulties of regulating such activities (Jernigan & Ross, 2020; Mart, 2017), which may subvert current alcohol marketing codes (Lobstein et al., 2017). It is also worth noting that marketing of alcohol on social media and in other digital channels occurs within a broader context. Bain et al. (2023) found that adolescents in Australia who were exposed to alcohol marketing across a range of contexts (including digital, television, sporting events) had increased alcohol consumption.

This intensive commercial activity suggests that, when we consider the new capacities that novel technological affordances offer 'users' of social media, it is important that we do not confine ourselves to end-users alone but equally explore advertisers as an important user group (Bucher & Helmond, 2017). Social media platforms continue to be programmable informational architectures built on an economic model that relies on connecting end-users to advertisers-as-users in increasingly sophisticated, efficient, and effective ways (Helmond, 2015; Meikle, 2016). As Carah and Shaul (2016) argue in their analysis of vodka brand Smirnoff (owned by Diageo), this suggests that brands have become crucial to "the ongoing experimentation that underpins the development of mobile social media platforms" (p. 69). Alcohol marketing is apparent across all major social media platforms; it is highly sophisticated and its content is continually changing based on this ongoing experimentation. In this way it can develop in ever-more effective ways to be embedded within young people's feeds and interactions in ways that make it normalised (and unable to be accessed by public health researchers interested in this content). Also, it is worth noting that while TikTok previously restricted alcohol marketing on its platform, this restriction was lifted in mid-2024.

Focused on maximising marketing opportunities, this experimentation has resulted in a number of novel developments that draw on the unique ability of social media platforms to algorithmically sort content. Rather than seeking to control the 'message', these work by stimulating and managing user engagement with branded content (liking, commenting, sharing, tagging), seeking to deeply embed brands in the everyday identity work and sociality of platform users (Carah et al., 2014). Via this process, users' expressions, movements, relationships, and leisure practices are rendered into data that can be algorithmically analysed to capture and direct user attention, make predictions about their likely consumer behaviours, and target advertisements towards them—thereby combining the data-driven and participatory affordances of platforms in powerfully productive ways for alcohol marketers (Carah & Brodmerkel, 2021). This unprecedented datafication captures and measures aspects of users' social lives that have never been quantified before (van Dijck et al., 2018), and in the process users *themselves* come to circulate and help construct alcohol marketing as an inherent part of developing their online drinking cultures. They can enjoy engaging with branded content that seamlessly appears as part of their individually tailored and tuned social media feeds (Lyons et al., 2023). As users engage with the interface in this manner, the line between user-generated and commercial content becomes fundamentally blurred (Atkinson et al., 2017; Goodwin et al., 2016).

By integrating itself so thoroughly with a technologically sophisticated and diverse social media ecology, alcohol marketing becomes progressively enmeshed in everyday life, and it is the smartphone that is particularly important to this process of real-world engagement across social settings (Carah & Brodmerkel, 2021; Lyons et al., 2017). For example, the vodka brand Smirnoff (owned by Diageo) creates purpose-built bars at cultural events like music festivals, replete with branding, and invites celebrities and musicians to party with consumers while there (Carah & Shaul, 2016). Photography via smartphones is encouraged, and hashtags promoted at the venue for coordinating the subsequent flow of images as they are uploaded by partygoers to Instagram. This attracts the attention of their followers, who then spread the content across the platform in ways mediated by Instagram's algorithms (algorithms that, over time, can be fine-tuned to aid this process). The reach of the "brand activation" (p. 74) at the festival can then be assessed by Diageo using various forms of user-generated data made available by the platform. As these interactive real-time campaigns develop, Diageo can learn about individual consumer lifestyles and preferences, and subsequently increasingly target those who are most likely to consume alcohol with further marketing. As the data-driven capacity for social media to organise and direct social life has advanced, such targeted marketing has become increasingly logistical, combining advertising exposure with the organisation of retail purchases and alcohol delivery via custom-built apps and websites that are seamlessly integrated with platforms (Carah & Brodmerkel, 2021).

These sophisticated commercial activities explicitly measure, access, and make use of users' differentiated forms of meaning making and diverse forms of sociality as they emerge and change across the social media ecology. The form of glamorous partying Smirnoff encourages in Carah and Shaul's (2016) analysis of music festivals fits well with the specific "repertoire" users associate with Instagram as "an environment for stylized self-presentation" (Boczkowski et al., 2018, p. 1). Smirnoff does not simply target the 'audience' on Instagram with promotional messages but rather helps to *co-produce* 'appropriate' uses of Instagram and its relative positioning within the social media ecology. Instagram becomes an environment where the stylised production of the self is enacted within and through specific forms of glamorous alcohol consumption, in a seamless manner. 'Appropriate' user-generated and commercial content on Instagram become mutually reinforcing and essentially indistinguishable, and this equally applies to the diverse platforms that are competitors to Instagram. Brand co-creation of repertoires on alternative platforms such as Facebook and Snapchat broadens marketing opportunities, as the goal becomes the viral circulation of commercial content appropriate for each specific platform and user base. In each case, quality time spent engaging with brands becomes the marketing focus, because it is the quality of engagement that is most useful as data for the algorithmic sorting and prioritising of marketing content. This brand co-creation also usually falls outside of marketing regulations in countries that have implemented a ban on digital alcohol marketing (Norman et al., 2024).

Alcohol marketing on social media draws on young people's identities in various ways, including how it engages users and enables multiple possibilities for interaction. The gendered nature of alcohol marketing is nothing new, and has been used heavily by the alcohol industry to segment markets and increase the sales of alcohol products for decades. However, for many young people, alcohol marketing is enmeshed in everyday life through their smartphone social media feeds in gendered ways. This marketing engages and encourages interaction with brands in ways that affect how people think about gender, women, and drinking, and how they construct their own gender identities (Atkinson et al., 2022). Additionally, a recent review of alcohol marketing that targets sexual and gender-diverse minorities found that, in socially liberal environments, it saturates these communities, and its reach has been extended through social media which allowed for more subtle ways of promoting alcohol products and normalising a culture of intoxication (Whiteley et al., 2023).

## Automated Alcohol Marketing as the Culmination of Data Capture and Algorithmic Processing

As more and more of users' social activities, online displays, and brand engagements are rendered into data to drive algorithmic processing, decision making within alcohol marketing strategies on social media becomes progressively managed in ways that require less human oversight or intervention. This involves more than simply exposure to a personalised marketing message—that is, more than algorithmic platform interfaces quantifying, measuring, and documenting user preferences and then microtargeting tailored alcohol advertisements towards them. Rather, this is simply the beginning of a process of continually optimising relationships between audiences and alcohol brands using tools like analytics dashboards, beacons, and pixels (Carah & Brodmerkel, 2021). These novel platform affordances help advertisers track the online actions of alcohol consumers after being exposed (tracking likes, comments, shares, click rates etc.), which in turn allows for combinations between ads and audiences to be "automatically generated, tested, and refined by the platform's advertising model (Carah & Brodmerkel, 2021, p. 21). Meta's algorithmic "Ads Manager" model, which organises and structures advertisers' access to both Facebook and Instagram, is perhaps the most advanced, feature-rich advertising system for this purpose in use today (Ali et al., 2019). Using Ads Manager, alcohol advertisers can hand over control to Meta's algorithms which then automatically place ads, closely measure objectives set for them (which include logistical outcomes like completing a retail alcohol purchase), work out the best way to achieve objectives through trialling different combinations of ads, ad formats, ad placements, and ad timing, and then "funnel campaign resources to make the most of this emergent, machinic knowledge in real-time" (Goodwin, 2022, p. 7). Within this automated system, alcohol advertisements are constantly modified, becoming highly dynamic variables in an experimental process that acts upon and reacts to young people's real-time actions in drinking cultures (Carah & Brodmerkel, 2021; Goodwin, 2022). The status of an advertisement as a discrete "text" with a stable personalised message refined by the advertiser for the targeted individual is challenged within this system.

While such automated developments are becoming the norm on social media, they do not undermine the pleasures many young people experience in youth drinking cultures, which remain spaces where they exercise considerable agency in identity performances and online sociality. Young people still make choices and are not coerced on social media, but automated marketing does threaten their autonomy through the experimental manipulation of their choice environment (Coeckelbergh, 2022). There is a potential here for commerciality to become ever more seamlessly integrated with sociality in youth drinking cultures in dynamic, changeable, and personalised ways that make young people's exposure to alcohol marketing messages less publicly visible, and therefore less accountable and less open to public debate (Carah & Brodmerkel, 2021).

The actual efficacy of these new marketing methods, which some argue are no more influential than older forms of marketing despite their novelties, remains a matter for ongoing debate (Samuel et al., 2021) and are difficult to test in observational research. Nevertheless, it is not yet clear that forms of automated marketing of addictive products like alcohol can be developed in ways that do not disproportionately harm vulnerable consumers or consumer groups (Goodwin, 2022). While a lack of transparency remains a crucial issue, the design of these systems does suggest an inevitable targeting of heavy consumers of alcohol with a greater proportion of campaign advertising. The issue here is not simply that advertising is now logistical, allowing for completion of a retail purchase, but that increasingly intensive data collection allows for algorithmically tuning content in ways that can influence young people's "affects, moods, emotions and desires in order to increase profits" (Lyons et al., 2023, p. 1). There is evidence, for example, that automated marketing worked to intensify advertising that was context, place, and time specific, and that played upon young people's anxieties and vulnerabilities, during the COVID-19 pandemic (Lyons et al., 2023).

Thomas and Kininmonth (2023) argue that developments in automated marketing on social media are just a small subset of a much wider shift to an automated media economy. This involves data collection and algorithmic processing that now enables automated decision making across a growing range of contexts, including, for example, content recommendation systems within and beyond social media, the generation of automated news stories, search engine results, and so on. The ultimate impact of these developments is up for debate, but it does seem undeniable that more intensive and powerful forms of automation are set to impact on online youth drinking cultures in a myriad of ways. As researchers we need to be aware of these changes, and carefully consider them with an open mind as we conceptualise, design, and develop our work around young people's alcohol consumption and drinking cultures.

## Conclusions

We have come a long way, in a relatively short period, in our understandings of the complex inter-relationships between young adults, drinking cultures, and social media. Alcohol content has been found to be pervasive within many young people's social media feeds and profiles, including alcohol marketing that is using increasingly sophisticated—and automated—technologies. All of these aspects of alcohol, youth cultures, and social media have been found to have social, cultural, and health consequences. A dynamic, real-time, mobile social media ecology has emerged that has implications for new forms of identity work, sociality, and social practices for young adults and their drinking cultures. Yet this is fundamentally a commercially driven environment in which vast profits are made by alcohol corporations, drawing on and using enormous datasets that include users' intimate content and daily routines. This all raises methodological implications for how best to study and therefore understand new forms of drinking cultures. We need to learn more about how specific alcohol content reaches particular subgroups of young people on social media. The way that social media platforms operate means that researchers cannot access the information that appears within people's social media feeds, unless users share it with them. There is a lack of full transparency of commercial alcohol promotion on social media platforms, and most platforms do not allow researchers to fully access commercial content (while Meta has an Ad library that can be reviewed, it is not possible to request and obtain all the data that goes into an alcohol promotion on Instagram, for example). Yet such data is crucial for developing alcohol policy and regulations that can help to limit harm from alcohol products. We also know very little about how young people appropriate, react to, or perhaps even subvert and resist, automated systems, and understanding and insight here need to be a much stronger aspect of our research agenda going forward.

## References

Alhabash, S., VanDam, C., Tan, P., et al. (2018). 140 characters of intoxication: Exploring the prevalence of alcohol-related tweets and predicting their virality. *Sage Open*, 1–15.

Ali, M., Sapiezynski, P., Bogen, N., & ... Riekle, A. (2019) Discrimination through optimization: How Facebook's ad delivery can lead to biased outcomes. In *Proceedings of the ACM on Human-Computer Interaction*, 3(CSCW), Article 199.

Atkinson, A., Ross-Houle, M., Begley, E., & Sumnall, H. (2017). An exploration of alcohol advertising on social networking sites: An analysis of content, interactions and young people's perspectives. *Addiction Research and Theory, 25*(2), 91–102.

Atkinson, A. M., Meadows, B. R., Emslie, C., Lyons, A., & Sumnall, H. R. (2022). 'Pretty in Pink' and 'Girl Power': An analysis of the targeting and representation of women in alcohol brand marketing on Facebook and Instagram. *International Journal of Drug Policy, 101*, 103547.

Atkinson, A. M., & Sumnall, H. R. (2016). 'If I don't look good, it just doesn't go up': A qualitative study of young women's drinking cultures and practices on Social Network Sites. *International Journal of Drug Policy, 38*, 50–62.

Auxier, B., & Anderson, M. (2021). Social media use in 2021. *Pew Research Center, 1*, 1–4.

Bain, E., Scully, M., Wakefield, M., Durkin, S., & White, V. (2023). Association between single-channel and cumulative exposure to alcohol advertising and drinking behaviours among Australian adolescents. *Drug and Alcohol Review, 42*(1), 59–67.

Bayer, J., Ellison, N., Schoenebeck, S., & Falk, E. (2016). Sharing the small moments: Ephemeral social interaction on Snapchat. *Information, Communication and Society, 19*(7), 956–977.

Bertel, T., & Ling, R. (2016). "It's just not that exciting anymore": The changing centrality of SMS in the everyday lives of young Danes. *New Media and Society, 18*(7), 1293–1309.

Beullens, K., & Schepers, A. (2013). Display of alcohol use on Facebook: A content analysis. *Cyberpschology, Behaviour and Social Networking, 16*(7), 497–503.

Boczkowski, P., Matassi, M., & Mitchelstein, E. (2018). How young users deal with multiple platforms: The role of meaning-making in social media repertoires. *Journal of Computer Mediated Communication*, 1–15.

Boyle, S., Earle, A., LaBrie, J., & Ballou, K. (2017). Facebook dethroned: Revealing the more likely social media destinations for college students' depiction of underage drinking. *Addictive Behaviours, 65*, 63–67.

Bucher, T. (2018). *If... then: Algorithmic culture and politics*. Oxford University Press.

Bucher, T., & Helmond, A. (2017). The affordances of social media platforms. In J. Burgess, T. Poell, & A. Marwick (Eds.), *Sage handbook of social media* (pp. 233–253). Sage.

Buehler, E. (2017) "You shouldn't use Facebook for that." Navigating norm violations while seeking emotional support on Facebook. *Social Media + Society*, 3(3), 1-11.

Carah, N., & Brodmerkel, S. (2021). Alcohol marketing in the era of digital media platforms. *Journal of Studies on Alcohol and Drugs, 82*(1), 18–27.

Carah, N., Brodmerkel, S., & Hernandez, L. (2014). Brands and sociality: Alcohol branding, drinking culture and Facebook. *Convergence, 20*(3), 259–275.

Carah, N., & Meurk, C. (2017). We need a media platform perspective on alcohol marketing: A reply to Lobstein et al. *Addiction, 12*, 370–373.

Carah, N., & Shaul, M. (2016). Brands and Instagram: Point, tap, swipe, glance. *Mobile Media and Communication, 4*(1), 69–84.

Cavazos-Rehg, P., Krauss, M., Sowles, S., & Bierut, L. (2015). "Hey everyone, I'm drunk." An evaluation of drinking-related Twitter chatter. *Journal of Studies on Alcohol and Drugs, 76*(4), 635–643.

Coeckelbergh, M. (2022). *The political philosophy of AI*. Polity.

Geusens, F., & Beullens, K. (2023). I see, therefore I am: Exposure to alcohol references on social media, but not on traditional media, is related to alcohol consumption via drinking and non-drinking identity. *Health Communication, 38*(2), 402–410.

Goodwin, I. (2022). Programmatic alcohol advertising, social media and public health: Algorithms, automated challenges to regulation, and the failure of public oversight. *International Journal of Drug Policy, 109*, 103826.

Goodwin, I., & Griffin, C. (2017). Neoliberalism, alcohol, and identity. In A. C. Lyons, T. McCreanor, I. Goodwin, & H. Moewaka Barnes (Eds.), *Youth drinking cultures in a digital world* (pp. 15–30). Routledge.

Goodwin, I., Griffin, C., Lyons, A. C., McCreanor, T., & Moewaka Barnes, H. (2016). Precarious popularity: Facebook drinking photos, the attention economy, and the regime of the branded self. *Social Media + Society, 2*(1), 1–13.

Griffiths, R., & Casswell, S. (2010). Intoxigenic digital spaces? Youth, social networking sites and alcohol marketing. *Drug and Alcohol Review, 29*(September), 525–530.

Hebden, R. (2023) *Embedded commercial technologies: The role of smartphones and alcohol marketing in young adult drinking cultures*. PhD thesis, Massey University, Palmerston North, New Zealand. Retrieved January 26, 2024, from https://mro.massey.ac.nz/items/3169bce3-f1ec-40a9-b7a3-dc2f8f4177a6

Helmond, A. (2015). The platformization of the web: Making web data platform ready. *Social Media + Society, 1*(2), 1–11.

Hendriks, H., den Putte, B., Winifed, A., & Moreno, M. (2018). Social drinking on social media: Content analysis of the social aspects of alcohol-related posts on Facebook and Instagram. *Journal of Medical Internet Research, 20*(6), 1–12.

Hutton, F., Griffin, C., Lyons, A. C., Niland, P., & McCreanot, T. (2016). "Tragic girls" and "crack whores": Alcohol, femininity and Facebook. *Feminism and Psychology, 26*(1), 73–93.

Jernigan, D., & Ross, C. S. (2020). The alcohol marketing landscape: Alcohol industry size, structure, strategies, and public health responses. *Journal of Studies on Alcohol and Drugs, Supplement*, (s19), 13–25.

Lindsay, J., & Supski, S. (2017). Curating Identity: Drinking, young women, femininities and social media practices. In A. C. Lyons, T. McCreanor, I. Goodwin, & H. Moewaka Barnes (Eds.), *Youth drinking cultures in a digital world* (pp. 49–65). Routledge.

Livingston, M., Taylor, N., Raninen, J., & Pennay, A. (2024). Youth drinking in decline: Recent developments and future priorities. *Drug and Alcohol Review, 43*(3), 593–595.

Lobstein, T., Landon, J., Thornton, N., & Jernigan, D. (2017). The commercial use of digital media to market alcohol products: A narrative review. *Addiction, 112*(1), 21–27.

Luomanen, J., & Alasuutari, P. (2022). The rising social media and declining alcohol use: The case of Finnish teenagers. *Contemporary Drug Problems, 49*(2), 213–227.

Lyons, A., McCreanor, T., Goodwin, I., & Barnes, H. M. (Eds.). (2017). *Youth drinking cultures in a digital world: Alcohol, social media and cultures of intoxication*. Taylor & Francis.

Lyons, A., & Willot, S. (2008). Alcohol consumption, gender identities and women's changing social positions. *Sex Roles, 59*(9-10), 694–715.

Lyons, A. C., Goodwin, I., Carah, N., Young, J., Moewaka Barnes, A., & McCreanor, T. (2023). Limbic platform capitalism: Understanding the contemporary marketing of health-demoting products on social media. *Addiction Research & Theory, 31*(3), 178–183.

Mackey, A. (2016). Sticky e/motional connections: Young people, social media, and the re-orientation of affect. *Safundi, 17*(2), 156–173.

Mart, S. (2017). New marketing, new policy? Emerging debates over regulating alcohol campaigns on social media. In A. C. Lyons, T. McCreanor, I. Goodwin, & H. Moewaka Barnes (Eds.), *Youth drinking cultures in a digital world* (pp. 218–219). Routledge.

McCreanor, T., Lyons, A. C., Griffin, C., Goodwin, I., Moewaka Barnes, H., & Hutton, F. (2013). Youth drinking cultures, social networking and alcohol marketing: Implications for public health. *Critical Public Health, 23*, 110–120.

Meikle, G. (2016). *Social media: Communication, sharing and visibility*. Routledge.

Mesman, M., Hendriks, H., & Van den Putte, B. (2020). How viewing alcohol posts of friends on social networking sites influences predictors of alcohol use. *Journal of Health Communication, 25*(6), 522–529.

Moewaka Barnes, H., McCreanor, T., Goodwin, I., Lyons, A., Griffin, C., & Hutton, F. (2016). Alcohol and social media: Drinking and drunkenness while online. *Critical Public Health, 26*(1), 62–76.

Moewaka Barnes, H., Niland, P., Samu, L., Sciasia, A. D., & McCreanor, T. (2017). Ethnicity/culture, alcohol and social media. In A. C. Lyons, T. McCreanor, I. Goodwin, & H. Moewaka Barnes (Eds.), *Youth drinking cultures in a digital world* (pp. 80–98). Routledge.

Nicholls, J. (2012). Everyday, everywhere: Alcohol marketing and social media – Current trends. *Alcohol and Alcoholism, 47*(4), 486–493.

Niland, P., Lyons, A. C., Goodwin, I., & Hutton, F. (2014). 'See it doesn't look pretty does it?' Young adults' airbrushed drinking practices on Facebook. *Psychology and Health, 29*(8), 877–895.

Niland, P., Lyons, A. C., Goodwin, I., & Hutton, F. (2015). Friendship work on Facebook: Young adults' understandings and practices of friendship. *Journal of Community and Applied Social Psychology, 25*(2), 123–137.

Niland, P., McCreanor, T., Lyons, A. C., & Griffin, C. (2017). Alcohol marketing on social media: Young adults engage with alcohol marketing on Facebook. *Addiction Research and Theory, 25*(4), 273–284.

Noel, J. K., Sammartino, C. J., & Rosenthal, S. R. (2020). Exposure to digital alcohol marketing and alcohol use: A systematic review. *Journal of Studies on Alcohol and Drugs, s19*, 57–67.

Norman, T., Anderson-Luxford, D., O'Brien, P., & Room, R. (2024). Regulating alcohol advertising for public health and welfare in the age of digital marketing: Challenges and options. *Drugs: Education, Prevention and Policy, 31*(1), 70–81.

Ortiz-Ospina, E. (2019). *The rise of social media*. Retrieved January 24, 2024, from https://ourworldindata.org/rise-of-social-media

Pegg, K. J., O'Donnell, A. W., Lala, G., & Barber, B. L. (2018). The role of online social identity in the relationship between alcohol-related content on social networking sites and adolescent alcohol use. *Cyberpsychology, Behavior, and Social Networking, 21*(1), 50–55.

Pennay, A., Caluzzi, G., Livingston, M., & MacLean, S. (2024). Risk and restraint – The key to understanding the decreasing use of alcohol for young people in high income countries? *Drug and Alcohol Review, 43*(3), 654–663.

Reddy, A., & Kumar, P. C. (2024, May). 'A Teaspoon of Authenticity': Exploring how young adults BeReal on social media. In *Proceedings of the CHI Conference on Human Factors in Computing Systems*, 907, 1–14.

Room, R., Greenfield, T. K., Holmes, J., Kraus, L., Livingston, M., Pennay, A., & Törrönen, J. (2020). Supranational changes in drinking patterns: Factors in explanatory models of substantial and parallel social change. *Addiction Research & Theory, 28*(6), 467–473.

Room, R., & O'Brien, P. (2021). Alcohol marketing and social media: A challenge for public health control. *Drug and Alcohol Review, 40*(3), 420–422.

Russell, A. M., Davis, R. E., Ortega, J. M., Colditz, J. B., et al. (2021). #Alcohol: Portrayals of Alcohol in Top Videos on TikTok. *Journal of Studies on Alcohol and Drugs, 82*(5), 615–622.

Samuel, A., White, G., Thomas, R., & Jones, P. (2021). Programmatic Advertising: An exegesis of consumer concerns. *Computers in Human Behavior, 116*, 1–9.

Sargent, J. D., & Babor, T. F. (2020). The relationship between exposure to alcohol marketing and underage drinking is causal. *Journal of Studies on Alcohol and Drugs, Supplement, (s19)*, 113–124.

Statistica. (2023). *Most popular social networks worldwide as of October 2023*. Retrieved January 24, 2024, from https://www.statista.com/statistics/272014/global-social-networks-ranked-by-number-of-users/

Sujon, Z., Viney, L., & Toker-Turnalar. (2018). Domesticating Facebook: The shift from compulsive connection to personal service platform. *Social Media + Society, 4*(4), 1–12.

Thomas, J., & Kininmonth, S. (2023). The automated media economy. In T. Flew, J. Holt, & J. Thomas (Eds.), *The Sage handbook of digital media economy* (pp. 82–101). Sage.

Thulan, E., Vilhelmson, B., & Schwanen, T. (2020). Absent friends? Smartphones, mediated presence, and the recoupling of online social contact in everyday life. *Annals of the American Association of Geographers, 110*(1), 166–183.

Thulin, E. (2017). Always on my mind: How Smartphones are transforming social contact among young Swedes. *Young, 26*(5), 1–19.

Truong, J. (2018). Attending to others: How digital technologies direct young people's nightlife. *Geographica Helvetica, 73*, 193–201.

van Dijck. (2013). *The culture of connectivity: A critical history of social media.* Oxford University Press.

Van Dijck, J., Poell, T., & De Waal, M. (2018). *The platform society: Public values in a connective world.* Oxford University Press.

Vanherle, R., Hendriks, H., & Beullens, K. (2023). Only for friends, definitely, not for parents: Adolescents' sharing of alcohol references on social media features. *Mass Communication and Society, 26*(1), 47–73.

Wahl-Jorgensen, K. (2018). The emotional architecture of social media. In Z. Papacharissi (Ed.), *A networked self and platforms, stories, connections* (pp. 77–93). Routledge.

Whiteley, D., Rickards-Hill, D., Dimova, E., & Emslie, C. (2023). *Performing solidarity? A scoping review of alcohol marketing to sexual and gender minorities* (pp. 1–9). *Education, Prevention & Policy.*

Zhao, X., Lampe, C., & Ellison, N. B. (2016). The social media ecology: User perceptions, strategies and challenges. In *Proceedings of the 2016 CHI Conference on Human Factors in Computing Systems* (pp. 89–100). Association for Computing Machinery.

# 13

# Friendship and Alcohol Use Among Young Adults: What Do We Know and Where Could Things Go?

Dom Conroy and Sarah MacLean

**Abstract** Links between young adult friendships and drinking practices are of interest from multiple disciplinary perspectives and methodological starting points. For example, alcohol has been studied in both survey and interview research as a catalyst for initiating friendships and developing intimacy within friendships. Using an inclusive, methodologically plural approach we draw together emergent findings from the diffuse empirical work relevant to this topic area. Research is critically discussed across two broad subsections: "How do friendships influence young adults' alcohol use (and non-use)?" and "How does alcohol use (and non-use) shape friendships?". A final chapter section draws on recent work

D. Conroy (✉)
Faculty of Arts and Social Science, The Open University, London, UK
e-mail: d.conroy@open.ac.uk

S. MacLean
Centre for Alcohol Policy Research, La Trobe University,
Melbourne, VIC, Australia
e-mail: S.MacLean@latrobe.edu.au



D. Conroy, F. Measham (eds.), *Young Adult Drinking Styles*, Sustainable Development Goals Series, https://doi.org/10.1007/978-3-031-98528-7_13

concerning friendship in the context of mental health interventions to present the case that friendships appear to be underutilised in alcohol harm reduction interventions. Specifically, we argue that closer attention to the fine-grained detail of interactions within specific friendship groups may provide an effective basis for challenging heavier drinking practices. Understanding links between young adult friendships and friendship groups, and drinking patterns and practices, is a growing area of interest across different national contexts for social scientists from diverse disciplinary backgrounds. From a broader cultural perspective, friendship and alcohol use among young adults seem to be intuitively fused, in that the practices of both friendship and alcohol consumption evoke associations with intimacy, liberation, transition, and collective identity. Five years on from writing our original chapter on links between alcohol consumption and friendship among young adults, the literature in this area remains fascinating and diverse yet persistently diverse. Drawing together the diverse body of theoretical and empirical work published in this area is difficult, partly given the varied ways in which the relationship between friendship and alcohol use/practice has been formulated and explored but also due to the rare 'centering' of friendship when exploring young adult drinking practices in research studies.

In psychology, this relationship has typically been explored from a social-cognitive perspective in which the influence of friendship has been operationalised as 'normative influence' of peer members on young adult drinking patterns. For psychologists, friendship is traditionally understood as something measurable at an intra-individual level, though psychology also has some examples of more contextualised efforts to consider how features of friendship might be linked to young adult drinking practices. Meanwhile, focusing on the influence of broader social change on young people's sociable alcohol use, sociologists have traced how new patterns of binge drinking among groups of young people have emerged in Western countries. In this context, heavy alcohol use has become a gendered part of how young women as well as young men engage with their friends. Thus, sociological (and also anthropological) writing on friendship in the context of alcohol consumption has focused on how alcohol use is knitted into young adult lives.

The international phenomenon of declines in young adults' alcohol consumption in many Western countries over the last two decades provides an important context to recent research. This has birthed studies of how friendships may be implicated in declining consumption, rather than always functioning to increase alcohol use among young adults.

## Literature Review Scope and Process

This updated chapter collates the current literature concerning links between friendship and alcohol use among young adults from a cross-disciplinary, methodologically plural perspective. We focus on research which has primarily concerned friendships between young adults, defined here as individuals aged between 18 and 30 years. Rather than systematically reviewing the literature, our process was (1) to identify prominent empirical work reporting different aspects relating to links between young adult drinking practices and emerging or established friendship(s); (2) to organise this body of work into appropriate and helpful themes; and (3) to consider what additional work might be needed in the future. Some work was omitted from this process. For example, work concerning peer influence or peer networks on drinking practices was understood as distinct from current interests. Excluded too were studies which focused on friendships in the context of particular subcultures (e.g. sports societies) on the basis that the main unit of focus in such studies tended to the subculture itself rather than friendship stemming from subcultural practices. Some important areas of focus are, for space reasons, excluded from this chapter. For example, we do not cover the role of alcohol corporations and their increasing interest in incorporating young people's relationships (especially intimate relationships like friendships) into their branding, advertising, and marketing strategies. Such discussion warrants a chapter in its own right and can be found elsewhere in this collection (Chapter 12).

We first define friendship with these processes and purposes in mind. We then present our review under two headings: 'How do friendships influence young adults' alcohol use (and non-use)?' and 'How does alcohol use (or non-use) shape friendships?' These headings are inevitably coarse in terms of how they group relevant studies, but they provide a meaningful, coherent way to disentangle key themes involved in research and discussion concerning friendship and alcohol use. Finally, we consider future areas for study and how research on alcohol use and friendship among young adults might be harnessed by practitioners, policymakers, and researchers to promote sustained, safe, and moderate alcohol consumption among young adults as a demographic group.

## Defining Friendship Among Young Adults

Friendship represents one type of intimate relationship between people, but is difficult to define. Rawlins (2008) usefully defines friendship as a relationship that is voluntary (the relationship cannot be forced), mutual, personal (people are interested in each other because of who they uniquely are), affectionate (we care about the person), and likely to be equal (entailing a possibility of interacting as equals). Unlike relationships with family members or spouses, friendship is not based on blood ties and is unlikely to be characterised by formal agreements which indicate how we should behave or specify how long the relationship should endure (O'Connor, 1998). Although cultural norms regarding the behaviour of friends do exist (Badhwar, 2008; Bryant & Marmo, 2012), friends need to negotiate the parameters of a friendship, for example, to establish the degrees of care and trust that are expected or acceptable (Rawlins, 1992).

Friendships arguably hold particular value and meaning for young adults during a period that may include several key life stage transitions such as living independently, developing first sexual/romantic relationships, starting paid work and perhaps engaging in further education. It has been suggested that young adults are more likely to feel close to important friends than to family members (Pulakos, 1989). Beyond these particular transitions, young adults may also be understood as working through issues relating to identity, values, and position in the world (see Arnett, 2000 for discussion of 'emerging adulthood'). Friendship may therefore have a distinctive role to play during young adulthood.

Because of this, understanding interactions between friendships and drinking practices are important for both theoretical reasons and practical and policy-related reasons. That is, to explain relationships between friendship and alcohol consumption, and to draw on relevant empirical work concerning alcohol and friendship to encourage less harmful drinking practices.

## 'How Do Friendships Influence Young Adults' Alcohol Use (and Non-Use)?'

Sociologists and anthropologists have shown that attitudes and practices concerning alcohol and other drug use are often shared and reproduced within friendship groups (Mayock, 2002; Pilkington, 2007; Rúdólfsdóttir & Morgan, 2009). Quantitative studies have identified relationships between drinking levels of individuals and those of friends and peers, both for teenagers (Ferguson & Meehan, 2010; Fujimoto & Valente, 2012a) and young adults (Louis-Jacques et al., 2012; Overbeek et al., 2011). In these quantitative research studies, the influence of friends over personal harmful drinking is typically operationalised in terms of the occurrence of harmful drinking among friends, or/and the extent to which friends endorse harmful drinking as an acceptable practice. In this way, the influence of friends and friendship on young adults' alcohol use is understood as a moderating factor which can either raise or reduce the likelihood of an individual's harmful drinking practices.

Psychological research has traditionally focused on modelling characteristics of particular types of, or qualities within, friendships as a moderating or mediating influence over alcohol and other drug use among young adults (Boman et al., 2013; MacKinnon et al., 2022). For example, MacKinnon et al. (2022) found that links between conflict within friendships and alcohol-related problems was mediated by coping-with-depression motives in their longitudinal survey of 174 same sex friendship dyads in Nova Scotia, Canada. Other studies have explored moderating effects of friendship on alcohol consumption in terms of whether and how individuals' ratings of friendship reciprocity (i.e., friendship dyads where both individuals appear to clearly view the other as a friend) may influence personal consumption levels. For example,

Giese et al. (2017) found that evidence of self-reported friendship reciprocity was associated with similar levels of alcohol consumption at relatively low levels but also found that binge drinking, by contrast, was similar only in situations where friendship was not reciprocated. These findings suggest that young adults may use alcohol more strategically than can be traditionally assumed and that heavy drinking practices may not be dependent on the perceived intimacy of the friendship.

Work discussed above illustrates the social-cognitive approach to exploring how friendship influences drinking behaviour and holds parallels with a broader tradition in psychological research of modelling the influence that peer and friendship groups have on individual behaviour. This is evident in terms like 'social contagion' (Fujimoto & Valente, 2012b), which often frame understanding in terms of the disruptive or pathological effect of groups/crowds on otherwise rational decision making on the part of the individual.

Relatively few studies explicitly explore the influence of friendship on alcohol use among young adults although recently research has suggested how the influential role of friendships may cascade in distinctive ways in differing cultural contexts. For example, Dumbili et al. (2022) interviews with 53 young adults aged 18–24 years living in Southern Nigeria underscored the importance of social drinking for enacting friendships, alcohol's role as a way of demonstrating maturity, and the role of subtle and overt pressures to consume alcohol within friendship groups. Dumbili et al. (2022) suggest that greater pressure may be required to encourage alcohol consumption within young adult friendship groups given the social-cultural and religious norms that constrain drinking in Nigerian culture and underscore how this may differ from drinking in Western cultural settings where young adults may consume alcohol in a relatively voluntary way. We should also note here that Dumbili et al's work on friendship and alcohol use among young adults is relatively unusual in that it is written in a non-Western context. This highlights the cultural imbalance in published research conducted in this area.

Decisions around whether to drink during a social occasion as a young adult may be conditional on whether drinking is perceived as likely to provide opportunities to initiate or deepen friendship bonds. For example, discursive research conducted among UK university students has suggested that student non-drinkers may be viewed as 'not joining in' with friends and that, relatedly, the possibility of not drinking might be rejected for fear of being understood as rejecting shared values when socialising with friends (Conroy & de Visser, 2013). This may be changing—see our discussion of Caluzzi et al.'s work (2020). Qualitative research can guide understanding of how friendship-linked qualities like sociability might underpin but also be contested within young adult drinking practices. Young adults aged 18–24 in MacLean (2016) discussed drinking at a similar pace to friends to 'keep up' and maintain a similar level of intoxication, suggesting that they would drink more in order to maintain a sense of connection with friends. At the same time, the bodily effects of alcohol made them able to engage with friends and generate a sense of intimacy. These findings suggest that research attention needs to explore not just the mere presence of friends (or particular types of friend) that may be important to alcohol practices, but also to attend to temporal and embodied aspects of drinking practices which may permit or accelerate a particular type of intimacy or bonding experience. This is an example of alcohol's influence on friendship, which we explore in the next chapter section.

## 'How Does Alcohol Use (or Non-use) Shape Friendships?'

To this point, we have largely considered how friendships might, in different ways, 'effect' distinct features of drinking practice among young adults including the overall quantity of alcohol consumed over time or the quantity of alcohol consumed during specific occasions. Models of cause and effect in psychological research can privilege one-way relationships in which intra-individual properties are understood to causally influence subsequent behaviour. Such accounts hold clear advantages, but risk losing much detail about social phenomena. Arguably, this is particularly true in the case of understanding alcohol–friendship relationships, where a growing body of evidence (both qualitative and quantitative) points to complex and, as discussed in the previous section, reciprocal or co-constituted 'effects' between friendship characteristics and dynamics and alcohol practices and patterns of consumption. Qualitative research exploring alcohol use in the context of friendship is considered in the remainder of this section. Studies adopting a qualitative design can partly be understood as a response to the typically individualistic approach described above and implicit within alcohol harm reduction strategies.

Social scientists have long been interested in identifying and understanding norms that guide people's actions and qualitative research has developed understanding of how these norms operate in the context of young adult friendships and drinking practices. For example, MacArthur et al. (2017) drew on interviews with 28 English young adults to show how an expectation to drink heavily can be policed within friendship groups but also how alcohol acted as a catalyst for fun and enjoyment and for building social and symbolic capital within friendship groups. Alcohol's use in producing intimacy between friends is also evident in research with Norwegian women, some of whom were slightly older than our definition of young adults here (27–34 years) (Vaadal & Dahl, 2021).

Normative expectations of gendered behaviour also strongly influence how young people drink with friends, with particular kinds of toxic or hyper-masculinity associated with alcohol consumption, aggression and violence (Peralta, 2007). Researchers have also shown how wider social and economic structures frame both alcohol consumption and friendships. Groups of friends enact gendered and classed subjectivities through drinking (Griffin et al., 2009; Measham, 2002; Measham & Brain, 2005) with the alcohol-dominated night-time economy providing the setting for many young adults' leisure practices.

Alcohol and its availability and price influence how young people socialise with their friends. Millennials in countries such as the UK, New Zealand, and Australia may structure a night out to enable the consumption of relatively cheaper off-licensed sales of alcohol at someone's house before they visit a licensed venue (termed 'pre-loading' or 'pre-drinking'). While saving money appears to have emerged as one important driver for pre-drinking in the UK, the opportunity to spend time with friends before going out is also important. This close relationship between the availability and pricing of alcohol and young adult's engagements with friends has been evidenced in a range of international settings including Australia (MacLean & Callinan, 2013) and New Zealand (McCreanor et al., 2016). For example, focus group research with 141 young adults between 2011 and 2012 has underscored how pre-loading applied to different practices and motivations including lower costs but also values and rituals involved in peer processes and friendships (McCreanor et al., 2016).

Research on pre-drinking and alcohol use in other settings has also demonstrated the opportunities and pleasures experienced among young adults when drinking with friends and within friendship groups and how this builds intimacy in friendships. For example, studies have shown how alcohol helps people generate and enjoy a sense of connection with others (e.g. Peralta, 2007; Törrönen & Maunu, 2007). Drinking practices have been recognised as an important catalyst for particular kinds of emotional connection that can emerge between young adults while socialising, and such connections can be closely linked with the quality of their relationships and interactions. Törrönen and Maunu (2011) explore how pride (a sense of attachment to friends) and shame (feeling excluded) experienced in relation to drinking can reinforce or undermine friendships and also serve to promote particular models and ways of talking about friendship. Friendships can be damaged or destroyed when people behave inappropriately when drunk; for example, requiring excessive levels of care, or demonstrating too much intimacy (MacLean, 2016; MacLean, Pennay, & Room, 2018).

Other research has helped develop understanding of how friendship contexts beyond the immediate boundaries of a particular drinking occasion warrant greater understanding and exploration. For example, accounts of hangovers experienced among Norwegian young adults aged 18–23 drew attention to how hangovers act as a narrative form of closure to the experience of a party which may hold implications for the emotional and social bonds that are forged within friendship groups (Fjær, 2012). This may be manifest in collective activities (e.g. all going out for breakfast together), which involve recollections, and evidence of teasing which has been discussed as a way of 'practicing intimacy' within friendships (Keltner et al., 2001, p. 236). Others describe how narrating drinking events through social media such as Facebook and Instagram reinforces friendship ties (Griffin et al., 2009; Tutenges & Sandberg, 2013). Thus, young adults use social media to disseminate a record of their friendships to others, with alcohol signifying the pleasure, intimacy, and sociability they shared.

Articulating how alcohol consumption is embedded in 'friendship practices' enables researchers to consider alcohol consumption and friendship making as co-constitutive in the production of social relationships and identities. For example, focus group research from New Zealand highlights the pleasures and sociability made possible by alcohol consumption among young adults, showing how discourses about the effects of alcohol and how alcohol should be consumed enable young adults to 'do' friendship (Niland et al., 2013). This discursive research suggested that positive features of drinking (e.g. enjoying friendships, supporting each other) were invoked rhetorically to offset negative aspects of drinking experiences. Such findings hold important implications for how health promotion/harm reduction messages are conceived and delivered. Specifically, findings here suggest that risk-focused, harm reduction health messages can fall short partly because they are effectively asking young adults to break strong and highly valued friendship bonds and may be unlikely to strike a chord with young adults who are motivated to neutralise and reject such undesired messages.

Building on this argument, MacLean (2016) argues that drinking alcohol together is a key means by which young people in the contemporary West produce and reproduce, friendships; or in other words that alcohol use is a crucible though which friendships are forged. Drawing on the sociological argument that friendships must be continually reproduced through sets of practices (Pahl, 2000)—she proposes that drinking enables young adults to generate a sense of intimacy and demonstrate trust in each other, both of which are hallmarks of contemporary friendship relationships. Young people are also able to negotiate the unclear parameters of friendship through alcohol use—by providing care for friends when they are out, with men and women sometimes holding different expectations about what this entails. The critical role of alcohol in constituting young adults' friendships may go some way towards explaining the persistence of heavy drinking within this demographic.

Research concerning alcohol abstinence has provided important insights into the status and symbolic power of alcohol as an often-present device relevant to contexts where young adults have opportunities to make friends or where there are opportunities to consolidate intimacy within established friendships or groups of friends. For example, interview research with UK undergraduates has suggested that not drinking can limit opportunities to forge new friendships during socially intense periods like 'Fresher's week' (Jacobs et al., 2018), but may also play a role in 'knowing which friends care about you' and therefore guide recognition of which friendships are worth pursuing (Conroy & de Visser, 2014). Discerning the genuineness of emerging friendships has been reported as a key concern for non-/light-drinking young adults when interacting with alcohol consuming peers in several qualitative studies involving university students (Conroy & de Visser, 2015; Jacobs et al., 2018). Frank et al. (2020) show how Danish young people need to provide one of a set of socially acceptable explanations to their friends to explain non- or light-drinking. Young people who don't want to drink alcohol at all are mindful that this may interfere with their capacity to develop and maintain friendships with others, a finding also drawn in the UK by Gambles et al. (2022) in a study of new university students. Non-drinking therefore provided a range of issues for young adults in terms of diminished opportunities to make friends or sustain friendships; but also in providing a basis for new standards or criteria about the kinds of friendship that might be desirable.

Rather than understanding alcohol's role as crudely 'shaping' friendships, recent research has given insights into how drinking practices provide a performative framework for enacting friendships and aspects of gendered identities during collective drinking occasions. For example, interviews completed with 18–25-year-old women in Newcastle, UK has highlighted alcohol's key role in constructing and negotiating both friendships and gendered identities in pre-drinking settings in the night-time economy of drinking in bars and clubs (Nicholls, 2020). Through analysis of interview data, Nicholls highlights the complexities of how alcohol use (and non-use) is woven into different aspects of friendship including its role in building trust and intimacy and 'friendship-cementing' during collectively experienced social occasions. Similar evidence has suggested how young people may work low-level alcohol consumption into their friendships in complex ways. Writing in Australia,

Caluzzi et al. (2020) observe a phenomenon of 'sober intimacy'—the sense of connection young abstainers and light-drinkers described through socialising without alcohol or in non-drinking environments. Light-drinking or abstinent young people emphasised that friendships were more authentic, where getting drunk together was not a dominant or important activity. They valued building and maintaining friendships where alcohol was not relied on to generate sociality or closeness (although some light-drinkers interviewed did also get drunk with friends occasionally). Indeed, evidence suggests that different styles of drinking behaviour may connect with different facets or stages of friendship. For example, Conroy et al. (2021) found in their interview research with ten 18–27-year-old UK university students that alcohol was identified as important for initiating or consolidating friendships yet simultaneously periods of sobriety were *also* important for developing intimacy at a certain stage in the formation of friendships (p. 11: Shaun's 'when I'm sober … I'm actually bonding with people').

While it is possible to trace unidirectional relationships between alcohol and friendship, with heavier drinkers engaged in different friendship practices (MacLean, Pennay, & Room, 2018) and friendships with heavier drinkers producing higher consumption levels in individuals, these relationships are inevitably complex and interactional. Alcohol and friendship-making have emerged in recent sociological research as part of a configuration of factors, including the night-time economy, work, family, education, social media, and discourses of selfhood, that inform young adult's contemporary experiences, understandings, and actions. One commitment for future qualitative research may involve maintaining an ongoing effort to explicitly acknowledge the inherent tension that drinking entails for young adult friendships, in that it both reinforces friendship bonds and threatenes them when people do things when they are drunk that are threatening, annoying, or disturbing to others (MacLean, 2016; MacLean, Pennay, & Room, 2018). Notably, one key advantage of qualitative methods over quantitative methods is that they allow us to tease out the complexity of interactions between features of friendship and patterns of drinking practices.

## Priorities for Future Research

In this revised chapter, we have aimed to highlight key characteristics of relevant empirical work in this area. Drawing on this diffuse body of work, we will next consider some of the priority areas for future work. Consolidating discussion of these priority areas, we will then focus on one particularly promising area for future research that would make friendships the focus of alcohol-related interventions. Priority areas for future work are as follows:

- ***Understanding friendships and alcohol use in non-Western cultures.*** Research reviewed in this chapter was overwhelmingly located in Western and English-speaking countries. Friendships clearly vary considerably in their dynamics and normative starting points within cultural settings (e.g. see Pinson's, 1985 work on drinking and drunkenness among Icelandic young adults and a more recent study set in Nigeria by Dumbili et al., 2022). We need to understand how the dynamics of friendship and alcohol use among young adults work in the context of low- and middle-income countries, for example.
- ***Exploring how increasingly diverse drinking styles impact on young adults' views of alcohol within friendships.*** Fewer young people drink than was the case in previous age cohorts (e.g. Pennay et al., 2015, and see also Chaps. 2 and 3 in this volume) and further research designed to explore how contemporary friendship operates among friendship groups reflecting heterogeneous styles of drinking practice (e.g. people who drink alcohol regularly and moderately; heavier drinkers; people who drink little or no alcohol) would be useful.
- ***Utilising methodologically plural methods for understanding reciprocal friendship–alcohol connections.*** The relationships between friendship, friendship groups, and alcohol practices are increasingly recognised as complex and multifaceted. Hard-defined 'causal pathways' between relevant variables risk a simplified understanding. Mixed methods and multi-modal research can help to explore reciprocal pathways between characteristics of friendship (e.g. historical

length of friendship; perceived quality of friendship) and different features of drinking belief and drinking practice.

- ***Taking a lifespan/transitions perspective to friendship and alcohol use.*** Future research concerning alcohol use over the lifespan might involve exploring alcohol's differential and/or similar role in friendships for individuals at different life stages. Such work provides an important reference point to guide the development of research which can link alcohol practices among young adults to alcohol practices at later points in life. For example, members of sexual minority groups maintain a higher average alcohol consumption as they move into middle age (MacLean, Savic, et al., 2018). One specific future research focus is to explore opportunities and impediments that might be found among gay, lesbian, or bisexual young adults for making connections within their communities with reduced reliance on alcohol.
- Likewise, very little is known about alcohol use among trans and gender-diverse young adults. Research considering how alcohol use is used to reinforce gender-related identity positions with friends (if indeed it is) may be useful.
- ***Measuring the impacts of interventions on friends, rather than just on directly targeted individuals.*** Studies tend to measure intervention impacts on people who participate in interventions rather than those around them. One study (Rulison et al., 2015) found that the odds of getting drunk for children 10–14 years old who did not have friends attending a programme were higher than for those who did. We didn't find comparable information about the effects of interventions that their friends engaged in on young people, which seems an avenue worth pursuing.
- ***Understanding digital spaces relevant to friendships and drinking practices.*** The alcohol industry creatively capitalises on the importance of alcohol in friendship practices in digital and non-digital spaces. For example, by inserting alcohol advertising into social media outlets typically used by young adults to interact (Nicholls, 2012; Niland et al., 2017). Understanding how to critically examine, identify, and disrupt industry practices relevant to the representation of alcohol use within young adult friendships is an imperative and growing research priority.

## Targeting Friendships Within Alcohol Harm Reduction Interventions

Empirical work discussed in the chapter, now updated for the revised edition of this book, has rarely focused on interventions that harness friendship in some way to reduce alcohol consumption. In this final section, we briefly consider how friendship has been approached in the context of mental health and adolescent substance use interventions to present the case that friendships appear to be underutilised in alcohol harm reduction interventions.

A recent systematic review of friendship in mental health interventions concludes that "there are compelling reasons to focus on friendships for adolescent mental health interventions given the prominence of these relationships for this age group" (Manchanda et al., 2023, p. 17). Some of the interventions described in the review focused on helping people build friendships to combat social isolation. Others provided adolescents with skills to provide support for friends experiencing mental health challenges. Again, involving adolescents rather than young people, another study shows that a school-based program aiming to reduce risk taking (i.e. bicycle safety, sports, alcohol and drug use) among friends and promote care within friendship groups was well-received by participants (Buckley et al., 2021). Although these strategies are not all directly applicable to alcohol use, they do signal potential to utilise the centrality of friendships to young people more extensively in alcohol interventions.

Intervention programmes might entail strategies to facilitate the education and teaching of young adults to talk about alcohol use problems within friendship groups, enact care to help friends manage substance use and support their friends to access supports to better manage alcohol. These approaches offer potential to benefit friends, in addition to a person targeted for an intervention. As noted above, interventions that change people's attitudes to substance use may also diffuse to their friends (Rulison et al., 2015). Programmes such as Circles of Support, developed in the disability field, can help friends and family of people with problematic alcohol or drug use to enhance their capacity to support others, while developing boundary-setting and self-care skills (Tari-Keresztes et al., 2023).

Clearly, interventions designed to reduce alcohol consumption by capitalising on aspects of one-to-one or group-level friendship could work in many ways. In addition, such programmes would need to be culturally nuanced, and demonstrate awareness of cultural differences in how friendship is enacted, and how alcohol consumption is predominantly viewed. One approach might involve alcohol's role within close friendships being challenged, or reframed, or simply monitored within the context of friendship occasions and dynamics over a standard time period. We hope that this brief section has inspired readers to consider how friendship-focused alcohol interventions might be explored in the future either within broader alcohol research programmes or as stand-alone pilot interventions.

## Conclusion

In this chapter, we have reviewed empirical work concerning friendships and alcohol practices/use among young adults via a cross-disciplinary, methodologically inclusive approach. Psychological studies have tended to test causal pathways or associations relating to friendships and alcohol practices, guiding understanding of the close nexus between friendships and individual drinking patterns. Sociological studies, many of which entail qualitative explorations, highlight the complex embeddedness of alcohol in social life and relationships in the contemporary era. Together, both approaches reinforce the importance of considering the impact of friendships on the reception and uptake of health promotion and the efficacy of other interventions such as restrictions on advertising and alcohol availability.

The chapter has highlighted a body of evidence underscoring the importance of friendship to the patterns and variations in drinking practices among adults. Given this evidence, we believe that friendships are underutilised in alcohol harm reduction interventions despite, tellingly, clear efforts to deliver targeted appeals to friendship in corporate messages and advertising designed to promote alcohol use among young adults during an era of declining alcohol use internationally. Working with young people in friendship groups may prove more effective than trying to change drinking practices in more distal groups of peers. We hope that this initial literature review will help to generate further work in this important but poorly integrated area of social science research.

## References


Arnett, J. J. (2000). Emerging adulthood: A theory of development from the late teens through the twenties. *American Psychologist, 55*(5), 469–480.

Badhwar, N. K. (2008). Friendship and commercial societies. *Politics, Philosophy & Economics, 7*(3), 301–326.

Boman, J. H., Stogner, J., & Miller, B. L. (2013). Binge drinking, marijuana use, and friendships: The relationship between similar and dissimilar usage and friendship quality. *Journal of Psychoactive Drugs, 45*(3), 218–226.

Bryant, E. M., & Marmo, J. (2012). The rules of Facebook friendship: A two-stage examination of interaction rules in close, casual, and acquaintance friendships. *Journal of Social & Personal Relationships, 29*(8), 1013–1035.

Buckley, L., Sheehan, M., Dingli, K., Reveruzzi, B., & Horgan, V. (2021). Taking care of friends: The implementation evaluation of a peer-focused school program using first aid to reduce adolescent risk-taking and injury. *International Journal of Environmental Research and Public Health, 18*(24), 13030.

Caluzzi, G., MacLean, S., & Pennay, A. (2020). Re-configured pleasures: How young people feel good through abstaining or moderating their drinking. *International Journal of Drug Policy, 77*, 102709.

Conroy, D., & de Visser, R. O. (2013). 'Man up!': Discursive constructions of non-drinkers among UK undergraduates. *Journal of Health Psychology, 18*(11), 1432–1444.

Conroy, D., & de Visser, R. O. (2014). Being a non-drinking student: An interpretative phenomenological analysis. *Psychology & Health, 29*(5), 536–551.

Conroy, D., & de Visser, R. O. (2015). The importance of authenticity for student nondrinkers: An interpretative phenomenological analysis. *Journal of Health Psychology, 20*(11), 1483–1493.

Conroy, D., Morton, C., & Griffin, C. (2021). 'Maturing Out' as dilemmatic: Transitions towards relatively light drinking practices among UK University students. *British Journal of Health Psychology, 26*(3), 902–916.

Dumbili, E. W., Okpan, S. O., Uwa-Robinson, K., & Azende, P. M. (2022). 'If you cannot beat them, you join them': Friendship, social influence and drinking to belong among Nigerian youth. In T. Thurnell-Read & L. Fenton (Eds.), *Alcohol, age, generation and the life course* (pp. 127–150). Springer International Publishing.

Ferguson, C. J., & Meehan, D. C. (2010). Original article: With friends like these…: Peer delinquency influences across age cohorts on smoking, alcohol and illegal substance use. *European Psychiatry, 26*, 6–12.

Fjær, E. G. (2012). The day after drinking: Interaction during hangovers among young Norwegian adults. *Journal of Youth Studies, 15*(8), 995–1010.

Frank, V. A., Herold, M. D., Schrøder, S., Bjønness, J., & Hunt, G. (2020). Legitimizing and negotiating abstinence: Young adults' narratives about practicing situational and long term abstinence in Denmark. *The International Journal of Drug Policy, 81*, 102655–102655.

Fujimoto, K., & Valente, T. W. (2012a). Decomposing the components of friendship and friends' influence on adolescent drinking and smoking. *Journal of Adolescent Health, 51*(2), 136–143.

Fujimoto, K., & Valente, T. W. (2012b). Social network influences on adolescent substance use: Disentangling structural equivalence from cohesion. *Social Science and Medicine, 74*(12), 1952–1960.

Gambles, N., Porcellato, L., Fleming, K. M., & Quigg, Z. (2022). "If you don't drink at university, you're going to struggle to make friends" prospective students' perceptions around alcohol use at universities in the United Kingdom. *Substance Use & Misuse, 57*(2), 249–255.

Giese, H., Stok, F. M., & Renner, B. (2017). The role of friendship reciprocity in university freshmen's alcohol consumption. *Applied Psychology: Health and Well-Being, 9*(2), 228–241.

Griffin, C., Bengry-Howell, A., Hackley, C., Mistral, W., & Szmigin, I. (2009). 'Every time I do it I absolutely annihilate myself': Loss of (self-)consciousness and loss of memory in young people's drinking narratives. *Sociology, 43*(3), 457–476.

Jacobs, L., Conroy, D., & Parke, A. (2018). Negative experiences of non-drinking college students in Great Britain: An interpretative phenomenological analysis. *International Journal of Mental Health and Addiction, 16*, 737–750.

Keltner, D., Capps, L., Kring, A. M., Young, R. C., & Heerey (2001). Just teasing: A conceptual analysis and empirical review. Psychological Bulletin, 127 (2), 229–248.

Louis-Jacques, J., Knight, J., Sherrit, L., Van Hook, S., & Harris, S. (2012). Do risky friends matter? Comparing the effect of a primary care alcohol intervention by whether friends drink. *Journal of Adolescent Health, 50*(2, Suppl), S13–S14.

MacArthur, G. J., Jacob, N., Pound, P., Hickman, M., & Campbell, R. (2017). Among friends a qualitative exploration of the role of peers in young people's alcohol use using Bourdieu's concepts of habitus, field and capital. *Sociology of Health & Illness, 39*(1), 30–46.

Mackinnon, S. P., Tougas, M. E., Kehayes, I. L. L., & Stewart, S. H. (2022). Friendship conflict, drinking to cope, and alcohol-related problems: a longitudinal actor-partner interdependence model. *Emerging Adulthood, 10*(3), 595–608.

MacLean, S. (2016). Alcohol and the constitution of friendship for young adults. *Sociology, 50*(1), 93–108.

MacLean, S., & Callinan, S. (2013). "Fourteen dollars for one beer!" Pre-drinking is associated with high-risk drinking among Victorian young adults. *Australian and New Zealand Journal of Public Health, 37*(6), 579–585.

MacLean, S., Pennay, A., & Room, R. (2018). 'You're repulsive': Limits to acceptable drunken comportment for young adults. *The International Journal of Drug Policy, 53*, 106–112.

MacLean, S., Savic, M., Pennay, A., Dwyer, R., Stanesby, O., & Wilkinson, C. (2018). Middle-aged same-sex attracted women and the social practice of drinking. *Critical Public Health*, 1–12.

Manchanda, T., Stein, A., & Fazel, M. (2023). Investigating the role of friendship interventions on the mental health outcomes of adolescents: a scoping review of range and a systematic review of effectiveness. *International Journal of Environmental Research and Public Health, 20*(3), 2160.

Mayock, P. (2002). Drug pathways, transitions and decisions: The experiences of young people in an inner-city Dublin community. *Contemporary Drug Problems, 29*(Spring), 117–156.

McCreanor, T., Lyons, A. C., Moewaka Barnes, H., Hutton, F., Goodwin, I., & Griffin, C. (2016). "Drink a twelve box before you go": Pre-loading among young people in aotearoa new zealand. *Kotuitui: New Zealand Journal of Social Sciences Online, 11*(1), 36–46.

Measham, F. (2002). "Doing gender" – "Doing drugs": Conceptualizing the gendering of drugs cultures. *Contemporary Drug Problems, 29*(2), 335–373.

Measham, F., & Brain, K. (2005). 'Binge' drinking, British alcohol policy and the new culture of intoxication. *Crime Media Culture, 1*(3), 262–283.

Nicholls, E. (2020). 'I feel like I have to become part of that identity': Negotiating femininities and friendships through alcohol consumption in Newcastle. *UK. International Journal of Drug Policy, 81*, 102524.
Nicholls, J. (2012). Everyday, everywhere: alcohol marketing and social media – Current trends. *Alcohol and Alcoholism, 47*(4), 486–493.
Niland, P., Lyons, A. C., Goodwin, I., & Hutton, F. (2013). 'Everyone can loosen up and get a bit of a buzz on': Young adults, alcohol and friendship practices. *International Journal of Drug Policy, 24*(6), 530–537.
Niland, P., McCreanor, T., Lyons, A. C., & Griffin, C. (2017). Alcohol marketing on social media: Young adults engage with alcohol marketing on facebook. *Addiction Research & Theory, 25*(4), 273–284.
O'Connor, P. (1998). Women's friendships in a post-modern world. In R. G. Adams & G. Allan (Eds.), *Placing friendship in context* (pp. 117–135). Cambridge University Press.
Overbeek, G., Bot, S. M., Meeus, W. H. J., Sentse, M., Knibbe, R. A., & Engels, R. (2011). Where it's at! The role of best friends and peer group members in young adults' alcohol use. *Journal of Research on Adolescence, 21*(3), 631–638.
Pahl, R. (2000). *On friendship*. Polity Press.
Pennay, A., Livingston, M., & MacLean, S. (2015). Young people are drinking less: It is time to find out why. *Drug and Alcohol Review, 34*(2), 115–118.
Peralta, R. (2007). College alcohol use and the embodiment of hegemonic masculinity among European American men. *Sex Roles, 56*(11/12), 741–756.
Pilkington, H. (2007). In good company: Risk, security and choice in young people's drug decisions. *The Sociological Review, 55*(2), 373–392.
Pinson, A. (1985). The institution of friendship and drinking patterns in Iceland. *Anthropological Quarterly, 58*, 75–82.
Pulakos, J. (1989). Young adult relationships: Siblings and friends. *The Journal of Psychology, 123*(3), 237–244.
Rawlins, W. K. (1992). *Friendship matters: Communication, dialectics, and the life course*. Aldine de Gruyter.
Rawlins, W. K. (2008). *The compass of friendship: Narratives, identities, and dialogues*. Sage.
Rúdólfsdóttir, A. G., & Morgan, P. (2009). 'Alcohol is my friend': Young middle class women discuss their relationship with alcohol. *Journal of Community & Applied Social Psychology, 19*(6), 492–505.
Rulison, K. L. P. D., Feinberg, M. P. D., Gest, S. D. P. D., & Osgood, D. W. P. D. (2015). Diffusion of intervention effects: The impact of a family-

based substance use prevention program on friends of participants. *Journal of Adolescent Health, 57*(4), 433–440.

Tari-Keresztes, N., Armstrong, N., Smith, J. A., Gupta, H., Goding, S., & Endemann, S. A. (2023). "You don't get that from professionals": A consumer-led peer recovery program for families and friends of individuals with alcohol and other drugs use issues in Darwin. *International Journal of Environmental Research and Public Health, 20*(8), 5514.

Törrönen, J., & Maunu, A. (2007). Light transgression and heavy sociability: Alcohol in young adult Finns' narratives of a night out. *Addiction Research & Theory, 15*(4), 365–381.

Törrönen, J., & Maunu, A. (2011). Friendship and social emotions in young adult Finns' drinking diaries. *Sociological Research Online, 16*(1), 4.

Tutenges, S., & Sandberg, S. (2013). Intoxicating stories: The characteristics, contexts and implications of drinking stories among Danish youth. *International Journal of Drug Policy, 24*(6), 538–544.

Vaadal, K., & Dahl, S. L. (2021). Maturing out of 'binge drinking': Young adult women's performance of age and gender in times of transition. *Journal of Youth Studies, 24*(10), 1326–1339.

# 14

# Into the Woods: Contextualising Atypical Intoxication by Young Adults in Music Festivals and Nightlife Tourist Resorts

Tim Turner and Fiona Measham

**Abstract** Drawing on extensive empirical evidence gathered at British music festivals and from ethnographic research with British tourists on the Balearic island of Ibiza, this chapter aims to provide an in-depth appreciation of the nature, extent and situated meaning of poly-drug use within bounded spectacular events. For many young people, music festivals and holidays represent a window of freedom, experimentation, transgression and transformation. As many of the usual rules and restrictions of everyday life are temporarily suspended, these spectacular events can be characterised by dramatic changes in usual patterns of consumption and leisure. We argue that the framing of some festivals as transformative, by festival production and festival-goers, can be likened to the fairy-tale

T. Turner (✉)
School of Social Sciences and Humanities, Coventry University, Coventry, UK
e-mail: t.turner@coventry.ac.uk

F. Measham
Department of Sociology, Social Policy and Criminology, University of Liverpool, Liverpool, UK
e-mail: f.measham@liverpool.ac.uk



D. Conroy, F. Measham (eds.), *Young Adult Drinking Styles*, Sustainable Development Goals Series, https://doi.org/10.1007/978-3-031-98528-7_14

narrative of a journey 'into the woods', where protagonists are plunged into strange new worlds before returning home with heroic stories to share (Yorke, 2013, p. xi). The chapter, structured around this journey metaphor, focuses on the relationship between poly-drug consumption and three inter-related dimensions of the event, as identified by Getz (2008, p. 414): motivation and expectations; the lived experience of 'being there'; and reflections on meaning and influences on future behaviour. The chapter concludes with implications for policy, practice and research. We argue that if young people are to emerge from the 'woods' unscathed, there is an urgent need to understand this temporal transgression and embed innovative harm reduction strategies within music festivals, tourist resorts and other spectacular spaces that can distort patterns of drug and alcohol use.

## Once upon a time in a faraway land…

The telling of stories and fairy tales is a universal feature of human society, their structure often shaped by the three-phase monomyth of *separation, immersion* and *return*. Leaving the safety of home to undertake a journey into the woods is the starting point for innumerable fables; the dark forest is a symbolic place of pleasure, risk, danger and subverted social rules. The magical realms of Lewis Carroll's *Wonderland*, C. S. Lewis's *Narnia* and Tolkien's *Middle Earth*, for example, represent "secondary worlds" of mischief and merriment, standing as "allegories of alternatives to the world we know" (Warner, 2014, p. xx). This chapter draws on this simple allegorical monomyth to explore young adult intoxication within the context of the magical, secondary worlds of UK outdoor music festivals and Ibizan nightlife tourist resorts. Like the dark forest, these leisure spaces represent carnivalesque realms that merge opportunities for transgressive pleasure with elements of risk, danger and subversion.

Drawing on a number of empirical studies by the authors, together and individually, of British young adults on holiday in the "freak zone safety net" (Power, 2013) of festivals and nightlife resorts, the authors consider how, for many of those entering these multi-day play spaces, their usual patterns of alcohol and other drug use can become distorted, with atypical and "extreme" intoxication integral to the immersive and transformational experiences on offer. The chapter outlines four types of atypical intoxication in these secondary worlds, utilising qualitative data drawn from Turner's ethnographic studies (Turner, 2018, 2023) with British tourists in Ibizan nightlife resorts, alongside quantitative data from Measham's annual English Festival Study (EFS), conducted onsite at a range of festivals from 2010 onwards (Measham et al., 2024). Participating festivals broadly aligned with Webster and McKay's (2018, p. 4) definition of "greenfield events, which predominantly programme music, often involve camping, open-air consumption and amplification". It is argued here that despite evidence of a broader decline in young adult drinking (discussed elsewhere in this edited collection), there are still pockets of excess which become even more risky for participants because of the *atypical* nature of these consumption patterns. For nearly half of festival-goers, for example, their polydrug consumption includes both the impermissible pleasures of drugs and the permissible pleasures of alcohol, with atypical intoxication spread across the course of the day and across multiple days, unlike at home. The aim here is to contextualise these atypical intoxication practices in the wider nightlife setting, characterising it as a metaphorical and, in many cases, also literal journey into the woods.

In alignment with the monomyth, the chapter is structured around three key sections. First, the issue of *Separation* is explored, as we consider the motivations, expectations and starting points for journeys into the hedonistic realms of festivals and nightlife tourist resorts. Second, under the title of *Immersion*, we consider the sensorial pleasures of intoxication within these secondary worlds, as well as the associated risks. What role does intoxication play in these hedonistic woodland wonderlands and how might young adult drinking and other drug use differ from everyday consumption patterns? Third, we examine our protagonists' *Return*, with a focus on the narratives and stories that young people bring back from their journeys into the "wild zones" of dark forest and white isle. We conclude that if young people are to emerge from their journeys into the "woods" unscathed, there is an urgent need to embed innovative and effective harm reduction strategies within the secondary worlds of music festivals, nightlife tourist resorts and other bounded play spaces where regular patterns of drinking and drug use and attitudes to risk can be rapidly, if temporarily, distorted. Thus, these secondary worlds embody an opportunity for engagement as well as for excess.

## Separation

In Joseph Campbell's seminal deconstruction of myth, *The Hero with a Thousand Faces*, the protagonist's epic journey begins with a "call to adventure" to faraway lands—a dark forest or jungle, a mysterious island or mountain, an underground kingdom—"places of strangely fluid and polymorphous beings, unimaginable torments, superhuman deeds, and impossible delight" (Campbell, 2008, p. 48). It is easy to see how the carnivalesque secondary worlds of music festivals and nightlife tourist resorts—where conventions are suspended in a social and spatial separation from home (Urry & Larsen, 2011, p. 12)—symbolise such magical realms of faraway adventure.

Similarly, in the classic novel *Heart of Darkness*, Joseph Conrad's hero's voyage into the African interior is a physical, psychological and metaphorical journey into an alien, primeval landscape focusing on central protagonist Marlow, following in ivory trader Kurtz' footsteps, immersing himself in Kurtz' slow reversion to brutality and degradation. During the geographical journey up the Congo River and into dense jungle, the layers of presumed civilisation are slowly peeled back and the local native culture increasingly embraced and, as Kurtz embarks on a brutal slaughtering of "savages", the reader is led to question the supposed gulf between colonial civilisation and native "savagery". In Ward's consideration of the relative importance of rational and emotive drivers for cruelty in colonial state crime, he draws together Conrad's novel and Katz' (1988) criminology of seduction, noting that "what Marlow cannot articulate but Conrad's narrative implies about Kurtz's relationship with the wilderness is better captured in a phrase by Jack Katz: it is a 'dialectic process through which a person empowers the world to seduce him to criminality' (Katz, 1988, p. 7)" (Kelly, 2005, p. 438). Thus, embarking on a journey into the woods or wilderness means offering oneself up to this seduction into transgression.

In Hayward's (2002) discussion of transgressive leisure, he notes that the thrill of transgression comes in part from this individual excitement to commit crime, Katz' (1988) seduction of the offender. However, for both Hayward and Ferrell, there is more to transgressive leisure than simply the individual thrill created by a break from monotony. For Ferrell, in the collective reaction to boredom, there are not only "ephemeral crimes committed against boredom itself—but larger efflorescences of political and cultural rebellion" (2004, p. 287) suggesting that music holidays—to forest festivals or Balearic superclubs—could be in themselves a form of cultural resistance to the monotony of the everyday. Additionally, Hayward (2002, p. xx) notes how transgressive leisure and carnivalesque pleasure offer an opportunity for escapism not just from boredom but also from the insecurity and "hyper-banalization" of everyday life in which people feel increasingly over-controlled not just by agents of the state but also in a cultural and economic sense.

Prior to the turn of the millennium, UK music festivals were relatively small in scale and few in number. Such festivals historically were countercultural in nature, if only for the brief period of their existence, inverting the usual social order to suffuse the tensions of everyday life (Presdee, 2000) and providing a "temporary autonomous zone" (Bey, 1985) from the outside world for a form of carnivalesque social anarchism. The threads of cultural resistance and commercial exploitation are increasingly intertwined, however, with both the carnivalesque "urban spectacles" (Gotham, 2005) and everyday licensed venues (Skandalis et al., 2024) proliferating as key sites of initiation and experimentation for young adults. For example, prior to the COVID-19 pandemic, Mintel. (2018) estimated that a total of 918 festivals operated across the UK, more than double that of a decade earlier, with CGA (2019) estimating that over 700 UK music festivals were attended by 7.1 million customers in 2018. Almost a quarter of UK adults reported going to a music festival in the previous year, while for young men aged 16–24, the figure increased to half (Mintel., 2018).

Clearly the pandemic has had a catastrophic impact on nightlife tourism, festivals and the wider hospitality and events industries around the world. Nevertheless, after a two-year shut down, Mintel (2022) estimated that ticket sales for 2023 would surpass pre-Covid levels, with almost half of 16–24 year olds returning to music festivals in the 12 months prior to March 2022. However, while the major players have survived in the wake of COVID, many of the smaller festivals and nightclubs have been less fortunate, further affected by the subsequent economic downturn and inflationary pressures on both the costs of infrastructure and customers' disposable income. For example, Barrett (2023) reports that one in six festivals has disappeared since the lifting of lockdown, while the Association of Independent Festivals raised the alarm at the prospect of 100 festivals facing cancellation in 2024 (Gutteridge-Hewitt, 2024). Nevertheless, there continues to be an insatiable demand for some of the major festivals in the annual festival calendar—Glastonbury 2024, for example, sold out in less than an hour, with a capacity of 210,000 at £360 per ticket (Pidd, 2023).

Given the growing financial significance of UK festivals for the events industry—estimated by Mintel (2022) to be worth £3.22 billion by 2026—festivals have replaced traditional European package holidays for many young people. Both festivals and nightlife resorts draw party-goers from across the world. In the UK, the average travel time to festivals is around four hours, while a third of adults are willing to travel abroad to festivals (Mintel, 2018). Nearly two-thirds (62%) of UK festival-goers travelled over 100 km to reach their festival of choice, while only 10% considered proximity to their home a major factor when deciding on which festivals to attend (CGA, 2019). This growing internationalisation of festivals and carnivals over the decades has seen their transition from indigenous cultural and counter cultural celebrations into "experience production systems" developed by international entrepreneurs (Ferdinand & Williams, 2013). The value of festival-goers as consumers is not lost on the hospitality and beverage industries: CGA (2019) estimates that £114m is spent on alcohol sales alone at UK music festivals each year and festivals are considered to be the number one marketing target for drinks suppliers, including alcohol industry-sponsored bars and stages, free samples and other promotional activities.

Within consumer culture, transgressive leisure is facilitated, commodified and rebranded for youth and young adult audiences as part of a growing "experience economy" (Pine & Gilmore, 1999) where people increasingly seek to purchase a meaningful, memorable and

'Instagrammable experience'. Thus, the experience economy exploits the tensions between capitalist consumerism and people's desire for authenticity, freedom and self-fulfilment. Haydock (2015), echoing Stallybrass and White (1986), notes an ambivalence at the heart of carnival precisely because of this combination of radicalism and conservatism, suggesting that it "makes little sense to fight out the issue of whether or not carnivals are intrinsically radical or conservative, for to do so automatically involves the false essentializing of carnivalesque transgression" (Stallybrass & White, 1986, p. 14). 'Instagrammable' festivals and nightlife resorts are now spectacular themed and branded environments curated and marketed for social media feeds and glossy magazine festival guides (Baxter-Wright, 2019), furnished with everything from forest art installations to brightly coloured dip-dyed sheep and ubiquitous giant-sized letters demanding social media attention. For the events industry, this means designing festivals and super-clubs with increasing innovation and differentiation (Sipe, 2018), to elicit "socially approved arousal of moderate excitement" with the end goal of "maximising profit through consumer enjoyment" (O'Sullivan, 2016, p. 3). For festival and club-goers, in their quest for experiential consumption within and yet potentially at odds with the highly structured nature of such leisure, this can lead to the hijacking of "brandfests" in the pursuit of more spontaneous, subversive and less sanitised excitement (O'Sullivan, 2016). "Excitement, even ecstasy (the abandonment of reason and rationale), is the goal" (Presdee, 2000, p. 7) and intoxication is a key vehicle for young adults to achieve this "controlled loss of control" within these performance zones (Hayward, 2002; Measham, 2002).

In general, prevalence of use of illegal drugs is higher amongst festival and club-goers than the general population. In the UK, 20.9% of festival-goers in a self-selecting online survey reported having taken any drugs at festivals that year (UKFA, 2017), compared with 9% of 16- to 59-year-olds and 19.8% of 16- to 24-year-olds in the general population, in the previous 12 months (Home Office, 2018). International surveys (Hesse & Tutenges, 2008; Lim et al., 2008; Martinus et al., 2010) also indicate that festival-goers have a higher prevalence of drug use than the general population. Similarly, attendance at dance clubs is consistently correlated with higher levels of drug use than in the general population, both in self-report studies of club-goers in the 1990s and 2000s (Measham et al., 2001; Measham & Moore, 2009), and in annual household surveys, with adults attending nightclubs four times or more in the previous month nearly six times more likely to report having taken drugs in the past year than those not attending nightclubs in the past month (Home Office, 2018). In relation to British holidaymakers, Bellis et al. (2003) Bellis et al. (2009) found that young adults going to Ibiza, a nightlife tourist destination with a much higher density of electronic dance music (EDM) superclubs than other Balearic islands, had significantly higher levels of drug use and lower levels of alcohol consumption and alcohol-related violence. The contrasting backdrop to festival and nightlife consumption is that in the general young adult population drug use (Home Office, 2018), along with drinking and drunkenness (Measham, 2008), has been stable or falling in the UK for over a decade (explored elsewhere in this collection).

This desire to seek the excitement of carnivalesque experiences is reflected in a continued demand for young-adult-orientated holidays, although it has shifted away from cheap package holidays—symbolised by the death of the iconic "Club 18-30" (Mackay, 2018), towards millennial preferences for festivals, adventure holidays and independent travel, creating photogenic experiences, health-conscious images and social kudos. Similarly, changes in leisure preferences towards gyms, restaurants and coffee shops, had already seen the value of the UK nightclub industry plummet by £200 million even before COVID lockdowns (Booth & Halliday, 2018). Festival and nightlife tourism, however, retain opportunities for young adult experimentation and excess as they escape the panoptic gaze of parents in the neon party enclaves of Spain, Greece, Croatia and Bulgaria, with the exotic, other-worldly EDM superclubs of Ibiza drawing young tourists from across the globe. For some, the *journey* to these secondary worlds is part of the appeal—leaving the humdrum routines of home and life in the "real world" (Dilkes-Frayne, 2016) for faraway adventures with friends and "randoms". In *Altered State*, the seminal account of Acid House by a promoter, Collin (1998, p. 51) identifies how for many young people such escapism represents "an extended vacation in an alternate reality … a peak experience that allows for utopian dreaming", echoed by our research participants:

> We save for this all year, we count down the days. It's a week where we don't have to think about anything apart from getting fucked up and having a laugh. (Harry, tourist, Ibiza)

> All year, you get up, go to work, come home. It's fucking boring, man. This is my ten days to get lost. It's what keeps me going for the rest of the year. (Rob, tourist, Ibiza)

> This is an escape. You can act differently here, no one knows who you are. (Alex, tourist, Ibiza)

For young people travelling to these secondary worlds, entering the "liminal travel space" (Pritchard & Morgan, 2006, p. 762) of airports, motorway service stations and train stations can be an important first stage of the journey which separates the everyday from the other-worldly. In the monomyth structure, this represents the "crossing of the first threshold" as the traveller begins to cross from "the veil of the known into the unknown" (Campbell, 2008, p. 67). These transitional travel hubs represent intriguing spaces defined by the performance of departure, arrival and mobility. The liminal traveller is "neither here nor there; they are betwixt and between", positioned in a liminal zone likened "to death, to being in the womb, to invisibility, to darkness, to bisexuality, to the wilderness, and to an eclipse of the sun or moon" (Turner, 1997, p. 95), out of time and out of place. Here, as social conventions begin to fall away, structure and order are replaced with a sense of "playfulness, chance and the possibilities of subversion" (Carlson, 1996, p. 24). As Turner (2023, p. 63) shows, for many young people these travel hubs represent the first stage of hedonistic intoxication:

> There were some lads on the plane who were really drunk. They kept falling over and stuff. They got told off by the aircrew. (Pacha Shirt, female tourist, Ibiza)

> I was slaughtered at the airport. (Jed, tourist, Ibiza)

> We only got here at 2am last night. We had to carry him off the plane cos he was so drunk [pointing at friend who was taken ecstasy and is laughing

> whilst digging at the sand with his hands]. We had to put him to bed and then me and my other mate went out. (George, tourist, Ibiza)

Allusions to the binge consumption of alcohol at airports, on flights and on lengthy car journeys were a common feature of interviews for this fieldwork. This seemed to be symbolic of social and spatial separation from "reality" (Turner, 1997) and a permissible prelude to the (often illegal) excesses of the experience ahead. Public transport travel hubs are ambiguous spaces, however, splicing notions of freedom with hyper-securitisation, control and surveillance, particularly at airports and train stations. Lengthy car journeys to festivals, by contrast, provide a final personal space within which friends can binge pre-load not only on alcohol but also illegal drugs for hours before parking up, queuing up and succumbing to the imposition of entry restrictions and potential 24/7 surveillance by festival staff, CCTV and increasingly drones once onsite. The condition of entry into wonderland entails running a gauntlet of security staff, metal detector gates, searches of one's person and possessions, and possibly even drug detection dogs. However, as Campbell (2008, p. 65) states, the rewards of crossing such thresholds are entry to the "regions of the unknown" and the untold pleasures of the secondary world. As Garratt (1998) noted, for many customers the experience of entering a dance club is akin to dropping into an adventure in Wonderland, a sentiment reflected by Turner (2023, p. 69) in relation to a participant's description of ketamine use in an Ibizan super-club:

> I took this big line of ket. To say it was euphoric isn't enough. It was like falling into another world. Down the rabbit hole, I was lost and falling, falling, falling. It was almost *beyond* happiness. (Maria, tourist, Ibiza)

# Immersion

## Suspension of Rules in the Secondary World

> Entering the grounds of the music festival was like entering another world for the day. Although the tickets say things about rules of the festival being

> like rules of the outside world, there is a sense that social rules and ways of relating to each other were quite different from the outside world, allowing people to engage with each other with a sense of freedom, free from the formality of being among strangers in the 'real world'. (Borlagdan et al., 2010, p. 97)

For many young people, the magical realms of festivals and nightlife tourist resorts feel like they exist outside the parameters of "real life"; reality no longer operates in quite the same way (Warner, 2014, p. 20). As in the mythological secondary worlds of Carroll, Lewis and Tolkien, many Ibizan research participants described a distorted sense of reality, as notions of space and time seemed to shrink and stretch (Turner, 2023, p. 50):

> I don't know how long I've been here. It feels like years, but it's just a few days. The whole place is just surreal. It's like nowhere else. (Ashley, tourist, Ibiza)

> I love it here. I don't want to leave. It's not real though. (Bianca, tourist, Ibiza)

The creeping sense of the surreal described within these narratives is enhanced by the deeply immersive spectacles that characterise such space. The late-night dance tents at festivals and the superclub dance floors of Ibiza are bound by their ability to create profoundly sensual *atmospheres* that can saturate space to completely transform the affective experience of those present (Edensor & Sumartojo, 2015; Shaw, 2013, p. 88). This is exemplified by Cambridgeshire's *Secret Garden Party* festival, claiming to be the first in the boutique festival genre, a "hedonistic woodland wonderland" (Time Out, 2023) with 24-hour forest raves in its "Lost Woods", quirky art installations and immersive entertainment; and the infamous *Shangri-La* sector of Glastonbury festival, described as a dystopian pleasure city that comes alive after midnight in "a great swell of music, art, drugs, joy, fear and wild abandonment" (Barton, 2012). For those present, this "magical alternate reality" (Braverman, 2000, p. 104) opens new possibilities of transgression as they step into a "temporary sphere of behaviour" (Shaw & Williams, 2004, p. 151), to combine alcohol with the illicit pleasures of drugs such as MDMA, cocaine, ketamine and LSD. In these "phantasmagoric realms" (Edensor, 2015, p. 332), the world of illegal drugs that usually operates on a veiled, subterranean level is inverted and woven into the consumer experience, blurring the boundaries between permissible and impermissible behaviours (Moore & Measham, 2012). As Steeves (2003, p. 185) suggests, in the hyper-real "fantasyscapes" of Disneyland, "a different kind of conscious engagement with the world is at work [and] one cannot help but be altered by the environment". Consequently, as our fieldwork in festivals and dance clubs consistently revealed, this created opportunities to engage in patterns of psychoactive consumption that were significantly different from their everyday lives back home (Measham, 2004a; Measham & Shiner, 2009, p. 507).

## Pushing the Boundaries: Intoxication in the Secondary World

What role does intoxication play in these spectacular performance zones and to what extent is this atypical of everyday consumption patterns? Consumption within festivals and nightlife tourist resorts can be both atypical and normal: a carnival of excess during a temporal and geographical dislocation from the usual constraints of work, home and family that is accepted, expected and even normalised within that space (Measham, 2004a; Measham et al., 2001; Turner, 2018; Turner, 2023). In-situ research with festival and club-goers offers an opportunity to shed light on intoxication at play embedded within these contexts.

The UK's largest ongoing study of festival alcohol and other drug use, conducted by Measham and colleagues, utilises an in-situ research design previously used in dance clubs (Measham et al., 2001, 2011), "High Street" nightclubs (Measham et al., 2012) and bars (Measham & Brain, 2005). The EFS includes annual convenience sample surveys, interviews, observations and focus groups with festival-goers and staff each summer from 2010 onwards at outdoor music festivals by teams of socially mixed (by gender, ethnicity, age, social class and sexual orientation) researchers (see McCormack et al., 2021 for further details of methodology). In 2018, 2250 respondents completed the annual survey at 11 UK music festivals chosen as contrasting examples of festivals in operation annually in the UK, ranging from urban parks to remote rural farms, from one to five days in length, from over-18s to family-friendly admission policies, and from specialist EDM to live music, comedy and theatrical entertainment. Short surveys averaging ten minutes in length were conducted with individuals across all show days and across the full footprint of each festival, including entertainment and camping areas, with over nine in ten surveys conducted between 12:00 and 18:00. Over half (51.1%) of respondents were identified as female and the mean age was 25.3 years.

Regarding alcohol consumption, nearly two-thirds (63.3%) of respondents in the 2018 festival survey had been drinking alcohol on the day of interview by late afternoon and they reported consuming an average of 7.6 units of alcohol (a UK unit of alcohol is equivalent to 10 ml of pure alcohol) by the time of interview. Female respondents had consumed an average of 6.2 units of alcohol and male respondents 8.8 units, meaning that both women and men had already exceeded binge drinking levels (NHS, 2019) by late afternoon and before the evening's entertainment had started. When including both those who had already consumed alcohol by the time of interview and those who intended to drink later, it rises to nearly nine in ten (86.8%) festival-goers either having had a drink or intending to drink that day. Indeed, a notable feature of festival and holiday consumption is the preponderance of people drinking alcohol throughout the day who would not usually drink alcohol in the daytime in their everyday lives. As one Ibizan nightlife respondent stated, "I only usually drink on Friday nights, but here, you just wake up and think, 'right, let's have a Stella'" (Rob, tourist, Ibiza).

If we explore festival drinking in more detail for different categories of respondents according to their self-reported usual drinking patterns, we can see that whilst more frequent drinkers are more likely to drink larger quantities of alcohol at festivals than their less frequent drinking peers, occasional drinkers also drank significant amounts of alcohol onsite. Looking at daily drinkers, 6.9% of festival-goers said that they usually drank alcohol every day in their regular lives and over eight in ten (81.1%)

of these daily drinkers already had had a drink on the interview day, consuming an average of 10.3 units of alcohol by late afternoon. At the other end of the spectrum are occasional drinkers (here defined as those who identify as drinkers but report usually drinking alcohol less than once a month): whilst only 2.9% of festival-goers considered themselves to usually drink alcohol less than once in a month, 60% of these already had had a drink by late afternoon and already had consumed on average 4.5 units of alcohol. When we look at consumption on both the fieldwork day and the previous day, this rises to over three quarters (76.9%) of occasional drinkers having consumed alcohol at the festival either that day or the previous day. This illustrates both the increased frequency of alcohol consumption and the increased quantity of alcohol consumed by young adults attending festivals, from daily drinkers through to occasional drinkers, by comparison with their usual drinking habits.

UK festivals can create atypical patterns of consumption not only in respect of alcohol, as above, but also illegal drugs, usually with alcohol and other drugs combined together. Drug use was strongly correlated with drinking: over half (52.4%) of festival-goers either already had taken or intended to take a drug at the festival on the day they were interviewed. Looking more closely at those reporting taking drugs "today or tonight", over nine in ten (91.8%) either already had drank alcohol or intended to later that day, compared with only 8.2% of drug users not planning on drinking. Drug users were also asked how typical their festival drug use was: over half (54.1%) said that they took a larger quantity of drugs than they usually consumed, and nearly a quarter (24.3%) said that they took a wider range of different types of drugs than they usually consumed.

## The Typical Repertoires of Atypical Intoxication

Regarding festivals as sites of atypical alcohol and other drug use, nearly half (46.9%) of festival-goers reported either already having consumed both alcohol and illegal drugs on the fieldwork day or said they intended to. Furthermore, 7.9% of all survey respondents reported that they *only* took drugs at festivals and over eight in ten (80.3%) of those either had already taken drugs or intended to that day.

As a character sketch, the average festival-goer who reported alcohol consumption to binge drinking levels on the fieldwork day was statistically significantly more likely to be younger, male, and in education rather than employment, but not of any specific ethnicity or sexual orientation. For male binge drinkers, the mean number of units consumed was 15.6 (by the median time of survey completion, 15:52 hours), while female binge drinkers had consumed a mean of 12 units (by the median time of survey completion, 16:07). Based on the widely used Department of Health definition[1] for 'sensible' drinking on a single occasion (6 units for women and 8 units for men), this means both women and men had consumed double the daily 'sensible' level of alcohol by around 16:00 hours. Binge drinkers were significantly more likely than non-binge drinkers to report already having taken or planning on taking any illegal drug on the fieldwork day (61.7% vs. 52.2%) and to be taking two or more illegal drugs (polydrug use, 51.6% vs. 39.2%). The most significant differences in which types of drugs were taken by binge drinkers compared with non-binge drinkers were for cocaine (34.2% vs. 18.3%) and for MDMA pills and crystal (46.1% vs. 31.9%). Of further interest is that there was no significant relationship between binge drinking and ketamine use (20.0% vs. 19.4%) on the fieldwork day, which is perhaps related to the heightened risk of combining ketamine with alcohol. This then represents a snapshot of the *typical* repertoires of *atypical intoxication* (Tables 14.1 and 14.2).

As to why this happens in these leisure spaces, the greater access and availability of illegal drugs at festivals and in nightlife resorts, as well as greater availability of holiday spending money and free time, all help to facilitate these atypical levels of consumption. As Turner (2023, p. 64) shows, for many young people, festivals and nightlife resorts are notable for the increased access to drugs and relatively open dealing compared to in everyday life.

[1] https://www.ons.gov.uk/peoplepopulationandcommunity/healthandsocialcare/drugusealcoholandsmoking/bulletins/opinionsandlifestylesurveyadultdrinkinghabitsingreatbritain/2017

**Table 14.1** Demographics for binge drinkers/non binge drinkers

| | Bingeing | Not bingeing | Chi2 | P | Cramer | P Bonferroni Corrected |
|---|---|---|---|---|---|---|
| Male | 246 (56.9) | 642 (46.6) | 13.607104140585000 | 0.000225 | 0.086729 | 0.0009 |
| Straight | 379 (89.0) | 1200 (88.8) | 0.06426616866937670 | 0.968378 | 0.006012 | 1.0 |
| White | 392 (91.4) | 1236 (90.2) | 0.5809998776511030 | 0.900768 | 0.017971 | 1.0 |
| Employed | 295 (68.9) | 761 (55.5) | 27.05982527380410 | 0.000006 | 0.122644 | 0.000024 |

**Table 14.2** Illegal drug use amongst binge drinkers / non-binge drinkers

| Today / Later | Bingeing | Not Bingeing | Chi2 | P | Cramer | P Bonferroni Corrected |
|---|---|---|---|---|---|---|
| Cocaine | 149 (34.2) | 254 (18.3) | 47.33568485233010 | 0.0 | 0.161228 | 0.0 |
| MDMA (pills or crystal) | 201 (46.1) | 442 (31.9) | 28.603879151388100 | 0.0 | 0.125331 | 0.0 |
| Any Illegal Drug | 269 (61.7) | 723 (52.2) | 11.675452092408800 | 0.000633 | 0.080072 | 0.003165 |
| Poly Drug | 225 (51.6) | 543 (39.2) | 20.401130305367000 | 6E-06 | 0.105845 | 3E-05 |
| Ketamine | 87 (20.0) | 268 (19.4) | 0.04339126033183560 | 0.83499 | 0.004881 | 1.0 |

Nevertheless, there is also a small but not insignificant group of festival-goers who do not take any psychoactive substances when they go to festivals: nearly one in ten (9.1%) festival-goers reported having consumed neither alcohol nor any other drugs on the fieldwork day and not planning to later.

In this section, we have demonstrated how alcohol and other drugs are intricately woven into the immersive secondary worlds of festivals and nightlife tourist resorts, with many participants describing patterns of usage that were very different to their everyday lives, characterised by researchers as "calculated hedonism", "determined drunkenness" (Measham, 2004b), "extreme drinking" (Martinic & Measham, 2008) and a "new culture of intoxication" (Measham & Brain, 2005). To understand the experiential context of these atypical patterns of intoxication, it is important to consider participants' narratives of pleasure, an issue that has been described by Hunt et al. (2010, p. 119) as "unseeable" in drugs research.

## Pleasure in the Secondary World

Researching pleasure, particularly the "impermissible pleasures" of intoxication (Moore & Measham, 2012), remains "the great unmentionable" (Hunt & Evans, 2008) in the drugs field and yet is essential to understanding and addressing drug use in the round (Nicholls & Hunt, 2025). The pull of professional self-preservation combined with the challenge of capturing psychoactive pleasure in print means that many researchers feel tempted to sidestep such narratives, fearing they may be condemned as unscientific, "pro-drugs", or both (Duff, 2008, p. 385; Moore, 2008, p. 355). Given that, for many people, pleasure is the principal motivation behind the atypical intoxication identified above, this obfuscates the entangled sensual pleasures of music, dancing, drugs, alcohol and risk within the secondary worlds of festivals and nightlife resorts, where alcohol and drugs represent an immersive component of the assembled space. Tutenges (2022, p. 417) situates this with the Durkheimian concept of "collective effervescence", defined as "a state of heightened intersubjectivity, a sort of raw vitality, which is characterized by turbulent, transgressive, and yet mutually attuned actions and emotions among individuals who are gathered in the same place". In his ethnographic study amongst tourists in the Bulgarian nightlife resort of Sunny Beach, Tutenges (2013) identifies how the combination of atmospheric components such as light, sound and alcohol can unify the crowd and the boundaries between self and others becomes blurred in a state of transgressive collective effervescence. Similarly, this reflects Deleuze and Guattari's (1998, p. 476) concept of assemblage, defined as an "amorphous collection of juxtaposed pieces that can be joined together in an infinite number of ways". This is demonstrated in the interview narratives below, reflecting recent scholarship on the embodied, affective and sensorial aspects of intoxication (see Bohling, 2015; Demant, 2013; Duff, 2008; Jayne et al., 2008; Tutenges, 2022; Turner, 2023):

> All I know, is I had the best time in there. It was so good. Loved it. Absolutely loved it. I saw Tiesto [superstar DJ]. I was in my element. It was the imagery on stage, his presence in the middle of it all, the visuals behind him and all the people around me. I was just so happy that these people were next to me. We all had our arms around each other, everyone on pills, everyone at the same level. (Jack, bar worker, Ibiza)

> The music, the pills, the DJs, the crowd, the whole aura. Everything was just perfect. Absolutely incredible. (Ella, ticket seller, Ibiza)

In these accounts, we see how intoxication can represent a key component of the immersive, effervescent atmosphere generated within festivals and nightlife resorts. In deconstructing the sensorial pleasures of psychoactive drugs, light and sound represent two crucial features of the assemblage. Light is an aspect of the sensory environment that can "envelop, guide, invite, deter and otherwise subtly influence our patterns of sociability" in urban space (Atkinson, 2007, p. 1907). The changing nature of cities at night has been explored within criminology, sociology and geography; however, recent scholarship has focused on the affective and atmospheric dimensions of night-time space (Shaw, 2013, p. 87; Turner, 2023). In our fieldwork, darkness was one of the most powerful precursors of atmosphere. As the sun goes down in the party spaces of music festivals and nightlife tourist resorts, the playful aspects of liminality and hyper-reality are intensified. Here, the temporal boundaries of light pull bodies in to create a "flexible atmosphere [...] intensified within a small time-space" (Shaw, 2013, p. 92). This alters the social relations between those present, with alcohol and other drugs becoming interwoven aspects of the assemblage.

Sound is also a powerful sensorial component of atmosphere and has been defined by Hill and Saroka (2010, p. 509) as the fourth dimension of the present. The "sonic ecology" (Atkinson, 2007) of atmosphere is important in understanding intoxication, because sound can break open practices of interaction and experimentation (Edensor & Sumartojo, 2015, p. 253). From Glastonbury to Ibiza, music defines both the meaning and the boundaries of themed space, sonically promoting culture, lifestyle and [drug] consumption (Hayward, 2012). Turner (2023, p. 75) highlights how the immersive symbiosis of sound and drugs featured regularly in Ibizan participant narratives:

> I took the best pill I've ever taken in my life in there [super-club]. The music was amazing. I had about two hours just next to the bass bins with my eyes closed. (Jack, bar worker, Ibiza)

> We did gold leaf [ecstasy]. It was so intense, so good, like dancing inside some claustrophobic sweatbox. I felt the bass through every part of my body, like it had passed through every one of us in the club. It connected us, like we were inside the music. (Maria, tourist, Ibiza)

The *connection* described here by Maria was a narrative of pleasure that emerged consistently in fieldwork. It seems that when we enter within these secondary worlds, the fear and distrust of strangers that we experience in the late modern landscapes of the "*soft city*" (Raban, 1974) ebb away. As Bauman (2000, p. 95) states:

> [T]he meeting of strangers is an event without a past. More often than not, it is also an event without a future ... a story most certainly 'not to be continued', a one-off chance, to be consummated in full while it lasts.

The pleasure of connection at festivals and nightlife resorts is of course enmeshed with the socialising effects of alcohol and other drug use. This desire for sociability has been described as a core aspect of the tourist experience, with fleeting temporary bonds formed during travel leaving indelible cherished memories (Harrison, 2003), as indicated in these excerpts:

> You get so loved up. It's unbelievable. We were dancing last night, and we all got in a circle and just starting hugging. (Paul, tourist, Ibiza)

> People you meet here are wicked. People you wouldn't meet every day at home. The best thing about being here has been meeting these [points to two friends made whilst on holiday]. (Matt, tourist, Ibiza)

Connection with friends is only one aspect, however. In reflecting Tutenges's (2022) application of the concept of collective effervescence, many respondents gave vivid accounts of moments where they felt deeply connected to themselves and to the crowd, as a consequence of the magical combination of dancing, music and intoxication. This "oceanic experience"—the feeling of deep connection to the crowd—may be rarely attained by music alone (Malbon, 1999, p. 110). Turner (2023, p. 118) shows that for some participants, it was their consumption of MDMA that intensified this oceanic state and led them to lose themselves in moments of empathic euphoria:

> I wandered through the different rooms in the club, and it was just like I was floating. I put my hand up for people to touch as they passed me. Everyone's just smiling at each other, everyone. Then I walk into this room and Primal Scream came on. I've never felt so happy. I just started dancing on my own—but not on my own—like the whole crowd is with me. (Carla, tourist, Ibiza)

## Risk and Rationalisation in the Secondary World

> Having traversed the threshold, the hero moves in a dream landscape of curiously fluid, ambiguous forms, where he must survive a succession of trials. (Campbell, 2008, p. 81)

In the monomyth structure, having crossed the threshold and entered the secondary world, down the rabbit hole into wonderland, the protagonist is open to the ambiguity of untold pleasures merging with trial, risk and danger (Campbell, 2008, p. 81). As Mark (tourist, Ibiza) stated:

> It's totally different here. It's unlike any other place I've ever been to, but it's hard work. It's an amazing experience, but it is *hard* work.

The sentiment expressed here demonstrates that whilst our participants were immersed in the transgressive sensorial pleasures of the secondary world, they were simultaneously exposed to a multitude of potential harms including exhaustion from lack of sleep; sunburn; dehydration; a substandard diet; sexual risk-taking; intoxication; drug-related harm; violent crime; theft; sexual assault; and intimidation from security, police or others.

Whereas mainstream criminology invariably foregrounds the risks of alcohol and other drug use for both offender and victim, it is important to maintain perspective and view this as only one aspect of several issues which potentially impact on the health, safety and well-being of young people acting within the boundaries of festivals and nightlife resorts. Furthermore, this exposure to harm is compounded by the way in which such contexts can rapidly distort perceptions of risk that characterise life in the "real world". As Turner (2023, p. 67) shows, for many participants, the hyper-reality of the secondary world instils an overwhelming sense of ambivalent well-being:

> You have to understand that getting hold of gear out here is like ordering a takeaway at home. I've got a list of numbers in this [hold up his mobile

> phone] that would have someone right here [West End, San Antonio] within five minutes. (Nick, bar worker/drug dealer, Ibiza)

> A lot of people will come out here and say, 'this is the first time I've ever taken a pill'. I met this couple here on holiday last week, they were so strait-laced at home, and here they'd been doing pills for the first time. It's just seen as acceptable out here. It's just the done thing. (Karen, PR Manager, Ibiza)

These excerpts reveal how interpretations of risk are not shaped in a cultural vacuum, rather they are grounded within the social milieu (Kelly, 2005, p. 1444). It is therefore important to appreciate how, for some young people, their usual patterns of psychoactive consumption may be rapidly transformed within the boundaries of festivals and nightlife resorts. This distortion is not necessarily founded on a lack of awareness about the risks of increased consumption, but rather the *perception* that they are unlikely to be harmed on holiday in wonderland, an issue which permeates the hyper-real, secondary world of Disney theme parks too, as Koenig (2006, p. 179) states: "guests get reckless, thinking, 'This is Disneyland. Nothing bad can happen to me'".

Perceptions of the potential consequences of intoxication therefore influence intent, both in terms of deciding to try certain drugs for the first time and in continuing to use them (Martins et al., 2011, p. 551). These perceptions are shaped by the bounded normalisation of illicit drugs within the socio-cultural context of festivals and nightlife resorts (Measham & Shiner, 2009). Gamma et al. (2005, p. 390) argue that one of the strongest behavioural determinants of drug use is witnessing immediate adverse effects. However, despite a number of MDMA-related deaths within the festivals and dance clubs which were our fieldwork sites (Cooney & Measham, 2023), the reactions of festival and club-goers to such fatalities on site were mostly nonplussed. Despite the cause of death being unconfirmed for many months, and the details of the incidents sketchy and unclear, drug users reassured themselves by utilising distancing strategies such as rationalising that they were not at risk because they had not made the same (presumed) mistake: for example, "I had the red pills, not the green pills, so I'm okay" or "I bought my drugs from my regular dealer not from the onsite dealer, so I'm okay". Turner (2023, p. 126) illustrates this sort of post hoc rationalisation on risk-taking in the following excerpts:

> I mean we read the paper about the lass dying [in a superclub], and not one person flinched. Not one of the group said 'oh I'm not going to have a pill tonight'. Then the group next to us started talking about it and they said the exact same thing, not one of them said they weren't going to have one that night. (Ben, tourist, Ibiza)

> We heard about the girl that died. One of my mates cut his finger in a club on a glass, and the paramedics took him away. They said gold leaf [pills] are fine, but to watch the red ones. We only got those the first day, we had a couple on the second day, but mostly we've been getting the ones called white females. They're better. (Male media student, tourist, Ibiza)

> I think you've got more chance of being struck by lightning twice than dying from pills. (Geordie male, tourist, Ibiza)

This apparent ambivalence did not mean that tourists were unaware of the potential harms associated with their use of drugs, but rather that they balanced perceived potential risks against already experienced pleasures (Kelly, 2005, p. 1454; Parker et al., 1998). Yet the spectre of the unknown content and strength of drugs in circulation in the illegal drug market hovered over them: over two-thirds (68.7%) of all respondents in the 2018 UK festival survey reported that they worried about the contents or strength of illegal drugs and, with public drug checking introduced to UK festivals two years earlier (Measham, 2019), 8.2% of respondents reported having used a festival drug checking service within the previous 12 months.

Despite this ambivalence around safety, it is important to recognise that young adult atypical intoxication within their time-limited immersion in the hedonistic spaces of festivals and nightlife resorts created multiple levels of additional risk by comparison with their everyday lives. As fieldwork frequently revealed, moments of danger punctured the atmosphere at times, whether it was explosions of violence, robbery, sexual assault, or alcohol or drug-related harm:

> A woman in her 20s collapses on the floor, and in that moment the spell of the club is broken. She looks terrible. Her eyes have rolled back, and her mouth hangs limply open. Those in the vicinity look shocked as two visibly shaken male friends grasp her under the shoulders and drag her limp body off the dance floor. As she disappears into the crowd, the group around me shake off their concern, turn to face the DJ and start dancing again. Out of sight and out of mind, the bubble is restored. (Tim Turner, field notes, Ibiza)

## Return

> I stood before a dark cave, wanting to go in [...] and I shuddered at the thought that I might not be able to find my way back. (Campbell, 2008, p. 85)

As the hero accomplishes their transcendental quest, so they must return home from the woodland wonderland and readjust to life in the "real world". As Campbell (2008, p. 189) states: "the first problem of the returning hero is to accept as real, after an experience of the soul satisfying vision of fulfilment, the passing joys and sorrows, banalities and noisy obscenities of life". Turner (2023, p. 64) illustrates how the difficulties of returning to the humdrum schedules of home after the hedonistic freedom of the secondary world was a recurring theme, exemplified in the following excerpts:

> It's so different from home. None of us want to leave. (Sarah, tourist, Ibiza)

> On the flight out, everyone is happy and wants to party. Coming back, they're all different. Everyone is tired and fed up about going home. (Dominika, cabin crew, Ibiza)

> I don't know how much I've spent. I haven't checked my balance once, and I've been waving my credit card around all week. The consequences are

> gonna kick me in the face when I get home ... financial consequences, health consequences. (Paul, tourist, Ibiza)

For many, the gradual transition back into the rhythms of everyday life seemed to be characterised by a brief but powerful stage of liminality—a temporal period of readjustment where the "stickiness" of their experience in the secondary world seemed to cross over and seep into normal life:

> When I got home, things were bad for a few days. I kept waking up in the middle of the night, I was convinced that the demon from 'Insidious' [a horror film] was in the room—*absolutely convinced*. And that was for three or four days. I couldn't shake it. (Alex, tourist, Ibiza)

> I swear I could still hear the music when I got home, I'd be in that weird state of half-sleep and I could hear the distant thud of techno. I'd wake up and be really confused, thinking I was still there. (Maria, tourist, Ibiza)

As this sense of being caught in-between reality and non-reality dissipated, our participants talked of the importance of stories that they could draw upon. These represented cherished memories, a key feature of a late modern experience economy that offers sensation-gathering opportunities that provide social kudos, identity and social bonds. In this respect, festivals and nightlife resorts represent experiential spaces where actors can generate "Instagrammable" stories of their transgressive interludes. These stories—retold and reshaped over a lifetime—can help to strengthen the social ties between those involved (Tutenges & Rod, 2009; Tutenges & Sandberg, 2013). Mythologised and exaggerated with each re-telling, such tales cement friendships and reveal much about the social meaning participants attach to their experiences within social worlds (Fleetwood & Sandberg, 2022). Intoxication is not simply for the fun of the moment, then, but "to create stories of transgression that they can later use as a form of entertainment and as a token of their capacity to modify and partly suspend their ingrown habits of self-censorship" (Tutenges, 2012, p. 147: Turner, 2023).

> We've had *the best time* here, so many memories to take home. (George, tourist, Ibiza)

> It's about the experience and the journey. It's a story to share with my friends—like, 'listen to what happened to me'—it's about getting away from boring, mundane life. You can be someone else for a while. (Christopher, tourist, Ibiza)

> It's all we come to do; we hope to come back with stories to tell. Good stories. It's like we come out here to be able to say, 'do you remember that moment we shared?' I think it builds relationships. I've got a huge cork board, like a half wall, dedicated to times on the island. Little mementoes, ticket stubs, stuff like that. I can pick out moments to draw back on to remember that time. (Alex, tourist, Ibiza)

The question here is, does this transgressive interlude, this atypical intoxication in festival fields and superclubs, result in any lasting change for young adult attitudes, values or behaviours? What do participants take back home with them from wonderland, aside from their stories, selfies and memories? In contrast to the career, skills and self-enhancement prospects of "serious leisure" (Sachsman, 2007), "casual leisure" at festivals and nightlife resorts requires relatively little planning or commitment, and instead, it is its very serendipity that offers sociability, creativity and potential self-discovery, as this Ibizan tourist noted:

> I think the place really opened my eyes. Big time. I'd experienced lots of things at home, but going there for the first time, it changed me. My eyes were well and truly opened. (Ben, tourist, Ibiza)

However, as noted by Sandberg and Tutenges (2015), drug stories and their journeys from the ordinary to the extraordinary and back again, can create, consolidate or challenge societal norms. Storytelling may be therapeutic, educational, entertaining, cautionary or unsettling. Most importantly, drug stories "constitute the glue that holds the culture together" (Sandberg & Tutenges, 2015, p. 169).

This chapter has presented previously unpublished data suggesting that festivals and nightlife resorts are an important feature of leisure time for over half of UK young adults, and for most of them, intoxication is an integral part of the experience within these deeply immersive secondary worlds. Festivals and nightlife resorts operate as performance zones for transgressive leisure bounded by time and space: within them, our research suggests, regular, everyday patterns of alcohol and other drug use are rapidly and drastically transformed. For nearly half of festival goers, these polydrug repertoires include both the impermissible pleasures of drugs and the permissible pleasures of alcohol, with *atypical* intoxication across the course of the day and across multiple days.

Not only do we see "extreme drinking" (Martinic & Measham, 2008), however, but also extreme drug use: with secondary world drug use notably different to everyday drug use in a number of ways. First, prevalence is higher amongst festival and club-goers than the general population; second, occasional users are more likely to make an exception and consume in these spaces; third, larger quantities of drugs are consumed; and fourth, wider repertoires of different drugs are consumed. These four features of atypical intoxication are likely to result in higher risk due to lower individual tolerance for alcohol and illegal drugs; more limited knowledge of current local drug markets; greater likelihood of drug transactions involving unknown street dealers rather than regular neighbourhood ones; and an associated greater likelihood of being unknowingly mis-sold unwanted products by onsite festival dealers compared to offsite dealers (Measham, 2019; Measham & Simmons, 2022). All these risk factors combine with binge drinking in an age group for whom the indicators suggest that these behaviours are all increasingly *atypical* features compared with their everyday lives, leading us to conclude that festivals and nightlife resorts are sites of particular concern for young adult health, well-being and safety. Despite and indeed because of the broader downturn in drinking, drunkenness and drug use, the risks of these pockets of excess are accentuated by their atypicality.

Furthermore, our research suggests, many young adults' usual attitudes to risk are suspended alongside their usual consumption patterns in their temporary immersion in nightlife space. Festival and club-goers protect themselves from acknowledging the risks of what they do with post hoc rationalisation and distancing strategies, despite not knowing the contents of their own illegal drugs or those of fatalities within those same events. It is important to note that most young adults *do* worry about the consequences of illegal, if not legal, drugs, and do engage with onsite harm reduction services, indicated by the demand for drug checking outstripping supply (Measham & Simmons, 2022). Therefore, if young adults are to emerge from their journeys into the "woods" unscathed, we suggest embedding non-judgmental and easily accessible harm reduction services within these immersive secondary worlds where psychoactive consumption, as well as wider attitudes to risk, are rapidly distorted in spaces where they are far away from the potential safety net of home. Our research highlights the value, therefore, in expanding the scale and range of care—including medical, welfare, sexual health, psychedelic support and drug checking services—located in or near points of consumption. Thus, these secondary worlds of atypical intoxication can provide sites of opportunity for engagement with support services, as well as cause for concern, regarding contemporary young adult consumption practices.

## References

Atkinson, R. (2007). Ecology of sound: The sonic order of urban space. *Urban Studies, 44*(10), 1905–1917.

Barton, L. (2012, June 13). Julien Temple: The dark side of Glastonbury. *The Guardian* [online]. Retrieved July 3, 2016, from https://www.theguardian.com/music/2012/jun/13/julien-temple-dark-side-of-glastonbury

Barrett, C. (2023). Covid-19 wiped out 17% of UK festivals. *Access All Areas*. https://accessaa.co.uk/covid-19-wiped-out-17-of-uk-festivals/

Bauman, Z. (2000). *Liquid modernity*. Polity Press.

Baxter-Wright, D. (2019, January 28). 10 of the most instagrammable UK festivals: Sequins, sunsets and glitter galore. *Cosmopolitan*. https://www.cosmopolitan.com/uk/entertainment/travel/g9930311/festivals-instagram/

Bellis, M. A., Hughes, K., Bennett, A., & Thomson, R. (2003). The role of an international nightlife resort in the proliferation of recreational drugs. *Addiction, 98*, 1713–1721.

Bellis, M. A., Hughes, K., Calafat, A., Montse, J., & Schnitzer, S. (2009). Relative contributions of holiday location and nationality to changes in recreational drug taking behaviour: A natural experiment in the Balearic Islands. *European Addiction Research, 15*, 78–86.

Bey, H. (1985). *TAZ: The temporary autonomous zone, ontological anarchy, poetic terrorism*. Autonomedia.

Bohling, F. (2015). Alcoholic assemblages: Exploring fluid subjects in the night-time economy. *Geoforum, 58*, 132–142.

Booth, R., & Halliday, J. (2018, December 31). UK's nightclubs suffer as young people seek less hedonistic pursuits: Games, food and even gyms are becoming more popular than hitting the dance floor. *The Guardian*. https://www.theguardian.com/music/2018/dec/31/uk-nightclubs-suffer-young-people-seek-less-hedonistic-pursuits

Borlagdan, J., Freeman, T., Duvnjak, A., Bywood, P. T., & Roche, A. M. (2010). *From ideal to reality: Cultural contradictions and young people's drinking*. National Centre for Education and Training on Addiction, Flinders University.

Braverman, B. (2000). Libraries and theme parks: Strange bedfellows. *Research Strategies, 17*, 99–105.

Campbell, J. (2008). *The hero with a thousand faces* (3rd ed.). New World Library.

Carlson, M. (1996). *Performance: A critical introduction*. Routledge.

CGA. (2019). *Your future in festivals: How to stand out from the crowd* [online]. https://www.cga.co.uk/wp/content/uploads/2019/05/YourFutureinFestivals-CGA-Insights.pdf.

Collin, M. (1998). *Altered state: The story of ecstasy and acid house*. Serpent's Tail.

Cooney, T., & Measham, F. (2023). Counting and accounting for drug-related deaths at UK music festivals 2017–2023: A commentary. *Drug Science, Policy and Law*. https://doi.org/10.1177/20503245231211444

Deleuze, G., & Guattari, F. (1998). *A thousand plateaus: Capitalism and schizophrenia*. University of Minnesota Press.

Demant, J. (2013). Affected in the nightclub. A case study of regular clubbers' conflictual practices in nightclubs. *International Journal of Drug Policy, 24*, 196–202.

Dilkes-Frayne, E. (2016). Drugs at the campsite: Socio-spatial relations and drug use at music festivals. *International Journal of Drug Policy, 33*, 27–35.

Duff, C. (2008). The pleasure in context. *International Journal of Drug Policy, 19*, 384–392.

Edensor, T. (2015). Light, design and atmosphere. *Visual Communication, 14*(3), 331–350.

Edensor, T., & Sumartojo, S. (2015). Designing atmospheres: Introduction to special issue. *Visual Communication, 14*(3), 251–265.

Ferdinand, N., & Williams, N. (2013). International festivals as experience production systems. *Tourism Management, 34*, 202–210.

Ferrell, J. (2004). Boredom, crime and criminology. *Theoretical Criminology, 8*(3), 287–302.

Fleetwood, J., & Sandberg, S. (2022). Narrative criminology and ethnography. In S. M. Bucerius, K. D. Heggerty, & L. Berardi (Eds.), *The Oxford handbook of ethnographies of crime and criminal justice* (pp. P246–P268). Oxford University Press.

Gamma, A., Jerome, L., Liechti, M. E., & Sumnall, H. R. (2005). Is ecstasy perceived to be safe? A critical survey. *Drug and Alcohol Dependence, 77*, 185–193.

Garratt, S. (1998). *Adventures in wonderland: A decade of club culture*. Headline.

Getz, D. (2008). Event tourism: Definition, evolution, and research. *Tourism Management, 29*(3), 403–428.

Gotham, K. (2005). Theorizing urban spectacles. *City, 9*(2), 225–246.

Gutteridge-Hewitt, M. (2024). *21 UK festivals cancelled, postponed or permanently cancelled, many more at risk, AIF reports*. DJMag.com https://djmag.com/news/21-uk-festivals-cancelled-postponed-or-permanently-cancelled-many-more-risk-aif-reports

Harrison, J. (2003). *Being a tourist: Finding meaning in pleasure travel*. University of British Columbia Press.

Haydock, W. (2015). Understanding English alcohol policy as a neoliberal condemnation of the carnivalesque. *Drugs: Education, Prevention and Policy, 22*(2), 143–149.

Hayward, K. (2002). The vilification and pleasures of youthful transgression. In J. Muncie, G. Hughes, & E. McLaughlin (Eds.), *Youth justice: Critical readings*. Sage.

Hayward, K. (2012). Five spaces of cultural criminology. *British Journal of Criminology, 52*, 441–462.

Hesse, M., & Tutenges, S. (2008). Music and substance preferences among festival attendants. *Drugs and Alcohol Today, 12*(2), 82–88.

Hill, D., & Saroka, K. (2010). Sonic patterns, spirituality and brain function: The sound component of neurotheology. *NeuroQuantology, 8*(4), 509–516.

Home Office. (2018, July). *Drug misuse: Findings from the 2017/18 crime survey for England and Wales*, Statistical Bulletin 14/18, Home Office.

Hunt, G., & Evans, K. (2008). 'The great unmentionable': Exploring the pleasures and benefits of ecstasy from the perspectives of drug users. *Drugs: Education, Prevention and Policy, 15*(4), 329–349.

Hunt, G., Moloney, M., & Evans, K. (2010). *Youth, drugs, and nightlife.* Routledge.

Jayne, M., Valentine, G., & Holloway, S. (2008). Emotional, embodied and affective geographies of alcohol, drinking and drunkenness. *Transactions of the Institute of British Geographers, 35*, 540–555.

Katz, J. (1988). *Seductions of crime*. Basic Books.

Kelly, B. C. (2005). Conceptions of risk in the lives of club drug-using youth. *Substance Use and Misuse, 40*, 1443–1459.

Koenig, D. (2006). *Mouse tales: A behind-the-ears look at Disneyland.* Bonaventure Press.

Lim, M., Hellard, M., & Hocking, J. (2008). A cross-sectional survey of young people attending a music festival: Associations between drug use and musical preference. *Drug Alcohol Review, 27*, 439–441.

Mackay, H. (2018, May 14). *Club 18-30: Are millennials responsible for its downfall?* BBC News [Online]. https://www.bbc.co.uk/news/uk-44109100.

Malbon, B. (1999). *Clubbing: Dancing, ecstasy, vitality*. Routledge.

Martinic, M., & Measham, F. (Eds.). (2008). *Swimming with crocodiles: The culture of extreme drinking, ICAP series on alcohol in society (Vol. 9)*. Routledge.

Martins, S., Carlson, R., Alexandre, P., & Falke, R. (2011). Perceived risk associated with ecstasy use: A latent class analysis approach. *Addictive Behaviours, 36*, 551–554.

Martinus, T., McAlaney, J., McLaughlin, L., & Smith, H. (2010). Outdoor music festivals: Cacophonous consumption or melodious moderation? *Drugs: Education Prevention and Policy, 17*(6), 795–807.

McCormack, M., Measham, F., & Wignall, L. (2021). The normalization of leisure sex and recreational drugs: Exploring associations between polydrug use and sexual practices by English festival-goers. *Contemporary Drug Problems, 48*(2), 185–200. https://doi.org/10.1177/00914509211009901

Measham, F. (2002). 'Doing gender'-'doing drugs': Conceptualising the gendering of drugs cultures. *Contemporary Drug Problems, 29*(2), 335–373.

Measham, F. (2004a). Play space: Historical and socio-cultural reflections on drugs, licensed leisure locations, commercialisation and control. *International Journal of Drug Policy, 15*(5–6), 337–345.

Measham, F. (2004b). The decline of ecstasy, the rise of 'binge' drinking and the persistence of pleasure. *Probation Journal, 51*(4), 309–326.

Measham, F. (2008). The turning tides of intoxication: Young people's drinking in Britain in the 2000s. *Health Education, 108*(3), 207–222.

Measham, F. (2019). Drug safety testing, disposals and dealing in an English field: Exploring the operational and behavioural outcomes of the UK's first onsite 'drug checking' service. *International Journal of Drug Policy, 67*, 102–107.

Measham, F., & Brain, K. (2005). 'Binge' drinking, British alcohol policy and the new culture of intoxication. *Crime, Media, Culture: An International Journal, 1*(3), 263–284.

Measham, F., & Moore, K. (2009). Repertoires of distinction: Exploring patterns of weekend polydrug use within local leisure scenes across the English night time economy. *Criminology and Criminal Justice, 9*(4), 437–464.

Measham, F., & Shiner, M. (2009). The legacy of normalisation: The role of classical and contemporary criminological theory in understanding young people's drug use. *International Journal of Drug Policy, 20*(6), 502–508.

Measham, F., & Simmons, H. (2022). Who uses drug checking services? Assessing uptake and outcomes at English festivals in 2018. *Drugs, Habits and Social Policy*, special issue on drug checking, 23 (3), 188–199. https://doi.org/10.1108/DHS-02-2022-0008

Measham, F., Aldridge, J., & Parker, H. (2001). *Dancing on drugs: Risk, health and hedonism in the British club scene*. Free Association Books.

Measham, F., Wood, D., Dargan, P., & Moore, K. (2011). The rise in legal highs: Prevalence and patterns in the use of illegal drugs and first and second generation 'legal highs' in South London gay dance clubs. *Journal of Substance Use, 16*(4), 263–272.

Measham, F., Moore, K., & Welch, Z. (2012). *Emerging drug trends in Lancashire: Nightclub surveys—Phase three report* (pp. 1–92). Lancaster University and Lancashire Drug and Alcohol Action Team.

Measham, F., McCormack, M., Simmons, H., & Wignall, L. (2024), Poppers, the politics of exemption and the characteristics of poppers users in the annual English Festival Study, 2014–2023, *British Journal of Criminology*. 65: 578–597. https://doi.org/10.1093/bjc/azae055

Mintel. (2022). *Rock on: UK music concerts and festivals sales set to surpass pre-COVID levels in 2023*. Mintel Group Ltd. https://www.mintel.com/press-centre/rock-on-uk-music-concerts-and-festivals-sales-set-to-surpass-pre-covid-levels-in-2023/

Mintel. (2018). *Music concerts and festivals—UK—August 2018*. Mintel Group Ltd.

Moore, D. (2008). Erasing pleasure from public discourse on illicit drugs: On the creation and reproduction of an absence. *International Journal of Drug Policy, 19*, 353–358.

Moore, K., & Measham, F. (2012). Impermissible pleasures in UK leisure: Explor-ing policy developments in alcohol and illicit drugs. In C. Jones, E. Barclay, & R. Mawby (Eds.), *The problem of pleasure: Leisure, tourism and crime* (pp. 62–76). Routledge.

NHS. (2019). *Binge drinking*. https://www.nhs.uk/live-well/alcohol-support/binge-drinking-effects/

Nicholls, J., & Hunt, G. (2025). Taking pleasure seriously: Should alcohol research say more about fun? *Addiction*, https://onlinelibrary.wiley.com/doi/pdf/10.1111/add.16747

O'Sullivan, S. (2016). The branded carnival: The dark magic of consumer excitement. *Journal of Marketing Management, 32*.

Parker, H., Aldridge, J., & Measham, F. (1998). *Illegal leisure: The normalization of adolescent recreational drug use*. Routledge.

Pidd, J. (2023, 19 Nov). Glastonbury tickets sell out in less than an hour. *The Guardian*. https://www.theguardian.com/music/2023/nov/19/glastonbury-festival-tickets-sell-out-in-less-than-an-hour

Pine, J., & Gilmore, J. (1999). *The experience economy: Work is theatre & every business a stage*. Harvard Business Press.

Power, M. (2013). *Drugs 2.0: The web revolution that's changing how the world gets high*. Portobello Books.

Presdee, M. (2000). *Cultural criminology and the carnival of crime*. Rout- ledge.

Pritchard, A., & Morgan, N. (2006). Hotel Babylon? Exploring hotels as liminal sites of transition and transgression. *Tourism Management, 27*, 762–772.

Raban, J. (1974). *Soft city*. Picador.

Sachsman, D. (2007). *Serious leisure: A perspective for our time*. Routledge.

Sandberg, S., & Tutenges, S. (2015). Meeting the Djinn: Stories of drug use, bad trips, and addiction. In L. Presser & S. Sandberg (Eds.), *Narrative criminology: Understanding stories of crime* (pp. 150–173). NYU.

Shaw, G., & Williams, A. (2004). *Tourism and tourism spaces*. Sage.

Shaw, R. (2013). Beyond night-time economy: Affective atmosphere of the urban night. *Geoforum, 51*, 87–95.

Sipe, L. (2018). Leveraging neo-localism for experience innovation: A case study of an urban park and entertainment venue. *Journal of Themed Experience and Attractions Studies, 1*(1), 29–37.

Skandalis, A., Banister, E., & Byrom, J. (2024). Spatial authenticity and extraordinary experiences: Music festivals and the everyday nature of tourism destinations. *Journal of Travel Research, 63*(2), 357–370.

Stallybrass, P., & White, A. (1986). *The politics and poetics of transgression*. Cornell University Press.

Steeves, H. (2003). Becoming Disney: Perception and being at the happiest place on earth. *Midwest Quarterly, 44*(2), 176–194.

Time Out. (2023, 18 April). *A hedonistic woodland wonderland in Cambridgeshire full of bands, DJs and cool installations*. https://www.timeout.com/london/things-to-do/secret-garden-party-1#

Turner, V. (1997). *The ritual process: Structure and anti-structure*. Transaction.

Turner, T. (2018). Disneyization: A framework for understanding illicit drug use in party zones. *International Journal of Drug Policy, 58*, 37–45.

Turner, T. (2023). *Disneyization of drug use: Understanding atypical intoxication in party zones*. Routledge.

Tutenges, S. (2012). Nightlife tourism: A mixed methods study of young tourists at an international nightlife resort. *Tourist Studies, 12*(2), 131–150.

Tutenges, S. (2013). Stirring up effervescence: An ethnographic study of youth at a nightlife resort. *Leisure Studies, 32*(3), 233–248.

Tutenges, S. (2022). Nightlife ethnography: A phenomenological approach. In S. M. Bucerius, K. D. Haggerty, & L. Berardi (Eds.), *The Oxford handbook of ethnographies of crime and criminal justice* (pp. 408–426). Oxford University Press.

Tutenges, S., & Rod, M. H. (2009). 'We got incredibly drunk … it was damned fun': Drinking stories among Danish youth. *Journal of Youth Studies, 12*(4), 355–370.

Tutenges, S., & Sandberg, S. (2013). Intoxicating stories: The characteristics, contexts and implications of drinking stories among Danish youth. *International Journal of Drug Policy, 24*, 538–544.

UK Festival Awards. (2017). *Market Report 2017*. UKFA. https://www.festivalawards.com/wp-content/uploads/2018/08/UK-Festival-Market-Report-2017.pdf

Urry, J., & Larsen, J. (2011). *The Tourist Gaze 3.0*. Sage.

Warner, M. (2014). *Once upon a time: A short history of fairy tale*. Oxford.

Yorke, J. (2013). Into the woods: *How stories work and why we tell them*. Penguin.

# 15

# Home Drinking and Solitary Home-based Drinking Practices among Young Adults

Dom Conroy and Emily Nicholls

**Abstract** The consumption of alcohol and solitary drinking within home spaces have come under recent scrutiny, raising the profile of home and solitary drinking as neglected fields for research and policy focus. Within scholarly discussion, renewed interest in drinking at home has contributed to understanding around current trends in domestic and public drinking practices, the role of physical spaces and time periods associated with drinking styles and how home as a reflective, intimate and personal space may shape or moderate alcohol consumption when drinking alone or with others. In this chapter we review the extant literature on home-based drinking. We then draw on interview data from our Drinking in Lockdown project conducted in the UK during the COVID-19

D. Conroy (✉)
Faculty of Arts and Social Science, The Open University, London, UK
e-mail: d.conroy@open.ac.uk

E. Nicholls
Department of Sociology, University of York, York, UK
e-mail: emily.nicholls@york.ac.uk



D. Conroy, F. Measham (eds.), *Young Adult Drinking Styles*, Sustainable Development Goals Series, https://doi.org/10.1007/978-3-031-98528-7_15

pandemic and associated lockdowns. We draw on data from our 'younger adult' (i.e., < 40 years) participants to contribute to the renewed interest in home-based drinking discussed above with a particular focus on drinking practices among this cohort. Participant talk around solitary home-based drinking highlighted factors that raise or diminish the likelihood of solitary drinking, reflecting attitudes towards and concerns about solitary home-based drinking during lockdowns and focusing on moderation/excess and framings of solitary drinking within home spaces and domestic relationships. This chapter contributes to a renewed, post-pandemic focus on solitary drinking's social acceptability and the sometimes dilemmatic connections between solitary drinking, domestic drinking and historic and current personal drinking.

## Introduction

Though historically a relatively neglected area of research, policy and public attention, domestic or home-based alcohol consumption has been the subject of growing scrutiny in recent years. Whilst the early 2020s' COVID-19 pandemic and associated social distancing and 'lockdown' measures may have triggered a renewed interest in domestic drinking practices (Callinan & MacLean, 2020), it is important to stress that domestic drinking—which is notably more affordable than consuming alcohol in licenced venues—was an embedded feature of drinking regimes before the pandemic (and continues to be in its aftermath). Indeed, over the last decade in particular, research and commentary on home-based alcohol consumption and alcohol-related harms has become a small but growing subfield in its own right—with relevant policy implications (Brierley-Jones et al., 2014; Foster & Ferguson, 2012; Foster et al., 2010; MacLean et al., 2024). Far from representing a 'blip' in consumption or a temporary shift, the move towards home drinking is part of a broader trajectory that is occurring alongside the closure—or perhaps more accurately the 'refashioning' and diversification—of licensed venues

(Thurnell-Read, 2021). Renewed interest in drinking at home has also contributed to scholarly discussion around themes including; existing trends in domestic and public drinking practices and their implications (Foster & Ferguson, 2012; Ally et al., 2016; Fenton et al., 2024), the spatial, contextual and temporal aspects of home drinking (Holloway et al., 2008; Wilkinson, 2017) and the ways in which the home as a reflective, intimate and personal space may shape or moderate alcohol consumption (Conroy & Nicholls, 2022; MacLean et al., 2022; Liu & Jayne, 2023).

In this chapter we review the extant literature on home-based drinking (with a particular focus on the UK context), highlighting the ways in which young people's drinking in particular tends to be associated with public space and framed as highly visible—and often problematic—whilst the domestic sphere is neglected. We then draw on data from our Drinking in Lockdown (DiL) project which involved interview and focus group research with UK-based drinkers—a number of whom were young (or 'younger') adults in their twenties and thirties. Specifically, we develop insights into DiL-derived data that concerned experiences of (and views concerning) drinking alcohol *alone*, in home spaces, a phenomenon we refer to as 'solitary home-based drinking' (SHBD). SHBD has been highlighted as a neglected phenomenon that may have grown during the COVID-19 pandemic era (Alcohol Focus Scotland, 2021). It remains overlooked in the alcohol literature despite research indicating a prevalence rate of 30–40% of solitary drinking, with the majority of this taking place at home (Skrzynski & Creswell, 2021). SHBD may also be associated with higher levels of alcohol consumption and harm and with specific forms of judgement or stigma not experienced when drinking with others (Cook et al., 2023). Drawing on illustrations from the DiL project work we will provide insights from our data into the perceived acceptability of SHBD among younger adults (defined as <40 years), what makes SHBD more or less likely among younger adults, and how SHBD may connect with domestic relationships and broader dilemmas surrounding individual consumption practices.

## Exploring the Emerging Home Drinking Literature

It is perhaps unsurprising that most policy, research, public and media attention around alcohol consumption in the United Kingdom has centred on public consumption (Eldridge, 2010), particularly around excessive drinking and intoxication. Such forms of drinking remain the most visible and the most explicitly associated with 'risk' in relation to crime, anti-social behaviour, violence and public (dis)order. There is also an expectation that it is entirely appropriate (or even necessary) and within the remit of government to subject public behaviour to various forms of regulation and policing. Public alcohol consumption is presented as a 'problem' of violence and crime (Fileborn, 2016), with a spotlight on late-night bars, clubs and pubs and a media and policy focus on public 'binge drinking' amongst groups including young people and students (Eldridge, 2010; Frost & Gardiner, 2005). As a result, the UK has seen attempts to simultaneously revive city centres at night and establish them as pleasurable sites of consumption (for young people in particular) (Chatterton & Hollands, 2002) yet this has prompted attempts to police and regulate these spaces and media and public concern about young people's supposed binge drinking and its consequences (Szmigin et al., 2008).

In contrast, domestic alcohol consumption takes place 'behind closed doors' where attempts to regulate may be difficult, ineffective or unpopular (the controversy around the introduction of Minimum Unit Pricing to regulate pricing for domestic sales of alcohol is a good example (Dobson & Hawkins, 2016)). In addition, Valentine et al. (2008) argue that the policy and media preoccupation with young people's public binge drinking has deflected attention away from everyday domestic drinking regimes. Where attention has been paid to domestic drinking, it has traditionally tended to focus on areas such as parental misuse of alcohol, 'problem' drinking and socially marginalised practices, rather than the 'everyday' practices of drinkers:

> ...noticeable for their absence are studies which examine the everyday domestic drinking practices of a broader diversity of social groups who would not consider themselves as having an alcohol problem, or to be suffering the consequences of other people's problematic drinking. (Valentine et al., 2008, p. 52)

This gap is increasingly stark because a significant—and increasing—proportion of alcohol consumption across all age groups now takes place in domestic settings, challenging "the contemporary geographical imaginary of drinking as a city centre issue" (Holloway et al., 2008, p. 537). In the UK, by 2018 over 70% of alcohol sold was purchased 'off-trade', that is, in supermarkets and via local or specialist shops for off-site consumption rather than in bars, pubs and restaurants (Institute of Alcohol Studies, 2018), whilst a 2021 survey reports that of those UK adults who reported that they had consumed an alcoholic drink in the past week, 80% of these had drunk at home, whilst only 36% had drunk in bars and pubs (Drinkaware, 2021). This picture is replicated across other high-income countries; for example a survey of over 2000 Australians in 2016 found that only 12% of their reported consumption took place in pubs, bars and nightclubs (Callinan et al., 2016) (it is, however, worth noting that younger adults are still more likely than older cohorts to drink alcohol in bars, pubs and restaurants (Drinkaware, 2021) or at family and friends' homes (Valentine et al., 2008)). Such findings only highlight the very real need for further research on alcohol consumption in domestic spaces.

Research must also pay attention to the unique affordances and contextual dimensions of 'home' as a site of consumption. The 'home' can be conceptualised in various ways; as a space of social reproduction, a site for the storing of meaningful material objects and a site of comfort and safety (for some at least) to name but a few examples (see Mallett, 2004 for an overview). Domestic alcohol consumption is more affordable—and more accessible, particularly with the rise of alcohol home delivery services (Colbert et al., 2023)—than public drinking, and may also offer consumers a greater degree of control over their space of consumption. For example, in a helpful move beyond the stereotype of focusing on youth public drinking, Wilkinson (2017) draws on the notion of 'drinkscapes' to consider the ways in which suburban indoor spaces are crafted and created by young drinkers (e.g., through the use of lighting and music) to facilitate their drinking practices. Home drinking may also provide opportunities to bond, socialise and build trust and intimacy for young people, whether this acts as an activity in its own right or as part of a 'pre-drinking' routine before moving to bar, pub and club spaces (Nicholls, 2019).

Domestic spaces may lack the environmental cues and social pressures of public drinking spaces (which may encourage high consumption levels through time-limited drink promotions such as 'happy hours', the reciprocal buying of 'rounds' in a friendship group and even architectural features (Tutenges & Bøhling, 2019; MacLean et al., 2024)). However, there may also be a comparative lack of policing of drinking within home spaces (by the self or others) (Conroy & Nicholls, 2022), and alcohol's affordability and accessibility may facilitate higher-risk drinking practices in these settings. As suggested above, domestic consumption has largely escaped public scrutiny, and with 'binge drinking' and problematic drinking conflated with high levels of public drinking by young people in urban spaces, Valentine et al. (2008) report research findings showing that even those who drank well above recommended guidelines in domestic spaces felt their practices were 'unremarkable' and of no concern. Furthermore, these types of consumption are not uncommon; evidence suggests that those who drink mainly at home tend to consume higher amounts overall than those who do *less* of their drinking at home (Foster & Ferguson, 2012, p. 355). Home-based drinking (particularly heavier consumption) clearly warrants greater research and policy attention given its association with a range of social and health harms including consistent evidence that alcohol use increases the risk and severity of domestic violence (Gilchrist et al., 2014; WHO, 2006).

## Solitary Home-based Drinking

The previous section highlighted how home-based drinking has hitherto been a comparatively neglected area of research focus. Renewed focus on home-based drinking in recent years has changed this somewhat and highlighted a range of considerations involved in home-based drinking, including solitary drinking. In this section, we first consider solitary drinking as a broader topic area of interest in the alcohol field and second, we explore published research that concerns solitary drinking in home-based settings.

A growing body of quantitative research has explored the incidence of solitary drinking and has provided an evidence base showcasing associations between drinking alone (whether at home or in bars/ public places) and relevant behavioural and psychological factors. Review work has demonstrated evidence of varied definitions and measures of solitary drinking (Skrzynski & Creswell, 2021). For example, measures of solitary drinking have focused on binary categories (solitary vs. social-only drinkers, e.g., Bourgault & Demers, 1997), while other studies have focused on the percentage of times that drinking occasions involve solitary drinking (e.g., Annis & Graham, 1995), the incidence of solitary drinking (e.g., Mohr et al., 2013) or measures concerning the location of solitary drinking occasions (e.g., Cooper et al., 1992). Explicit focus on the presence of other people is apparent in some solitary drinking measures including Rabinowitz and Marjefsky's (1998) single-item solitary drinking measure assessing presence or absence of a drinking partner (notably, presence/absence of a non-drinking person or partner is not incorporated into this measure). Time span has varied considerably between different solitary drinking studies, with some studies focusing on the incidence of solitary drinking over the last month, the last year, or in someone's lifetime. Other empirical work has guided understanding of how the relative likelihood of an individual to engage in solitary drinking may in itself be associated with more harmful patterns of drinking behaviour. For example, meta-analytic evidence based on 18 datasets has demonstrated small, positive associations between solitary drinking incidence and alcohol consumption levels, and between solitary drinking and alcohol-related problems (Skrzynski & Creswell, 2021). The COVID-19 pandemic and abrupt curtailment of opportunities to drink in public spaces also appeared to generate some renewed interest in attempts to 'measure' solitary drinking and associated harms. For example, cross-sectional research conducted during a Canadian lockdown and based on a sample of 320 adult drinkers demonstrated independent associations between solitary drinking and increased alcohol consumption and between solitary drinking and self-reported alcohol-related problems (Wardell et al., 2020).

We turn now to consider solitary drinking within a specific space and return to the notion of 'solitary home-based drinking' (SHBD) introduced at the start of the chapter. We use this term inclusively rather than categorically to refer to drinking alcohol in domestic space where the alcohol consuming individual is 'drinking alone' either given their location in the home space (e.g., drinking alone in a room in the house) or 'drinking alone' given their company (e.g., drinking alcohol at home where any others present are *not* consuming alcohol for part or all of the drinking occasion). During the COVID-19 pandemic in particular, this could include drinking whilst socialising with others online. There is limited recent data on the prevalence of home-based drinking but a general increase in home drinking is recognised, underpinned by many factors including convenience, cost and safety (Foster & Ferguson, 2012). Increased SHBD among younger adults also seems highly plausible given the context of a considerable surge in the availability and use of digital technologies in a post-pandemic world (De et al., 2020), which may facilitate drinking 'together apart' with friends online.

Insights into links between SHBD and drinking styles and harmful outcomes have been provided in recent years. Survey and interview data collected pre-pandemic with a convenience sample of Australian light and heavy drinkers has recently highlighted the prevalence of and perceptions surrounding SHBD, showing that 27% of heavy drinkers indicated that solitary drinking only occurred when they were alone in their own home (Cook et al., 2023). In this study, interviewees' expressed a view that solitary drinking involved or signified personal inadequacy and harmful patterns of alcohol consumption, yet it was also perceived as pleasurable and relaxing (and of course, may be the easiest or only option available at times to those who live alone). Importantly, these findings suggest that SHBD might present as a drinking practice that carries complex stigmatisation, and which may be more likely to reflect potentially harmful styles of personal drinking. In the next section, we turn to explore data that concerned solitary drinking from interviewees participating in the DiL project. This focused on drinking practices among UK-based individuals during the first national lockdown between April and July 2020.

## Examining Solitary Home-based Drinking: An Empirical Illustration

We turn to develop discussion of SHBD illustratively by presenting and discussing relevant interview data from the DiL interview project data. The data we present in this section concerned, in different ways, SHBD understood following the inclusive definition provided previously in this chapter. Interestingly, our data rarely contained accounts of *personal* in-depth experiences of SHBD; rather, it concerned viewpoints around the perceived solitary drinking undertaken by participants or other people as something that had become more noticeable and pertinent under the lockdown circumstances. Whilst some data concerned solitary drinking linked to the pandemic, other material involved broader reflections on drinking habits including pre-pandemic SHBD.

Extracted from a broader sample of 20 participants, we draw on data from six individuals, generated via four semi-structured interviews and one focus group interview (see Table 15.1 for demographic, occupational and alcohol consumption details). Interviews took place 62–118 days following 26th March 2020 (the start of the first legally enforced UK lockdown). All participants formally consented prior to interviews and are identifiable using appropriate pseudonyms. All participants were white and British. Individuals were and identified as 'younger adults' (aged between 26 and 39, Mean age = 33.2 years) including 26–32-year-old young adults (Jess, Lucie, Kriss) and 37–39-year-old younger middle-aged individuals (Damien, Kayla, Mel). Interview data were transcribed verbatim and subjected to an inductive form of thematic analysis (Braun & Clarke, 2006). Here, we present findings and examples around; the requirement to adopt and negotiate new SHBD practices during the pandemic (Kriss extract), the social permissibility (or otherwise) of SHBD (Damien extract) and how SHBD links to broader concerns about

**Table 15.1** Sample demographic and alcohol consumption details

| Participant demographic details | Occupational and domestic details | Approximate drinking patterns during lockdown | |
|---|---|---|---|
| | | Days per week | Units per occasion |
| Kayla, female, 39 | Part-time student and full-time worker in creative design (initially furloughed but now full-time work); lives with husband | 4<br>4 | 15 (initial 3 weeks)<br>8 (last 3–4 weeks) |
| Damien, male, 38 | Full-time student; lives alone | 2 | 14 |
| Mel, female, 37 | Project manager; lives with husband and young daughter | 5–6 | 10–20 |
| Kriss, male, 32 | Employed; lives with female partner; | 6–7 | 2–6 |
| Jess, female, 27 | Student and support worker; doing PhD, lives with Lucie | 1–2 | 9–10 |
| Lucie, female, 26 | Teacher; lives with Jess | 1–2 | 9–10 |

drinking behaviours, relationships and social encounters (Kayla, Jess and Lucie and Mel extracts).

The first aspect of SHBD apparent from the data was that many participants adopted relatively novel or entirely new drinking practices because of the pandemic and subsequent government-enforced 'lockdowns'. Several younger adult participants had relatively active pre-pandemic social lives involving activities (and alcohol consumption) that took place beyond the domestic space. As a result, they had a frame of reference for experiencing the sudden shift to home-based drinking during the UK's first 2020 lockdown as something relatively novel, and were required to reframe their historic drinking practices while being almost entirely home-based during the lockdown:

> Before lockdown I would never drink indoors [at home] … my partner doesn't drink so errm it's not really the same sitting there on your own having a beer … maybe one but not having 5 or 6 … so previously the only time I would have drunk indoors is if people would have come round y'know maybe after being in the pub or y'know for dinner and we'll have some drinks, play some games etc. … whereas that's changed. (Kriss, Male, 32)

Pre-pandemic, alcohol consumption for Kriss happened almost exclusively on Saturdays in connection with watching sports with friends and daytime drinking (see Palmer, 2011). Consumption would usually take place away from domestic space and would only occur 'indoors' (i.e., at home) when friends were visiting (often after drinking in the pub); a practice that was no longer possible during the pandemic due to social distancing requirements. Lockdown had meant that Kriss had to establish for himself whether his typically relatively heavy drinking style at weekends would or could continue outside of its usual context. Kriss lived with his girlfriend, who was a non-drinker, so alcohol consumption of any quantity would involve him drinking 'alone' in the sense that, though sharing the same home space, Kriss drank alcohol without being in the company of other drinkers. Indeed, Kriss's "on your own" phrasing is interesting here as during lockdown he was not physically or literally 'on his own' but sharing domestic space with his partner. Rather, it is the act of *drinking* alone that is the concern; Kriss is 'on his own' in relation to alcohol consumption and a practice that used to be inherently social is now only available to him as a solo pursuit.

Kriss' reasons for being unwilling to engage in SHBD beyond perhaps a single alcoholic drink were not made explicit. However, the sense from his interview was that consuming many alcoholic drinks and subsequently being in some state of intoxication at home whilst drinking alone was not an attractive option given that the pleasure and enjoyment afforded by alcohol was conditional on being in the company of other drinkers. This reflection is also interesting in relation to attempts to construct oneself as a 'moderate' and 'responsible' drinker. If drinking alone is undesirable—or even potentially *problematic*—then limiting consumption to "a beer" (but never "5 or 6") might help to mitigate the potential stigma of solitary home drinking (particularly for younger adults who may be more likely to drink in bars, pubs and clubs than older cohorts. In this sense, the shift to drinking at home *and* alone was something Kriss was forced to navigate, with the notion of drinking moderate or even minimal amounts positioned as a way for him to manage this.

A second aspect of solitary home-based drinking concerned participant talk around the social permissibility of solitary drinking (to excess):

> If you tell someone "yeah, I got pissed on a bottle of wine last night on my own" people don't generally worry about that ... like if I said "I did four lines of coke and passed out", well you've got a drug problem ... but why isn't it a drinking problem? Why is it so acceptable to consume alcohol as almost a dependency? Like because if you're not classified as an alcoholic then no one worries about it ... but you know, I think if someone's drinking five pints of beer every night and couldn't go a night without doing that ... there's something wrong there in my eyes, but actually in society's eyes it's like "oh cool, but we need to drink you know", it's just not treated the same way. (Damien, Male, 38)

SHBD, particularly involving alcohol consumption in large volumes, was identified by Damien as a practice of concern. Here, Damien casts the spotlight on excessive SHBD, flagging the double standards involved in the relative acceptability of heavy, solitary alcohol consumption juxtaposed to other types of excessive substance use. Solitary drinking is entangled with drinking large quantities of alcohol here, as illustrated in Damien's hypothetical example of drinking a bottle of wine 'on one's own'. Importantly, he distinguishes solitary, excessive drinking as something that falls under the radar by virtue of someone not being "classified as an alcoholic", implying that society and communities set a high bar of permissibility to behaviour that could reasonably be viewed as near-equivalent to an addiction or dependency to alcohol.

As with the extract from Kriss, the phrase "on my own" is the sole identifier for solitary drinking in this extract but plays an important role in Damien's construction of solitary (and excessive) drinking practices. Damien constructs a hypocritical normative acceptability surrounding behaviour (alcohol consumption that is excessive and solitary) that would be considered dangerous and anti-social in the context of other types of substance use (cocaine). The "we need to drink" phrasing in the final sentence of the extract produces a rhetorical effect that carries an imperative—alcohol consumption should be understood as a basic important everyday activity of life for younger adults (i.e., < 40 years), whether it is consumed to excess or not, or in company or as a solitary activity (see Griffin et al., 2009). This extract is interesting because whilst Damien positions excessive SHBD as something that is socially accepted, this practice is simultaneously positioned as involving, at the least, double standards reflecting a more permissive societal approach to drinking practices than other kinds of substance use. Notable here is that other participants did not view excessive SHBD as quite as normalised or accepted as Damien suspects.

A third aspect of SHBD involved reference to how it linked to broader concerns about drinking behaviour and, interestingly, as something that must be considered in relation to relationships with others (particularly in the household) and social encounters. This was apparent in Kayla's extract below which concerned SHBD in the context of Internet-mediated social encounters:

> There was a day that I felt particularly unwell ... realised that my alcohol consumption had increased ... I thought "you know this needs to stop, need to keep this in check"... I've now gone back to my pre-pandemic drinking behaviours ... I don't drink on my own, so if my husband is away from for work errm I don't drink on my own ... I don't have (online) conversations with friends drinking ... that's not a social activity I've engaged in ... I find it a bit weird ... maybe because it is abnormal or maybe normal for now for some ... I know there's a lot of people eating dinner together via zoom ... I'm not saying it's wrong, it's just not something I've ever thought about doing. (Kayla, Female, 39)

Immediately following her reflections on a period of (for her) heavier alcohol consumption, Kayla explicitly underscores that at no point had she engaged in SHBD. The rhetorical effect here was, again, interesting as it constructs the impression that while her recent drinking practices may include one qualifier for 'problem drinking' (i.e., relatively high consumption levels) another potentially relevant qualifier (solitary drinking) is *not* present ("I don't drink on my own") and would not even be considered.

Several interviews also provided insights into the relative attractiveness of SHBD in the context of relationships with other people. Jess and Lucie were co-habiting friends and material from their focus group interview gave a more explicit sense of how decisions to drink alone (or not) might take place over the period of an evening or a week:

> I (Lucie) sometimes do drink by myself … you (Jess) don't do that as much … before lockdown I would sometimes drink by myself if I was home alone and having a glass of wine, or having a glass while I was watching something but more often than not with friends … even though I could, if I wanted to get drunk mid-week, I'd rarely go more than beyond like two glasses of wine, whereas at a weekend I will quite happily polish off a bottle … and that's something [different] because we're drinking together on a weekend aren't we, we're drinking more … but I don't really have any desire to drink a full bottle of wine by myself … because I guess for me, I do enjoy being drunk and I guess if I did live by myself I probably would some nights just drink a bottle of wine, but I'd actually much rather get drunk with you, because we're together. (Jess, Female, 27 & Lucie, Female, 26)

Material presented in the extract above seemed to encapsulate a wide range of drinking practices including alcohol consumption to different degrees of volume and involving (or not) the presence of other people. For Lucie, SHBD held some appeal to a point but—as with Kriss above—only within clearly defined parameters ("rarely beyond two glasses of wine", "(no) desire to drink a full bottle by myself"). The pleasures afforded by relatively heavy alcohol consumption ("enjoy being drunk") were far more preferable—and perhaps permissible—when they took place in the company of others. In this way, the socially contextualised role of pleasure afforded by alcohol consumption was one feature of this extract ("I'd actually much rather get drunk with you"). Another feature was the symbolic role of alcohol within a close relationship. Lucie identifies that she clearly *could* engage in SHBD more often ("I could get drunk mid-week") and might in other circumstances ("if I did live by myself") but acknowledges her preference to drink more heavily when she is with her housemate Jess. This highlights the key entanglements of alcohol, friendship and socialising, whereby (heavy) drinking is inherently framed as a social practice (de Visser et al., 2013) and—as implied throughout this section—SHBD to excess might be positioned as indicative of a more 'problematic' relationship with alcohol (or at the very least as something undesirable or unappealing). Such findings are interesting as previous research by Valentine et al. (2008) suggests that those living alone are 'significantly' less likely to drink at home than other groups.

In several of these examples, domestic alcohol consumption is actively shaped by others (in Kriss' case by his partner's non-drinking and for Lucie and Kayla by the presence—or absence—of others they live with). This was also the case in the final extract below, which showcases how Mel's drinking is shaped by the absence of her partner and represents the clearest example of experiences of personal SHBD, its associated thoughts and feelings and its connection with other people:

> (My partner) doesn't drink a lot so I can't drink much because he doesn't drink that much and I feel guilty about it … I drink more when he's working nights than any other time … I'm a terrible person … (I drink more) because it doesn't matter as he's not here … I don't get lairy in his face [laughter] … I don't know, I just feel like I can get away with it when he's not here … I should not be so much of a fiend. (Mel, Female, 37)

Here, Mel describes mixed feelings about SHBD. Freed from feeling compelled to drink in a certain way when her partner was away, Mel tended to drink more on her own ("it doesn't matter as he's not here"). However, this didn't necessarily feel wholly positive, positioned more as something Mel can "get away with" rather than as an actively pleasurable experience. There is also potentially a gendered dynamic here in that SBHD allows Mel to drink more heavily without getting 'lairy' in front of others (i.e., acting in a loud and potentially abrasive and 'unfeminine' manner) (Day et al., 2004). This type of SHBD also held important repercussions, including feelings of shame and guilt and a suggestion that somehow heavy consumption positions Mel as "a terrible person" or a "fiend" who "should not" drink so much or in this way (implying a moral dimension). This echoes the sentiment expressed across the data presented in this chapter, whereby heavy SHBD continues to be regarded with some ambivalence and at times positioned as undesirable or even 'wrong'.

## Discussion

In this chapter, we have reviewed the growing evidence base concerning home-based drinking, highlighting the role of domestic spaces, and the relationships and dynamics operating within these spaces, as a neglected area of alcohol research which warrants greater attention. We then presented relevant data concerning views and experiences of SHBD from our DiL project. Drawing on relevant illustrations from the DiL project we have presented interview data concerning attitudes towards and concerns about shifting towards SHBD during the lockdown period, broader reflections about SHBD, themes relating to moderation/excess involving solitary drinking, and reflections on the role of domestic relationships and presence or absence of others in relation to SHBD. The interview data also highlighted the range of associations and practices linked to solitary drinking and particularly highlights the sensitivities and potential stigma associated with solitary drinking as a practice. Notably, solitary drinking was talked about cautiously by participants as something that was to an extent socially accepted yet still involving double standards relative to public drinking or consumption of other substances (e.g., by Damien) and as something undermining the function of alcohol consumption as a fundamentally *social* practice (Kriss, Mel and Lucie).

Whilst the pandemic and lockdown presented new challenges and demanded reconfigurations of drinking, these extracts expose wider tensions and ambivalences around the acceptability—or otherwise—of SHBD more broadly. One interpretation of the limited *in-depth* accounts of personal SHBD experiences is that talking about drinking alcohol alone, at home, still carries a degree of stigma and an association with 'problem drinking' which make talking about it far from straightforward. This absence/omission is arguably significant in its own right and should be explored in greater detail in future qualitative research. Nonetheless, these findings enhance our understanding of younger adults' attitudes towards and perceptions of SHBD and suggest that stigma remains—at least to an extent—around heavy SHBD. Our empirical illustration concerns SHBD among a small sample of 'younger adults' aged between 26 and 39 that included late Millennials (i.e., born late-1980s roughly) rather than Generation Z individuals (i.e., born 1997–2012). Understanding how stigma, or anything else, links to solitary drinking among younger adults as a stand-alone group, and relative to middle aged or older adults (i.e., aged 40+ years), is important. It is also possible that new social affordances of the digital age (e.g., enhanced access to opportunities to socialise online) mean that younger adults may feel *less* inhibited about solitary drinking to a modest level (e.g., drinking alcohol 'together apart' whilst physically alone but socialising or interacting with friends online). Experiences of stigma may also be closely tied to the spatial context in which solitary drinking occurs (whether in home-based, public, digital or hybrid geographical spaces). While our interviewees did not discuss solitary drinking occurring in a public context, previous interview research with 60 Australian younger adults has highlighted the culturally contingent nature of experiences of drunkenness which can serve to reinforce stigmatising identities (including gendered stigma) linked to being alone and drunk in public spaces (MacLean et al., 2018).

Whilst findings presented here draw on a small-scale study that was conducted during the exceptional circumstances of the COVID-19 pandemic and associated lockdowns, they nonetheless contribute to a wider but still developing body of literature on home-based drinking, solitary drinking and the intersections of the two, and have clear implications for understanding SHBD in a post-pandemic context. Future research could build on this to further explore the drinking practices of a younger cohort where overall declines in drinking are more pronounced, access to technology and online socialising is embedded within everyday practices and alcohol consumption (even with others) is increasingly associated with a number of 'risks' rather than perceived primarily as a tool to enable pleasure, relaxation or sociability (Whitaker et al., 2023). With alcohol being (re)framed in these ways, it will be interesting to explore the extent to which practices such as SHBD are adopted, rejected, accepted or stigmatised amongst those who are coming of age in a post-pandemic context.

## References

Alcohol Focus Scotland. (2021). Alcohol sales and consumption in Scotland during the pandemic. https://www.alcohol-focus-scotland.org.uk/news/alcohol-sales-and-consumption-in-scotland-during-the-pandemic/

Ally, A. K., Lovatt, M., Meier, P. S., Brennan, A., & Holmes, J. (2016). Developing a social practice-based typology of British drinking culture in 2009–2011: Implications for alcohol policy analysis. *Addiction, 111*(9), 1568–1579.

Annis, H. M., & Graham, J. M. (1995). Profile types on the Inventory of Drinking Situations: Implications for relapse prevention counseling. Psychology of Addictive Behaviors, 9(3), 176–182.

Bourgault, C., & Demers, A. (1997). Solitary drinking: A risk factor for alcohol-related problems? *Addiction, 92*, 303–312.

Braun, V., & Clarke, V. (2006). Using thematic analysis in psychology. *Qualitative Research in Psychology, 3*(2), 77–101.

Brierley-Jones, L., Ling, J., McCabe, K. E., Wilson, G. B., Crosland, A., Kaner, E. F., & Haighton, C. A. (2014). Habitus of home and traditional drinking: A qualitative analysis of reported middle-class alcohol use. *Sociology of Health & Illness, 36*(7), 1054–1076.

Callinan, S., & MacLean, S. (2020). COVID-19 makes a stronger research focus on home drinking more important than ever. *Drug and Alcohol Review, 39*(6), 613–615.

Callinan, S., Livingston, M., Room, R., & Dietze, P. (2016). Drinking contexts and alcohol consumption: How much alcohol is consumed in different Australian locations? *Journal of Studies on Alcohol and Drugs, 77*(4), 612–619.

Chatterton, P., & Hollands, R. (2002). Theorising urban playscapes: Producing, regulating and consuming nightlife city spaces. *Urban Studies, 39*(1), 95–116.

Colbert, S., Thornton, L., Wilkinson, C., Feng, X., & Richmond, R. (2023). 'The convenience is a double-edged sword': Qualitative interviews with people who use online alcohol delivery services. *Drug and Alcohol Review, 43*(2), 425–433.

Conroy, D., & Nicholls, E. (2022). 'When I open it, I have to drink it all': Push and pull factors shaping domestic alcohol consumption during the COVID-19 pandemic UK Spring 2020 lockdown. *Drug and Alcohol Review, 41*(6), 1275–1283.

Cook, M., MacLean, S., & Callinan, S. (2023). Home alone: Patterns and perceptions of solitary home alcohol consumption in an Australian convenience sample. *Drug and Alcohol Review, 42*(5), 1018–1027.

Cooper, M. L., Russell, M., Skinner, J. B., & Windle, M. (1992). Development and validation of a three-dimensional measure of drinking motives. *Psychological Assessment, 4*, 123–132.

Day, K., Gough, B., & McFadden, M. (2004). "Warning! alcohol can seriously damage your feminine health" a discourse analysis of recent British newspaper coverage of women and drinking. *Feminist Media Studies, 4*(2), 165–183.

De, R., Pandey, N., & Pal, A. (2020). Impact of digital surge during Covid-19 pandemic: A viewpoint on research and practice. *International Journal of Information Management, 55*, 102171.

de Visser, R. O., Wheeler, Z., Abraham, C., & Smith, J. A. (2013). 'Drinking is our modern way of bonding': Young people's beliefs about interventions to encourage moderate drinking. *Psychology & Health, 28*(12), 1460–1480.

Dobson, L., & Hawkins, B. (2016). The idea of freedom in the policy debate on the minimum unit pricing of alcohol. *Journal of Social Philosophy, 47*(1), 41–54.

Drinkaware. (2021). Alcohol consumption UK. https://www.drinkaware.co.uk/research/alcohol-facts-and-data/alcohol-consumption-uk#drinkingpreferences

Eldridge, A. (2010). Public panics: Problematic bodies in social space. *Emotion, Space and Society, 3*(1), 40–44.

Fenton, L., Fairbrother, H., Whitaker, V., Henney, M., Stevely, A. K., & Holmes, J. (2024). Geographies of alcohol and generation: Examining the decline in youth drinking in England through a spatial lens. *Drug and Alcohol Review, 43*(3), 675–684.

Fileborn, B. (2016). *Reclaiming the night-time economy: Unwanted sexual attention in pubs and clubs*. Palgrave Macmillan.

Foster, J. H., & Ferguson, C. S. (2012). Home drinking in the UK: Trends and causes. *Alcohol and Alcoholism, 47*(3), 355–358.

Foster, J., Read, D., Karunanithi, S., & Woodward, V. (2010). Why do people drink at home? *Journal of Public Health, 32*(4), 512–518.

Frost, J., & Gardiner, S. (2005). Binge drinking: the latest moral panic? *Safer Communities, 4*(4), 5–9.

Gilchrist, L., Ireland, L., Forsyth, A., Laxton, T., & Godwin, J. (2014). *Roles of alcohol in intimate partner abuse*. [Alcohol Research UK report] https://s3.

eu-west-2.amazonaws.com/files.alcoholchange.org.uk/documents/FinalReport_0117.pdf?mtime=20181128155801

Griffin, C., Bengry-Howell, A., Hackley, C., Mistral, W., & Szmigin, I. (2009). 'Every time I do it I annihilate myself': Loss of (self-)consciousness and loss of memory in young people's drinking narratives. *Sociology, 43*(3), 457–476.

Holloway, S. L., Jayne, M., & Valentine, G. (2008). 'Sainsbury's is my local': English alcohol policy, domestic drinking practices and the meaning of home. *Transactions of the Institute of British Geographers, 33*(4), 532–547.

Institute of Alcohol Studies. (2018). *The alcohol industry.* Factsheet. https://www.ias.org.uk/uploads/pdf/Factsheets/FS%20industry%20012018.pdf

Liu, C., & Jayne, M. (2023). 'At home' with alcohol: New insights into young people's domestic practices in China. *Social & Cultural Geography, 24*(10), 1827–1845.

MacLean, S., Pennay, A., & Room, R. (2018). 'You're repulsive': Limits to acceptable drunken comportment for young adults. *International Journal of Drug Policy, 53*, 106–112.

MacLean, S., Room, R., Cook, M., Mugavin, J., & Callinan, S. (2022). Affordances of home drinking in accounts from light and heavy drinkers. *Social Science & Medicine, 296*, 114712.

MacLean, S., Caluzzi, G., Cook, M., Room, R., & Callinan, S. (2024). Drinking alcohol at home feels different from drinking in public places: A qualitative study of midlife Australians. *Health & Place, 86*, 103179–103179.

Mallett, S. (2004). Understanding home: A critical review of the literature. *The Sociological Review, 52*(1), 62–89.

Mohr, C. D., Brannan, D., Wendt, S., Jacobs, L., Wright, R., & Wang, M. (2013). Daily mood—Drinking slopes as predictors: A new take on drinking motives and related outcomes. *Psychology Addictive Behaviour, 27*, 944–955.

Nicholls, E. (2019). *Negotiating femininities in the neoliberal night-time economy: Too much of a girl?* Palgrave Macmillan.

Palmer, C. (2011). Key themes and research agendas in the sport-alcohol nexus. *Journal of Sport and Social Issues, 35*(2), 168–185.

Rabinowitz, J., & Marjefsky, S. (1998). Alcohol & drug abuse: Predictors of being expelled from and dropping out of alcohol treatment. Psychiatric services, 49(2), 187–1189.

Skrzynski, C. J., & Creswell, K. G. (2021). A systematic review and meta-analysis on the association between solitary drinking and alcohol problems in adults. *Addiction, 116*(9), 2289–2303.

Szmigin, I., Griffin, C., Mistral, W., Bengry-Howell, A., Weale, L., & Hackley, C. (2008). Re-framing 'binge drinking' as calculated hedonism: Empirical evidence from the UK. *International Journal of Drug Policy, 19*(5), 359–366.

Thurnell-Read, T. (2021). 'If they weren't in the pub, they probably wouldn't even know each other': Alcohol, sociability and pub based leisure. *International Journal of the Sociology of Leisure, 4*(1), 61–78.

Tutenges, S., & Bøhling, F. (2019). Designing drunkenness: How pubs, bars and nightclubs increase alcohol sales. *International Journal of Drug Policy, 70*, 15–21.

Valentine, G., Holloway, S. L., Jayne, M., & Knell, C. (2008). *Drinking places: Where people drink and why*. Joseph Rowntree Foundation.

Wardell, J. D., Kempe, T., Rapinda, K. K., Single, A., Bilevicius, E., Frohlich, J. R., et al. (2020). Drinking to cope during COVID-19 pandemic: The role of external and internal factors in coping motive pathways to alcohol use, solitary drinking, and alcohol problems. *Alcoholism: Clinical and Experimental Research, 44*(10), 2073–2083.

Whitaker, V., Curtis, P., Fairbrother, H., Oldham, M., & Holmes, J. (2023). Young people's explanations for the decline in youth drinking in England. *BMC Public Health, 23*(1), 402.

Wilkinson, S. (2017). Drinking in the dark: Shedding light on young people's alcohol consumption experiences. *Social & Cultural Geography, 18*(6), 739–757.

World Health Organisation (WHO). (2006). Intimate partner violence and alcohol. https://www.who.int/violence_injury_prevention/violence/world_report/factsheets/fs_intimate.pdf

# Part V

## Young Adult Drinking Styles Since COVID-19: Policy and Practice

# 16

# What the COVID-19 Pandemic Taught Us about Violence Associated with Alcohol Consumption

Carly Lightowlers

**Abstract** In the UK, COVID-19 restrictions significantly altered alcohol availability, with periods in which access to on-trade premises was limited or closed off entirely, and saw drinking broadly confined to the home. The impact of these restrictions on young people's alcohol drinking have been studied. Yet, few have considered how these changes in drinking impact upon trends in alcohol-related violence, including domestic violence. This chapter explores evidence about the alcohol–violence relationship, including insights gleaned before, during, and after the pandemic, to challenge the assumption that the alcohol-related violence problem is wholly driven by young people, on-licensed premises and the NTE in which they cluster.

C. Lightowlers (✉)
Department of Sociology, Social Policy and Criminology, University of Liverpool, Liverpool, UK
e-mail: C.Lightowlers@liverpool.ac.uk



D. Conroy, F. Measham (eds.), *Young Adult Drinking Styles*, Sustainable Development Goals Series, https://doi.org/10.1007/978-3-031-98528-7_16

## Overview/Synopsis

It appears that alcohol drinking is only constructed as a public policy problem when certain populations are engaged in certain types of drinking and with certain outcomes. For example, in the late 1990s and the early 2000s, owing in part to the growth of the night-time economy (NTE), the volume of alcohol consumed in individual drinking sessions increased (binge-drinking), as did levels of alcohol-related harm amongst young people. Increased consumption by young people in these settings also proved to be a particular cause for concern. The public nature of these drinking practices saw young people and NTE settings identified as populations and sites of risky drinking practices. Policy consequently focused on governing and policing NTE settings and on curtailing public drunkenness and associated crime and disorder.

From 2020, COVID-19 responses and restrictions varied globally, and some significantly altered alcohol availability. This chapter reflects upon the UK context, where there were periods in which access to on-trade premises (e.g. pubs and restaurants) was limited or closed off entirely, meaning that during these periods, all occurrences of alcohol-related violence were linked to consumption of off-trade alcohol.[1] Also, lockdowns and other restrictions affected individuals' off-trade purchases and broadly confined their drinking of alcohol to home settings. This posed a novel opportunity to examine how alcohol-related violence is associated with off-trade alcohol availability.

It is important to contextualise changes in alcohol drinking and violence during the pandemic within broader pre-existing trends in relation to both. For example, violence has been thought to be declining and even before the pandemic occurred, more drinking was taking place in the home, and the pandemic merely accelerated this trend. In addition to health implications, including the rise in alcohol-related deaths over this period, increased drinking in the home impacted the types of violence commonly assumed to be related to alcohol consumption and the mechanisms behind them (e.g. differences between NTE stranger and domestic violence). And despite the prominence previously given in both research

[1] Notwithstanding illegal/unlawful operation of on-premises sites.

and policy to the contribution of the off-licensed trade in alcohol-related violence, the pandemic cemented understanding about the similar impact of the off-trade on violence.

This chapter explores emerging evidence about the alcohol–violence relationship, including insights gleaned before, during, and after the pandemic, to challenge the overwhelming policy assumption that the alcohol-related violence problem is wholly driven by young people, on-licensed premises and the NTE in which they cluster. The chapter will argue that in order to assess the impact of alcohol consumption on violence, and to disentangle its impact on domestic violence in particular, it is important to disaggregate alcohol sales according to premises (on- and off-licensed). In turn, this invites us to question the validity of framing alcohol-related violence as a problem predominantly associated with young people and to conduct further research on this topic.

## Construction of Alcohol, Crime and Disorder as a Problem of Young People

Alcohol drinking can be implicated in crime in various ways. Whilst alcohol is never the sole *cause* of violence, its presence can exacerbate its severity (Graham et al., 2011; Taylor et al., 2010). And some crime types are more commonly associated with alcohol drinking, such as violence (Bennett & Holloway, 2005, 2010; Dingwall, 2006). Recent estimates in England and Wales suggest that around two in every five violent crimes are thought to be alcohol-related (Stripe, 2021). Alcohol also plays a key contributory role in domestic violence, with an estimated 25–50% of all domestic violence taking place when the perpetrator has been drinking (Bennett & Bland, 2008) and around a third (32%) of violent incidents occurring around the home thought to be alcohol-related (Stripe, 2021). Owing to the widespread presence of alcohol in violent incidents, the criminal justice system has long been concerned with preventing and responding to such incidents.

In the UK, policy preoccupation with alcohol-related violence reached a peak at the turn of the century, in response to widespread moral panic about 'binge-drinking' culture and associated crime and disorder (Measham, 2006). The 'problem' to be addressed was constructed as one of young people engaging in hedonistic and risky leisure pursuits in NTE districts (Measham & Brain, 2005; Finney, 2004). This framing of the problem has since dominated both the public and criminological imagination. The focus on the NTE setting, it is argued here, has resulted in heightened and exaggerated attention being paid to young people's drinking as well as siloed thinking by policymakers and academics which has diminished the attention that ought to be paid to the role alcohol plays in other forms of violence, such as domestic violence.

In the late 1990s and in the early 2000s, owing in part to the growth of the NTE, the volume of alcohol consumed in individual drinking sessions increased (binge-drinking), as did levels of alcohol-related harm amongst young people (Parker, 1998; Measham, 2006; Measham & South, 2012). These trends were accompanied by "broader attitudinal change in terms of the culturally acceptable and desirable state of intoxication for drinkers" (Measham & Brain, 2005, p. 268), leading to policy concern about public drunkenness, violence, anti-social behaviour, accident and injury as well as about increased alcohol consumption by young women (Measham & South, 2012).

The patterns of alcohol consumption and acute intoxication observed at this time were thought to characterise 'weekday restraint and weekend excess', with young people tending to abstain from drinking during the week, when work was prioritised, and indulging in hedonistic excesses at the weekend in NTE settings to 'make up' for a hard-working week (Measham, 2006). It was no coincidence that violent incidents were also concentrated on weekend evenings in areas surrounding late-night entertainment venues (see evidence reviewed by Bottoms & Wiles, 1997; Maguire & Brookman, 2005).

Identification of young people's drinking as problematic stemmed from evidence that suggested heavier drinkers were more likely to be 'risk-taking', that is, getting very drunk, trying drugs and being arrested (Parker, 1998). Those who displayed criminal or publicly disruptive drunken behaviour were seen as problematic, owing to their decision to consume alcohol and get drunk as a form of leisure activity. Their public and visibly drunken behaviour—particularly unconsciousness, vomiting and violence—attracted a higher level of social opposition and saw young people and NTE settings identified as populations and sites of risky drinking practices. As such, young people engaging in drinking heavily were constructed as 'folk devils' (*cf.* Cohen, 1972) and seen as a threat to moral order in public and NTE settings.

The UK policy responses that ensued focused on governing and policing NTE settings and curtailing public drunkenness and associated crime and disorder, and they increased enforcement powers for police to respond to intoxicated individuals and to control spaces and premises (Hadfield et al., 2009; Measham, 2006; Measham & Brain, 2005). But these measures did not go as far as to stem the tide of alcohol flowing freely in these settings.

Several studies of population-wide levels of consumption have highlighted that those who are older and more affluent drink more (Blazer & Wu, 2009; Han et al., 2017; Collins, 2016), thus challenging the idea that only young people are engaged in problematic alcohol consumption. However, these insights did not translate into concerns around associated crime and violence. Rather, young 'folk devils' remained centre stage in efforts to reduce alcohol-related crime, and binge drinking became synonymous with young people drinking in public, as Jayne et al. (2012, p. 357) allude to when they say:

> *Binge drinking (and associated drug cultures), although technically referring to periods of episodic heavy alcohol consumption, has come in cultural terms to mean dangerous drinking by uncouth youth in the streets, an often labelled as 'The British disease'.*

Sociologists and criminologists are keenly aware that alcohol drinking is seemingly only constructed as a public policy problem when certain populations are engaged in certain types of drinking and with certain outcomes (Critcher, 2008; Nicholls & Berridge, 2020; Staddon, 2015), and they are also aware of the stigmatising effects that result from identifying the problem with certain groups or individuals and labelling them as problematic, especially when the drinking of other groups is seemingly deemed socially acceptable. This applies, for example, to the disproportionate criminalisation of populations, such as the young and homeless, owing to their more public drinking practices (explored further below). This focus also diverts attention away from unhealthy drinking practices amongst other groups (e.g. older adults) who may be linked with increased drinking and associated harms, including violence, in domestic settings. As well as attributing the blame for alcohol-related violence to particular populations, drinking practices and outcomes have also been associated with certain sites of 'risky' drinking, as we shall explore next.

## Construction of the NTE as a Site of Risky Drinking Practice

It is important to consider the interplay between people and place when it comes to drinking and harmful outcomes, including violence. People drink and behave very differently depending on their environment and in different social settings, as the review by Plant et al. (2002) and the seminal study by MacAndrew and Edgerton (1969) highlight.

Indeed, around the turn of the century, we "witnessed increased sessional consumption by a wider social spectrum of young people with a wider choice of drinks, drinking establishments and drinking times, fuelled by economic deregulation of the drinks industry and increasingly sophisticated and targeted marketing strategies" as well as the transformation of city centres (Measham & Brain, 2005, p. 276). The social processes associated with the liberalisation and deregulation of the alcohol industry and the NTE in the early twenty-first century saw the latter grow exponentially, and it was promoted as a liminal space (Hayward & Hobbs, 2007) in which drinking to excess (Measham, 2004; Measham & Brain, 2005) and transgressive behaviour as part of the 'pursuit of pleasure' (Measham, 2004, p. 309) and 'carnivalesque' experience were marketed to young people (Presdee, 2000). This widespread development of the urban and NTE and the active promotion of 'consumer excess and intoxication' therein (Measham & Brain, 2005, p. 275) were accompanied by an increase in alcohol-related crime and disorder. Consequently, public drunkenness and associated crime and disorder (as opposed to drinking/violence in the home) have dominated the focus of policy and crime prevention efforts ever since.

Young people frequenting NTE settings were perceived as a threat to social order, playing into more general constructions of this population as risky (see France, 2007) as well as a drain on public resources (Szmigin et al., 2008). Exaggerated media representations likewise represented and reinforced constructions of young people as 'drinking devils' (McPherson, 2017), city centres as 'no-go' areas at night (Frost & Gardiner, 2005) and alcohol consumption (e.g. binge drinking) as a pressing public policy and policing concern. Subsequently, 'irresponsible consumers' drinking to excess in these settings were criminalised and sites were controlled through initiatives such as drinking banning orders/zones etc. (e.g. Hadfield & Measham, 2015; Pennay, 2012).

Public settings are an understandable focus of policing efforts, in the sense that city centres and NTE environments can more easily be policed/patrolled, and incidents can be responded to as and when they are identified by police, patrons, by-standers and employees of the NTE. Indeed, to assist with the volume of such incidents, privatised policing of NTE venues has been seen in the form of 'bouncers' and security staff, which may be prescribed as a licensing condition. Their function is to assist with curtailing the carnivalesque and disorderly behaviour which is commonly associated with drinking in these settings (*cf.* Hobbs et al., 2005). Public spaces such as parks and open spaces are also patrolled and policed, for example through the introduction of public drinking laws. These have been found to disproportionately criminalise the drinking of young people and the homeless (see Pennay, 2012). However, for those whose victimisation occurs in the home—where alcohol consumption can occur unbridled—no such 'protection' is afforded, nor are perpetrators identified and dealt with as readily. Violence in these settings is more likely to see women and children victimised. Indeed, the legislative and economic policy landscape allows for the continued free flow of alcohol for home consumption environments, despite concerns about its associated harms (e.g. the deaths associated with alcohol consumption during the pandemic; Boniface et al., 2022; PHE, 2021).

This framing of the drinking-crime problem as one exclusively pertaining to the NTE has thus seen young people become the disproportionate target of crime prevention efforts and resultant criminalisation. This tendency is exacerbated by the fact that young people's drinking practices may be more likely to centre around social activities that take place in public settings, such as parks and NTE settings, compared to older age groups who may drink more in domestic settings. Moreover, given that the NTE is a site typically associated with alcohol-related *stranger* (and to a lesser extent *acquaintance*) violence (Budd et al., 2003; Graham & Wells, 2003; Finney, 2004), young people have been identified as the typical perpetrators in these environments. The age profile of alcohol-related *domestic* violence is likely older; yet these sites and populations are more challenging to study and 'observe'. They thus avoid the public and political scrutiny afforded to young people in public settings. Moreover, young people may indeed be more *at risk* than *risky* when we note the drinking that occurs in domestic settings.

This is not to deny that public disorder and violence are experienced in NTE settings. Nor is it to deny the widespread strain such incidents put on health and criminal justice agencies. It is rather to highlight how the 'moral failings' of a specific group have been disproportionately focused on and represented in irresponsible ways, singling out a cohort of 'folk devils' upon which to focus the blame and to target for intervention. Doing so has allowed the wider problem of the free-flow of alcohol in these settings—made available by increasing self-regulating licensing regimes and alcohol industry—to evade further scrutiny and governance. Indeed, as Critcher (2008, p. 1141) notes:

> *Constructed as a discursive field, defined as a risk and requiring regulation is the issue of illegitimate pleasure in public places—as opposed to the heavy drinking characteristic of other sections of the population which takes place in private (undoubtedly including politicians, judges and police officers).*

The UK policy focus on public drunkenness and associated crime and disorder (as opposed to drinking/violence in the home) persists to date (Wilson et al., 2022), despite the known association and significant proportion of alcohol-related violence in the home (e.g. domestic abuse/violence) (Leonard, 2005; Bryant & Lightowlers, 2021) and the widespread concerns voiced about the potential amplification and increase in domestic violence during and in the wake of the Covid pandemic (Wilson et al., 2022).

## Trends in Alcohol Consumption and Violence Predating the COVID-19 Pandemic

Not only might the conception of public spaces as the only risky site in terms of alcohol-related violence be contestable, but so is the idea that alcohol-related violence is only a problem of young people occupying these settings. Not least as parallel declines in both youth drinking and violence have both been observed.

Indeed, in the past couple of decades, young people are drinking less. Youth alcohol consumption in England has decreased (Oldham et al., 2018; Whitaker et al., 2023) and is driven by changes in heavy drinking in particular (Oldham et al., 2020). More young people (16–24-year-olds) are choosing to abstain, and those who do drink are doing so "less often and in smaller quantities" (Oldham et al., 2018, p. 3). Internationally, survey evidence spanning the UK, Europe, North America and Australasia similarly point to a decline of youth engagement in alcohol use since the early 2000s, in terms of reduced volume and frequency of consumption as well as delayed age of initiation (Oldham et al., 2020; Whitaker et al., 2023). Meanwhile, previous generations of heavier drinkers are aging and continuing to drink (Kuerbis et al., 2014; Barry & Blow, 2016).

We know that drinking practices and associated health and crime harm are influenced by social change and economic conditions. Efforts to understand the reasons behind the sustained youth 'drinking decline' phenomenon and its drivers have included hypotheses such as changing social norms around drinking; better parenting; increased emphasis on education, health and well-being; reduced affordability of alcohol; changing social (including internet-based) interactions; and better policy intervention to prevent underage sales, amongst others (Bhattacharya, 2016; Oldham et al., 2018). And the decline in young people's drinking around the turn of the century has also been linked to "economic recession and associated job insecurities, whilst amongst older age groups and professional occupations increased home drinking, wine drinking, and weekday drinking are all increasing (Jayne et al. 2008; Valentine et al 2007; Measham and Østergaard 2009)" (Measham & South, 2012, p. 709).

However, there is limited evidence to support a single definitive explanation, and reasons behind the drinking decline remain a topic of ongoing scholarly enquiry, with scholarship around sobriety, abstinence and moderation running in parallel (Banister et al., 2019). These focus on the interactions between multiple factors, and it is thought that "changing practices of socialisation, decreased alcohol affordability and changed attitudes toward risk and self-governance may be key explanations" of the youth drinking decline (Whitaker et al., 2023, p. 1), but that these are understood and experienced differently by different groups of young people based on their age, gender and socio-economic status (Whitaker et al., 2023). Moreover, it is broadly accepted that "there is a perceived cultural shift between generations of young people, manifesting in terms of their spaces and places of socialisation, and shifting attitudes towards risk, self-governance and the future" that is influencing young people's drinking choices and behaviours (Whitaker et al., 2023, p. 11). In parallel, the criminal justice demands resulting from public drunkenness and associated problems have also decreased (Measham & South, 2012, p. 709).

Whatever the drivers, this change in the age profile of drinkers challenges the assumption that alcohol drinking is a normalised leisure activity among young adults and it is of interest when considering associated trends in crime and violence, not least as NTE violence has typically been associated with young males and heavy episodic drinking practices (Finney, 2004; Richardson & Budd, 2003; Lightowlers et al., 2014). As such, it has been hypothesised that the decline in drinking amongst young people, particular heavy drinkers, has resulted in decreases in associated violence. However, few studies have examined this explicitly.

## Links with Violence

In many countries in the Global North, a concurrent declining trend in violence (and crime more generally)—coined the 'crime drop' of the late twentieth century has been observed over roughly the same period (Farrell et al., 2014).[2] As identified by Bryant (2023a), in England and Wales, National Statistics (ONS, 2021) also show a specific decline in alcohol-related violence. Moreover, there has also been a decline over a similar period in risky behaviour (defined as smoking, substance use, sexual initiation and crime) more generally amongst young people in high-income countries (Ball et al., 2023).

Bryant (2023a) thus prompts us to consider downward trends in both young people's alcohol consumption and alcohol-related violence over the last decade and suggests that declines in youth drinking might be contributing to observed declines in stranger and acquaintance violence related to alcohol intoxication in England and Wales, such as those in NTE settings. Bryant (2023a, p. 2) suggests that reduced consumption amongst young people in particular could reduce violent incidents, "as intoxication increases the risk of engaging in such incidents (e.g. Dawson 1997)". If this is the case, it would also challenge the usefulness of the widespread scrutiny, surveillance and criminalisation that has been a feature of alcohol-related violence control and prevention strategies focused on the NTE, and the heightened attention paid to young people's drinking therein.

In the first exploratory study of its kind, Bryant (2023a) poses the question as to whether these trends in youth drinking could explain a parallel reduction in alcohol-related violence observed over the same period. She notes: "violence is a broad category, and while any instance of aggression may share some drivers, it is widely accepted that different kinds of violence—e.g. domestic as opposed to stranger violence—may have their own distinct drivers. Therefore, it is essential we examine trends in such alcohol-related violence subtypes" Bryant (2023b). Her exploratory analyses of the Crime Survey for England and Wales (CSEW) highlight that whilst there have been downward trends in stranger and

[2] Since the 1990s.

acquaintance violence related to alcohol intoxication, this is not the case when it comes to alcohol-related domestic violence. Indeed, "changing patterns in youth drinking are identified as a potential contributor to this violence decline" (Bryant, 2023a, p. 17). But it is of note that the proportion of domestic violence involving alcohol intoxication has been relatively stable between 2009/10 and 2019/20 and "should not be discounted as a policy priority" (Bryant, 2023a, p. 16). These findings challenge the assumption that alcohol-related violence is a crime predominantly associated with the behaviours of young people. And, as the decline in alcohol-related violence "remains unexplained and generally unexamined" (Bryant, 2023a, p. 4), the academic research community is thus encouraged to pursue further research to further analyse the victim and perpetrator age profiles of such incidents. This has the potential to shed further light on the mechanisms and drivers of age-cohort changes in drinking and associated crime.

## Changes to Drinking Practices and Associated Violence During the COVID-19 Pandemic

Alcohol patterns shifted owing to the COVID-19 pandemic and the associated stay at home directives, as well as widespread changes in alcohol availability, including periods when access to on-trade premises (e.g. pubs and restaurants) was limited or closed off entirely (Boniface et al., 2022). "In response to the 2020 COVID-19 outbreak, many countries imposed restrictions on outlets selling alcohol to reduce virus transmission. In England, while shops selling alcohol were deemed 'essential', multiple restrictions were imposed on licensed outlets such as pubs and bars" (Reynolds, 2022, p. 1). Despite the confusing and sometimes contradictory nature of decisions concerning the operation of licensed premises during the pandemic (Reynolds, 2022), drinking in managed on-trade environments diminished dramatically and pushed drinking further into the home, amplifying pre-existing shifts towards at home drinking and off-licensed purchasing of alcohol (Boniface et al., 2022; Foster & Ferguson, 2012; Foster et al., 2021) and polarising drinking across the UK, with moderate drinkers generally consuming the same or less, and heavier drinkers on average consuming at more harmful levels (Boniface et al., 2022). The extent of alcohol's impact on violence was more hidden as a result, but did continue (Lightowlers & Bryant, 2023; 2025). Harms and adverse health outcomes associated with alcohol drinking were also observed, such as the rise in alcohol-related deaths over this period (Boniface et al., 2022; PHE, 2021).

The significant alterations to alcohol availability during the pandemic meant that there were periods when all alcohol-related violence was linked to consumption of off-trade alcohol and so not necessarily a problem associated with NTE drinking. This posed a novel opportunity to examine how alcohol-related violence is associated with off-trade alcohol availability. Lightowlers & Bryant (2023; 2025) used police-recorded violent crime data to exploit this opportunity and assess the contribution of off-trade alcohol availability on trends in alcohol-related violence during periods of on-trade closures over the pandemic period. Using growth curve models, they explored changes in the proportion of alcohol-related (1) violence as well as (2) domestic violence and found rates of alcohol-related violence to be higher in periods when on-licensed premises were open. Interestingly, they observed no significant differences in levels of alcohol-related domestic violence, nor in the proportion of domestic violence which was recorded as alcohol-related during periods of on-trade closures and suggest this points to the important contribution of the off-trade makes to such incidents. The authors are, however, also careful to caution that as well as changes to alcohol availability the situation was complicated by other effects of the pandemic. Indeed, given that social contact outside the home was limited, this confined people both to drink more in the home but also exerted considerable pressure on domestic relationships and family life this likely also impacted upon the probability of violence occurring in the home, which may have been further impacted by economic stressors such as job losses during this period (see WHO, 2020). These findings add weight to earlier calls to take seriously the contribution alcohol plays to domestic violence both in social policy and academic scholarship (Wilson et al., 2022) and cement knowledge about the similar contribution the off-licensed trade plays in alcohol-related violence, including domestic violence, as it is methodologically challenging to parse out the contributions of the on- and off-trade when both usually operate in parallel (Lightowlers & Bryant, 2023; 2025). Additionally, despite widespread concerns about domestic violence during the pandemic, little consideration was extended to the compounding role alcohol may play for those who were confined to their homes. These recent findings challenge the assumption that young people, on-licensed premises and the NTEs in which they cluster are the sole drivers of the alcohol-related violence problem. They also raise further questions to be answered about the age profile of victims and offenders. Such evidence has the potential to dispel myths about the populations and sites perceived to be at risk of alcohol-related violence. These myths have dominated the political imagination thus far and they have been evoked to regulate and criminalise irresponsible consumers of the NTE.

## Future Directions for Research, Policy and Practice

This chapter has explored evidence about the alcohol–violence relationship, including insights gleaned before, during, and after the pandemic in the UK context. It has charted a shift in young people's drinking, suggesting that the likely perpetrators of alcohol-related violence are older than hitherto assumed, especially if we duly acknowledge the domestic setting as a site of such violence. In so doing, the chapter has challenged the assumption that young people, on-licensed premises and the NTEs in which they cluster are the sole drivers of the alcohol-related violence 'problem'. It has argued that in order to assess the impact of alcohol consumption on violence, and on domestic violence in particular, it is important to disaggregate alcohol sales according to premises (on- and off-licensed) (see Holmes et al., 2014).

In explicitly inviting the research community to pursue further research to understand the age profile of those involved in alcohol-related violence, the perspective presented here offers an opportunity to broaden the forms of violence that are included as objects of academic and policy analysis and to break away from dominant criminalising discourses about young people and their drinking. It also offers an opportunity to broaden the types of environments in which drinking and associated violent incidents are considered to occur, focusing not only on NTE environments but also on other public as well as on private settings. This represents an invitation to broaden our collective sociological imagination (Mills, 1959) to more accurately represent the mechanisms, actors and challenges associated with alcohol-related violence and to respond more effectively to its social impact.

Indeed, consideration of public health approaches and upstream intervention that may have the potential to disproportionately safeguard populations 'at risk' from alcohol related harm, such as women and children, is encouraged, rather than enabling the persistence of responses rooted in moral panic associated with anxieties around young people's binge drinking in the NTE. Avoiding the pitfalls of these siloes—evident in the disciplines of criminology and alcohol studies alike and cemented in violence reduction and alcohol policy—is key to developing our understanding and development of meaningful efforts to reduce alcohol-related harm and prevent violence. So, whilst age remains an important determinant of drinking behaviours, the above invitation provides us with the opportunity to offer young people redemption from being vilified as irresponsible alcohol consumers and being criminalised as a result.

## References


Ball, J., Grucza, R., Livingston, M., ter Bogt, T., Currie, C., & de Looze, M. (2023). The great decline in adolescent risk behaviours: Unitary trend, separate trends, or cascade? *Social Science & Medicine, 317,* 115616. https://doi.org/10.1016/j.socscimed.2022.115616

Banister, E., Conroy, D., & Piacentini, M. (2019). Non-drinkers and non-drinking: A review, a critique and pathways to policy. In D. Conroy & F. Measham (Eds.), *Young adult drinking styles: Current perspectives on research, policy and practice*. Palgrave Macmillan.

Barry, K. L., & Blow, F. C. (2016). Drinking over the lifespan: Focus on older adults. *Alcohol Research Current Reviews, 38*(1), 115–120.

Bennett, L., & Bland, P. (2008). *Substance abuse and intimate partner violence.* VAWnet, National Resource Center on Domestic Violence/Pennsylvania Coalition Against Domestic Violence.

Bennett, L., & Holloway, K. (2005). *Understanding drugs, alcohol and crime.* Open University Press.

Bennett, T., & Holloway, K. (2010). Chapter 29: Drug and alcohol-related crime. In F. Brookman, M. Maguire, H. Pierpoint, & T. Bennett (Eds.), (pp. 579–597). *Handbook on crime*, Willan Publishing.

Bhattacharya, A. (2016). *Youthful abandon: Why are young people drinking less?* The Institute of Alcohol Studies.

Blazer, D. G., & Wu, L. (2009). The epidemiology of at risk and binge drinking among middle-aged and elderly community adults: National survey on drug use and health. *American Journal of Psychiatry, 166*, 1162–1169.

Boniface, S., Card-Gowers, J., Martin, A., Retat, L., & Webber, L. (2022). *The COVID hangover: Addressing long-term health impacts of changes in alcohol consumption during the pandemic.* Institute of Alcohol Studies.

Bottoms, A. E., & Wiles, P. (1997). Environmental criminology. In M. Maguire, R. Morgan, & R. Reiner (Eds.), *Oxford handbook of criminology* (pp. 305–359). Oxford University Press.

Bryant, L. (2023a). Patterns in alcohol-related violence: Exploring recent declines in alcohol-related violence in England and Wales. Retrieved November 3, 2023, from https://www.ias.org.uk/wp-content/uploads/2023/02/Patterns-in-alcohol-related-violence-IAS-February-2023.pdf

Bryant, L. (2023b). Patterns in alcohol-related violence: Exploring recent declines in alcohol-related violence in England and Wales. IAS blog Retrieved November 6, 2023, from https://www.ias.org.uk/2023/02/27/patterns-in-alcohol-related-violence-exploring-recent-declines-in-alcohol-related-violence-in-england-and-wales/

Budd, T., Tedstone, C., & Curry, D. (2003). *Alcohol related assault: Findings from the British Crime Survey.* Home Office.

Bryant, L., & Lightowlers C. (2021). The socioeconomic distribution of alcohol-related violence in England andWales. *PLoS ONE, 16*(2), e0243206. https://doi.org/10.1371/journal.pone.0243206

Cohen, S. (1972). *Folk devils and moral panics: The creation of the mods and rockers.* Routledge.

Collins, S. E. (2016). Associations between socioeconomic factors and alcohol outcomes. *Alcohol Research: Current Reviews, 38*(1), 83–94.

Critcher, C. (2008). Moral panic analysis: Past, present and future. *Sociology Compass, 2*, 1127–1144.

Dingwall, G. (2006). *Alcohol and crime*. Willan Publishing.

Farrell, G., Tilley, N., & Tseloni, A. (2014). Why the crime drop? *Crime and Justice, 43*(1), 421–490.

Finney, A. (2004). *Violence in the night-time economy: Key findings from the research*. Home Office.

Foster, J. H., & Ferguson, C. S. (2012). Home drinking in the UK: Trends and causes. *Alcohol and Alcoholism, 47*(3), 355–358.

Foster, J. H., Martin, C. R., & Davis, J. P. (2021). Alcohol consumption during the covid-19 lockdown period: Predictors of at-risk drinking at different AUDIT-C cut-off thresholds. *International Journal of Environmental Research and Public Health, 18*(24), 13042.

France, A. (2007). *Understanding youth in late modernity*. Open University Press.

Frost, J., & Gardiner, S. (2005). Binge drinking: The latest moral panic? *Safer Communities, 4*(4), 5–9.

Graham, K., & Wells, S. (2003). 'Somebody's gonna get their head kicked in tonight!' Aggression among young males in bars—A question of values? *British Journal of Criminology, 43*(3), 546–566.

Graham, K., Bernards, S., Wilsnack, S. C., & Gmel, G. (2011). Alcohol may not cause partner violence but it seems to make it worse: A cross national comparison of the relationship between alcohol and severity of partner violence. *Journal of Interpersonal Violence, 26*, 1503–1523.

Hadfield, P., & Measham, F. (2015). The outsourcing of control: Alcohol law enforcement, private-sector governance and the evening and night-time economy. *Urban Studies, 52*(3), 517–537.

Hadfield, P., Lister, S., & Traynor, P. (2009). 'This town's a different town today' policing and regulating the night-time economy. *Criminology & Criminal Justice, 9*(4), 465–485.

Han, B. H., Moore, A. A., Sherman, S., Keyes, K. M., & Palamar, J. J. (2017). Demographic trends of binge alcohol use and alcohol use disorders among older adults in the United States, 2005–2014. *Drug and Alcohol Dependence, 170*, 198–207.

Hayward, K., & Hobbs, D. (2007). Beyond the binge in 'booze Britain': Market-led liminalization and the spectacle of binge drinking. *British Journal of Sociology, 58*(3), 437–456.

Hobbs, D., Hadfield, P., Lister, S., & Winlow, S. (2005). *Bouncers: Violence and governance in the night-time economy*. Oxford University Press.

Holmes, J., Guo, Y., Maheswaran, R., Nicholls, J., Meier, P. S., & Brennan, A. (2014). The impact of spatial and temporal availability of alcohol on its consumption and related harms: A critical review in the context of UK licensing policies. *Drug and Alcohol Review, 33*(5), 515–525.

Jayne, M., Valentine, G., & Holloway, S. (2012). Chapter 20: Consumption and context. In T. Kolind, B. Thom, & G. Hunt (Eds.), *The Sage handbook of drug and alcohol studies: Social science approaches* (pp. 352–363). Sage Publications Ltd.

Kuerbis, A., Sacco, P., Blazer, D. G., & Moore, A. A. (2014). Substance abuse among older adults. *Clinics in Geriatric Medicine, 30*(3), 629–654.

Leonard, K. E. (2005). Alcohol and intimate partner violence: When can we say that heavy drinking is a contributing cause of violence? *Addiction, 100*, 422–425.

Lightowlers, C., Elliot, M., & Tranmer, M. (2014). The dynamic risk of heavy episodic drinking on interpersonal assault in young adolescence and early adulthood. *British Journal of Criminology, 54*(6), 1207–1227.

Lightowlers, C., Coomber, K., & Quigg, Z. (2023a). The impact of COVID-19 and associated public health restrictions on trends in police-recorded violence in an English police force area. *BMC Public Health, 23*, 1448.

Lightowlers, C., Pina-Sánchez, J., & McLaughlin, F. (2023b). The role of deprivation and alcohol availability in shaping trends in violent crime. *European Journal of Criminology, 20*(2), 738–757.

Lightowlers, C., & Bryant, L. (2023). *Off-trade alcohol availability and violence: Assessing the impact of on-tradeoutlet closures*. London: Institute of Alcohol Studies.

Lightowlers, C., & Bryant, L. (2025). Alcohol and violence: Isolating the impact of the Off-Trade. *The British Journal of Criminology*, azaf045. https://doi.org/10.1093/bjc/azaf045

MacAndrew, C., & Edgerton, R. (1969). *Drunken comportment: A social explanation*. Aldine Publishing.

Maguire, M., & Brookman, F. (2005). Violent and sexual crime. In N. Tilley (Ed.), *Handbook of crime prevention and community safety* (pp. 516–562). Willan Publishing.

Measham, F. (2006). The new policy mix: Alcohol, harm minimisation, and determined drunkenness in contemporary society. *International Journal of Drug Policy, 17*, 258–268.

Measham, F., & Brain, K. (2005). 'Binge' drinking, British alcohol policy and the new culture of intoxication. *Crime, Media, Culture, 1*(3), 262–283.

Measham, F., & South, N. (2012). Drugs, alcohol and crime. In M. Maguire, R. Morgan, & R. Reiner (Eds.), *The Oxford handbook of criminology* (5th ed.). Oxford University Press.

Mills, C. (1959). *The sociological imagination*. Oxford University Press.

McPherson, R. (2017). "Fifteen: 'Binge' drinking devils and moral marginality: young people's calculated hedonism in the Canterbury night-time economy". In Youth Marginality in Britain. Bristol, UK: Policy Press. Retrieved Nov 6, 2023, from https://doi.org/10.51952/9781447330530.ch015

Measham, F. (2004). The decline of ecstasy, the rise of 'binge' drinking and the persistence of pleasure. *Probation Journal, 51*(4), 309–326. https://doi.org/10.1177/0264550504048220

Nicholls, J., & Berridge, V. (2020). Chapter 2: Substance use, dangerous classes and spaces: A historical perspective. In S. MacGregor & B. Thom (Eds.), *Risk and substance use: Framing dangerous people and dangerous places*. London: Routledge.

Office for National Statistics (ONS). (2021). *The nature of violent crime in England and Wales: Year ending March 2020; Table 9a: Proportion of violent incidents where the victim believed the offender(s) to be under the influence of alcohol or drugs*. Office for National Statistics.

Oldham, M., Holmes, J., Whitaker, V., Fairbrother, H., & Curtis, P. (2018). *Youth drinking in decline*. The University of Sheffield.

Oldham, M., Callinan, S., Whitaker, V., Fairbrother, H., Curtis, P., Meier, P., Livingston, M., & Holmes, J. (2020). The decline in youth drinking in England—Is everyone drinking less? A quantile regression analysis. *Addiction, 115*(2), 230–238.

Parker, H. (1998). Illegal leisure: alcohol, drugs and the regulation of modern youth. In P. Carlen & R. Morgan (Eds.), *Crime unlimited: Questions for the 21st century* (pp. 144–165). Palgrave Macmillan.

Pennay, A. (2012). 'Wicked problems': The social conundrum presented by public drinking laws. *Drugs: Education Prevention and Policy, 19*(3), 185–191.

Plant, M., Plant, M., & Thornton, C. (2002). People and places: Some factors in the alcohol-violence link. *Journal of Substance Use, 7*(4), 207–213.

Presdee, M. (2000). *Cultural criminology and the carnival of crime*. Routledge.

Public Health England (PHE). (2021). Monitoring alcohol consumption and harm during the COVID-19 pandemic: Report. https://www.gov.uk/government/publications/alcohol-consumption-and-harm-during-the-covid-19-pandemic

Reynolds, J. (2022). Framings of risk and responsibility in newsprint media coverage of alcohol licensing regulations during the COVID-19 pandemic in England. *Drug and Alcohol Review, 42*(1), 213–224.

Richardson, A., & Budd, T. (2003). Young adults, alcohol, crime and disorder. *Criminal Behaviour and Mental Health, 13*, 5–16.

Staddon, P. (2015). *Women and alcohol: Social perspectives*. Policy Press.

Stripe, N. (2021). *The nature of violent crime: Appendix tables. Year ending March 2020*. Office for National Statistics.

Szmigin, I., Griffin, C., Mistral, W., Bengry-Howell, A., Weale, L., & Hackley, C. (2008). Re-framing 'binge drinking' as calculated hedonism: Empirical evidence from the UK. *International Journal of Drug Policy, 19*(5), 359–366.

Taylor, B., Irving, H. M., Kanteres, F., Room, R., Borges, G., Cherpitel, C., Greenfield, T., & Rehm, J. (2010). The more you drink, the harder you fall: A systematic review and meta-analysis of how acute alcohol consumption and injury or collision risk increase together. *Drug and Alcohol Dependence, 110*, 108–116.

Whitaker, V., Curtis, P., Fairbrother, H., et al. (2023). Young people's explanations for the decline in youth drinking in England. *BMC Public Health, 23*, 402.

Wilson, I. M., Lightowlers, C., & Bryant, L. (2022). Home drinking during and post-COVID-19: Why the silence on domestic violence? *Drug and Alcohol Review, 42*(5), 1013–1017.

World Health Organization (WHO). (2020). *COVID-19 and violence against women*. World Health Organization.

# 17

# Alcohol and Mental Health in Young Adults

**Laura Goodwin, Jo-Anne Puddephat, and Patricia Irizar**

**Abstract** The co-occurrence of alcohol and mental health problems in the general population is well-documented. Among young adults, evidence suggests that most of those with an alcohol problem are also suffering with a mental health problem. The transition from childhood to adolescence is a critical point for the development of both alcohol and mental health problems. Young adults who experience alcohol and mental health problems concurrently have worse outcomes than those with one problem alone, and treatments for co-occurring problems are

L. Goodwin (✉)
Department of Health Research, Lancaster University, Lancaster, UK
e-mail: l.goodwin1@lancaster.ac.uk

J.-A. Puddephat
Department of Psychology, Edge Hill University, Ormskirk, UK
e-mail: jo-anne.puddephatt@edgehill.ac.uk

P. Irizar
Department of Psychology, Liverpool John Moores University, Liverpool, UK
e-mail: p.irizar@ljmu.ac.uk



D. Conroy, F. Measham (eds.), *Young Adult Drinking Styles*, Sustainable Development Goals Series, https://doi.org/10.1007/978-3-031-98528-7_17

complex. In this chapter, we discuss (1) key theories regarding co-occurring alcohol and mental health problems, (2) evidence on the extent of these issues, and (3) current treatments.

Alcohol and mental health problems commonly co-occur in the general population (Bell & Britton, 2014; Conway et al., 2016; Lai et al., 2015; Puddephatt et al., 2022), with evidence from clinical practice suggesting that most adolescents and young adults with a substance use problem (including alcohol use disorders [AUD]) also have a co-occurring mental health problem (Erskine et al., 2015). The onset of most mental health problems occurs during the transition from childhood to adolescence (Patel et al., 2007), and this time-period is also often a turning-point for when occasional substance use can become more regular and potentially problematic (Jordan & Andersen, 2017). Among most adolescents and young adults with co-occurring problems, the presence of a mental health problem usually precedes the onset of problematic alcohol use, though some will develop an AUD before suffering with poor mental health (Merikangas et al., 2010). Both mental health and alcohol problems are significant contributors to health-related disability in young adults (Gore et al., 2011; Sawyer et al., 2012).

Across many Western countries, alcohol use is declining in young adults (Holmes et al., 2022; Kraus et al., 2020; Vashishtha et al., 2020), with many choosing to completely abstain from alcohol (Corre et al., 2023). In adult populations, there is a J-shaped relationship between alcohol and mental health, whereby both abstinence from alcohol and harmful drinking are more common in those with a mental health problem (El-Guebaly, 2007; Fat et al., 2014; Goodwin et al., 2017; Puddephatt et al., 2021). Evidence from the early 2000s identified poor social and mental health outcomes among young abstainers (Hoel et al., 2004; Laukkanen et al., 2001), yet more recently, abstinence has been found to be associated with multiple mental and physical health benefits for young adults (Conroy & de Visser, 2018; de Visser et al., 2014; Larm et al., 2018). Despite reduced alcohol use among young adults in recent years, the prevalence of mental health problems are rising (Patalay & Gage, 2019; Pitchforth et al., 2019). The COVID-19 pandemic further exacerbated this, with the negative effects on the mental health of young adults now being widely known (Kauhanen et al., 2023).

It is important to understand the extent of and reasons for co-occurring alcohol and mental health problems, as people with co-occurring problems are more likely to experience adverse outcomes compared to those with only one problem (Erskine et al., 2015; McCarthy & Petrakis, 2010). The management and treatment of co-occurring problems are also complicated, with lower treatment engagement and poorer outcomes (Tomáš & Lenka, 2023), and many clinicians feel unable to adequately support young adults with co-occurring problems (Blumenthal et al., 2001). In this chapter, we will (1) outline several key theories which can be used to explain the coexistence of these problems, (2) present epidemiological evidence regarding the relationship between alcohol use and mental health among young adults, and (3) current guidance on treating those with a co-occurring alcohol and mental health problem. The literature in this chapter primarily focuses on populations spanning from adolescents to young adulthood.

## Theorising the Relationship Between Alcohol and Mental Health

Reasons for drinking are complex and influenced by a combination of cultural, economic, and social factors. Early motivational theories argue that people are motivated to use alcohol to cope, for social reasons, or to fit in (Cooper, 1994; Cox & Klinger, 1988). The incentive-motivation model argues that the decision to drink alcohol is determined by the incentives associated with drinking alcohol outweighing the benefits of not drinking alcohol (Cox & Klinger, 1988). This decision may be further influenced by the desire to either increase positive affect or decrease negative affect either towards themselves or towards others (Cooper et al., 1995). An extension of the incentive-motives model is the drinking motives model (Cooper, 1994), which argues that there are four main reasons for drinking; social (drinking to obtain social rewards), enhancement (drinking for pleasure), conformity (drinking to avoid negative social consequences), and coping (drinking to avoid negative emotions). For those with a mental health problem, evidence shows that alcohol is used to cope with symptoms (Puddephatt et al., 2024; Puddephatt et al., 2023) and drinking to cope motives mediate the relationship between mental health symptoms and alcohol use (Bakhshaie et al., 2021; O'Hare & Sherrer, 2011). However, drinking to cope may differ depending on the type of mental health problem and the symptoms experienced within these (Puddephatt et al., 2023).

Abstinence can be common in some groups but, like alcohol use, motivations are complex and likely differ across different population groups. Theories of abstinence include the sick-quitter hypothesis (people stop drinking due to declines in their health) (Goldman & Najman, 1984), promotion of health campaigns (e.g., Dry January), normalisation of abstinence (Raninen et al., 2021), economic factors, social media, and changes in alcohol policy. Indeed, some of these reasons may differ depending on the characteristics of groups. For example, age is associated with increased risks of health conditions, therefore, it could be theorised that abstinence is common among older age groups due to pre-existing health conditions. However, among young adults, evidence indicates that there has been a decline in the uptake of alcohol (Ng Fat et al., 2018). Previous work suggested that this could be due to a range of reasons, such as legal enforcement, financial constraints, alternative behaviours through the rise in technology, and changes in social norms (Bhattacharya, 2016). However, these theories have seldom been empirically tested.

The relationship between alcohol (including abstinence) and mental health problems are complex. There are four main theories: (1) heavy drinking causes declines in mental health (substance-induced enhancement theory (Kushner et al., 1990)), (2) declines in mental health cause increases in the uptake of alcohol (self-medication hypothesis (Khantzian, 1987, 1997)), (3) shared genetic and environmental factors (Castillo-Carniglia et al., 2019), (4) stopping drinking to manage health (sick-quitter hypothesis (Goldman & Najman, 1984)). The substance-induced enhancement theory argues that heavy drinking and experiencing withdrawal frequently cause biological changes which induce symptoms related to mental health problems. Whereas the self-medication hypothesis states that people with a mental health problem use substances to alleviate stress. Elsewhere, it is argued that alcohol and mental health problems share common genetic and environmental risk factors, such as trauma, genes, and parent–child relationship (Castillo-Carniglia et al., 2019). While the sick-quitter hypothesis argues that people stop drinking due to declines in health. Evidence which has tested the directionality of the first three theories have found stronger evidence for the self-medication hypothesis (Bell & Britton, 2014; Treur et al., 2021).

## Theorising the Relationship Between Alcohol and Mental Health in Young Adults

Theories around drinking (or abstinence) and mental health among young adults are largely similar to those in the general population. However, theories such as the social learning theory (Bandura & Walters, 1977) and social norms theory (Berkowitz, 2003), provide additional insights relating to this population. The social learning theory suggests that patterns of behaviour are acquired either by direct experience or through observation of other people, and its consequences for them (Bandura & Walters, 1977). In the context of alcohol use, this theory argues that individuals may be more likely to drink alcohol if this is commonly observed as a behaviour of others and where there are positive consequences. The social norms theory suggests that individuals incorrectly perceive the attitudes or behaviours of others to different from their own, and in the context of drinking, individuals overestimate the consumption and frequency of drinking which can facilitate increases in drinking while also providing justification for doing so (Berkowitz, 2003). However, context may be an important factor for young adults, for example the setting in which drinking is taking place or whether individuals observe peers or parents' drinking (Preston & Goodfellow, 2006).

As previously discussed, there have been notable changes in the uptake of drinking among young adults. The normalisation thesis proposed by Parker and colleagues argues that certain substances can become socially and culturally accepted in young people's lives, though this process is dynamic and varies across substance type and contexts (Parker et al., 1999). Caluzzi and colleagues argue that the normalisation theory can be used to explain the decline in youth drinking through two ways (Caluzzi et al., 2022). First, denormalisation of drinking where drinking becomes less accepted and less commonly observed among peers, therefore, there may be less experimentation with alcohol and alcohol may become less accessible. Second, normalisation of non-drinking where abstinence becomes more accepted and this practice is more socially and culturally more accepted though, contrary to the former, drinking is still acceptable.

However, there are additional factors to consider when we attempt to understand alcohol use among young adults. For example, there has been substantial research which has explored the role of adverse childhood experiences (ACE) on alcohol and other drugs. ACEs refer to a traumatic event or experience during childhood which can be physical, emotional or sexual. Evidence has shown that the risk of AUDs during adulthood increases with increasing number of ACEs experienced by a young person (Anda et al., 2002), while a recent systematic review and meta-analysis showed strong associations between ACEs and health behaviours and conditions, particularly mental health problems and AUDs (Hughes et al., 2017). Parental alcohol use is also a contributing factor. It has been established that young adults whose parents drink or have an AUD may be at risk of developing alcohol and/or mental health problems (Kuppens et al., 2020). This is thought to occur through a family environment lens whereby parental alcohol use or alcohol problems create a negative family environment impacting on parent–child relationships (Kuppens et al., 2020).

Other factors which are of relevance to young adults are the role of digital technology, global pandemics, and changes in the priorities of young adults. Young adults have grown up in a world where technology has been increasingly used. In the context of alcohol use, technology (including social media) may promote or discourage the uptake of drinking through advertisements, and sharing views on drinking (including the encouragement of non-drinking) (Atkinson et al., 2024) through a public forum (Caluzzi et al., 2022; Griffiths & Casswell, 2010). However, this may be dependent on the way in which people interact with social media, for example, the increased use of online spaces mean that alcohol is less of a central feature to socialising (Caluzzi et al., 2022). During the COVID-19 pandemic, there were physical distancing restrictions globally which impacted individuals' ability to physically interact with others which likely had an impact on health and lifestyle behaviours, including the way in which people drank alcohol. Elsewhere, there are suggestions that young adults are more health conscious and those with mental health problems prefer not to drink alcohol because of the impact it has on their symptoms (Sumnall et al., In Preparation), with the latter reflecting findings in adult population (Puddephatt et al., 2023).

In terms of co-occurring alcohol and mental health problems among young adults, the proposed mechanisms are similar to that mentioned previously, though there may be more developmental impacts given the biological changes occurring during this time (Otasowie, 2021). For example, we have previously discussed shared genetic and environmental factors and co-occurring alcohol and mental health problems. Young adults may be particularly at risk of experiencing co-occurring problems due to the way in which alcohol can impact the brain and the way in which young adults may be particularly affected by their familial environment (Otasowie, 2021). Due to this potentially increased vulnerability, young adults may increase the risk of experiencing co-occurring problems through a positive feedback loop (Khokhar et al., 2018). While these theories uphold when considering co-occurring alcohol and mental health problems among young people, there is limited evidence regarding the direction of the relationship among adolescents (Otasowie, 2021).

Taken together, the relationship between alcohol use (and abstinence) and mental health among young adults is complex. Existing theories have attempted to explain the directionality of this relationship but there are likely a range of different ways in which alcohol and mental health problems manifest within young adults and the factors likely involved in this relationship, particularly given the changing landscape of drinking among young adults.

## Evidence on the Relationship Between Alcohol and Mental Health in Young Adults

Global evidence shows that in most adolescents and young adults with a substance use disorder (including AUD), the presence of a co-occurring mental health problem is extremely common, with many having more than one co-occurring mental disorder (Erskine et al., 2015). In the United States (US), epidemiological evidence from community samples suggest that among adolescents (aged 13–18 years) with a substance use disorder, 55–80% also have a co-occurring mental health problem (Merikangas et al., 2010). These estimates are even greater within clinical samples (Chan et al., 2008). A range of problems commonly co-occur with substance use disorders in adolescents, including mood disorders, conduct disorders, trauma-related disorders (Chan et al., 2008), and attention deficit/hyperactivity disorder (ADHD) (Gudjonsson et al., 2012; Molina et al., 2007). More recently, research indicates that AUDs are often prevalent among adolescents with autism (Pijnenburg et al., 2023; Sinclair et al., 2023).

Similar patterns are apparent across the globe. Australian research found that adolescents (aged 13–17 years) with severe mental health issues were four times more likely to drink to harmful levels (Lima et al., 2020). This study found evidence of a bidirectional relationship, whereby the presence of one problem almost doubled the likelihood of having a co-occurring problem. A further longitudinal study found that heavier use of substances (alcohol and/or cannabis) was associated with symptoms of psychosis at two-year follow-up (Thompson et al., 2021). Cross-sectional studies have shown that hazardous and/or harmful alcohol use is associated with higher levels of depression in young men and women aged 20–24 years, and higher levels of anxiety in men only (Caldwell et al., 2002). An additional study of students, aged 18–24 years, found that 44% met criteria for hazardous or harmful drinking, and these individuals were 20% more likely to report psychological distress compared to those with lower levels of alcohol consumption (Tembo et al., 2017). Taken together, there is clear evidence that alcohol and mental health problems commonly occur among young adults.

Co-occurring alcohol and mental health problems are also associated with the use of additional substances. Research on 18-year-olds living in the west of England examined the relationship between alcohol use, mental health, and drug use, finding that those reporting co-occurring depression and hazardous drinking were four times more likely to use cannabis, compared to those who report only one problem (Sumnall et al., in preparation). When looking at younger age groups, one study found that having a mental health problem was associated with an increased likelihood of substance use (among those aged 13–15 years) and greater involvement with any one substance increased the likelihood of using another (Boys et al., 2003). These findings are concerning, as co-occurring problems have detrimental consequences for adolescents and young adults. UK data for approximately 7000 adolescents (aged 12–18 years) obtained through Hospital Episode Statistics, found that, among those with an alcohol-related emergency admission, those with a co-occurring mental health diagnosis, another substance use diagnosis, or a diagnosis of self-harm at index admission, were more likely to be readmitted within four years (Hoy, 2017).

Despite these findings, youth drinking has been declining across the Western world since the early 2000s, with rates of abstinence increasing among young adults (Holmes et al., 2022). For example, in the UK, the proportion of young adults who reported abstinence increased from 18% in 2005 to 29% in 2015, and this was largely driven by increases in the proportion of people who have never drank alcohol, that is, "lifetime abstainers" (Ng Fat et al., 2018). In contrast to research in the adult general population, recent research into young adults indicates that increases in abstinence are more common in healthier people (e.g., non-smokers, those with high physical activity, and good mental health) (Ng Fat et al., 2018). Similarly, a literature review of non-drinking in young adults found that non-drinkers have better mental health outcomes for a range of measures, including well-being, life satisfaction, and confidence (Corre et al., 2023). This also contrasts earlier research into young adults, from 2006 to 2008, whereby low physical activity and long-standing illnesses were associated with greater odds of being a non-drinker (Ng Fat & Shelton, 2012). Qualitative research provides some potential mechanisms with explanations pointing to the avoidance of alcohol-related harm, pursuing healthy lifestyles (incorporating physical and mental health, as well as social well-being), and the unaffordability of alcohol (Caluzzi et al., 2021; Whitaker et al., 2023). There is some evidence to suggest that young adults drink less due to the displacement of alcohol by other studies, which may relate to affordability, as other substances may be considered cheaper (Whitaker et al., 2023). Most notably, it is thought that the decline in youth drinking is well-established and is unlikely to reverse (Holmes et al., 2022).

## Sociodemographic Differences

The relationship between alcohol use and mental health among young adults may differ depending on sociodemographic characteristics, such as socioeconomic status, gender, or ethnicity. Though some studies have explored the role of socioeconomic status when investigating co-occurring alcohol and mental health problems in adult populations (Boniface et al., 2020; Puddephatt et al., 2021), few have focused specifically on young adults. However, one Australian study of mothers and their offspring at age 21 established that those with co-occurring problems were more likely to have experienced socioeconomic disadvantage than those with a single problem (Salom et al., 2014). Similarly, there is a dearth of literature into ethnic differences in the relationship between alcohol and mental health among young adults, though there is some evidence to suggest that students from white ethnic groups consume more alcohol than students from ethnic minority groups (Bhatti et al., 2020), whereas students from ethnic minority groups are more likely to report poor mental health than their white counterparts (Weitzman, 2004). This is reflected in the adult population, whereby ethnic minority groups are less likely to drink alcohol, however, within certain ethnic minority groups (e.g., Indian and Black African), those with a mental health problem are more likely to drink hazardously than those without a mental health problem (Puddephatt et al., Preprint).

In terms of gender differences, research suggests that girls may be more likely to suffer from co-occurring substance problems and internalising disorders (e.g., depression, anxiety), whereas boys are more likely to report co-occurring externalising disorders (e.g., conduct disorder, ADHD) (Otasowie, 2021). A population-based study of 9000 young people in Norway found that anxiety and depression symptoms were related to higher levels of binge-drinking in girls only (Strandheim et al., 2009). Similarly, in Sweden, a smaller study of young people determined that girls with low well-being and poor mental health were more likely to have had alcohol experiences (e.g., tried alcohol, been intoxicated) (Boson et al., 2016). In contrast, cross-sectional data indicates a positive association between hazardous and/or harmful alcohol use with depression in both young men and women, but with higher levels of anxiety in men only (Caldwell et al., 2002). Further, a study of Norwegian adolescents found little evidence of any substantial gender differences in the association between mental health and substance use (Skogen et al., 2014). There has been limited research into gender minorities, though there is some evidence to suggest that transgender young people experience high rates of depression, suicidality, and substance use (Newcomb et al., 2020) and are more likely to be victims of alcohol-related sexual assault (Coulter et al., 2015).

## The Impact of the COVID-19 Pandemic

The COVID-19 pandemic and associated control measures (e.g., lockdowns) which were implemented to mitigate the spread of the virus, had an impact on both alcohol use and mental health among young people, with a global systematic review finding that adolescents experienced higher rates of anxiety and depression, and more frequent alcohol use (Jones et al., 2021). The impact of the pandemic on alcohol use among young adults varied depending on the type of drinking pattern measured (e.g., binge-drinking, quantity and frequency of drinking), where and when drinking took place, and other factors such as mental health symptoms (Coakley et al., 2021; Creswell et al., 2024; Patrick et al., 2022). A longitudinal analysis of a UK student sample found an increase in symptoms of depression but a reduction in alcohol use, during the first lockdown (Evans et al., 2021). Similarly, the proportion of people drinking five or more drinks on a typical day decreased during the first UK lockdown, and this decrease was most marked amongst young people, falling from 32% to 9% (Niedzwiedz et al., 2021). Contrary to this, cross-sectional research observed that a higher proportion of 18–34-year-olds reported increased alcohol consumption compared to older age groups, and increased alcohol consumption was associated with poor mental health in the whole sample (Jacob et al., 2021). Further research is needed to understand the lasting impact of the COVID-19 pandemic on mental health and alcohol use among young people, as this may have important implications for the treatment of co-occurring problems in the context of post-pandemic recovery.

## Current Guidance for the Treatment of Co-occurring Problems

Treatment for people with co-occurring problems is complicated by the fact that the individual has two related health conditions, which are typically treated separately by different providers. Interventions range from preventative approaches (e.g., interventions to prevent onset of mental health problems or heavy drinking in schools/universities (Teesson et al., 2020)), to screening and identification (e.g., assessment of alcohol use in mental health services (Levy et al., 2016)), to pharmacological and psychological treatment approaches tailored for co-occurring problems (e.g., integrated interventions for people with post-traumatic stress disorder [PTSD] and AUD (Roberts et al., 2022)). The treatment landscape for young people is more complex (particularly during the transition from adolescence to adulthood) as they may not be eligible for children's services, yet adult services may not always be appropriate, and alcohol problems may not yet have been identified or reported (Otasowie, 2021). Guidance for the treatment of co-occurring problems outlines three different pathways, comprising serial (when someone receives treatment for one problem before the other), parallel (treatment is received separately from different services, but at the same time) and integrated (when the same treatment provider treats both problems concurrently) treatment models (Hobden et al., 2018). Our public involvement work has identified limitations for each of these treatment models, including long delays between serial treatments, for example, waiting for mental health treatment after attending alcohol treatment, meaning that someone is more likely to relapse. Complications of parallel and integrated models relate to information sharing between mental health and alcohol treatment providers and concerns from service users about not wanting to address both of their problems at the same time.

A combined school-based preventive programme targeting anxiety, depression and substance use in adolescents in Australia, theorised that addressing psychopathologies in isolation may not be as effective as a multidimensional approach given the common predisposing risk factors for these conditions (Teesson et al., 2020). Schools were randomised to either receive the substance use only programme, the mental health only programme, a combined programme or to a control arm without intervention. Alcohol use, heavy episodic drinking and anxiety symptoms increased less in the adolescents who received the integrated intervention, but there wasn't a significant difference for depression (Teesson et al., 2020). There is opportunity to further explore the utility of integrated interventions which support young people to develop positive coping responses to stress and mental health problems.

One of the key factors negatively affecting outcomes for this population is poor identification of the co-occurring problem (Yule & Kelly, 2019). Screening and assessment approaches to improve identification can include mental health services asking a young person about their alcohol use, using an existing structured questionnaire, with recommendations promoting early identification of problematic alcohol use to reduce the development of future problems (Levy et al., 2016). However, this assessment may be more complicated in young people, resulting from presumptions that substance use behaviours may be recreational in nature and clinicians report concerns about upsetting parents by raising the issue (Otasowie, 2021). Reviews have shown that single-item screens about frequency of use can be effective in young people and the Alcohol Use Disorder Identification Test (AUDIT) appears to be the most valid screening tool for this population (Toner et al., 2019). Conversely, screening for mental health problems in alcohol and drug services can ensure that someone gets the support they need earlier and this may help them to reduce their alcohol use. Mental health screening in the context of an alcohol service can use short validated measures to assess common mental health symptoms, such as depression and anxiety, but assessment for severe mental health conditions is more difficult and can require clinical assessment (Marel et al., 2022). There is debate as to whether specialised mental health treatment is always required for co-occurring common mental health problems (Office for Health Improvement & Disparities, 2023) and this may depend on the type of mental health problem someone is experiencing, the extent that their symptoms are related to their alcohol use and the support that someone has through their family. Young people with co-occurring problems may not always present to the relevant mental health and alcohol service providers and so screening in other settings (e.g. primary care, community services, criminal justice system) could be beneficial.

Recommendations promote the use of integrated treatment models for co-occurring problems (Marel et al., 2022). Whilst there is some evidence for the benefits of integrated treatment approaches in adult populations (Mehta et al., 2021), the findings in young people have been mixed. For example, an intervention for college students with heavy episodic drinking and depression found that a combined CBT and brief motivation interviewing intervention (which also addressed alcohol use) was not more effective than the stand-alone CBT intervention for depression (Pedrelli et al., 2020). Furthermore, a web-based intervention for college students who met criteria for hazardous drinking and depression did not find evidence that an integrated intervention was more effective in reducing alcohol use and symptoms of depression compared to the interventions arms with a single focus (i.e. only mental health or alcohol) (Geisner et al., 2015).

Guidance on improving care for those with co-occurring problems recommends a 'no wrong door approach' and outlines that care should be everyone's responsibility, which means that people shouldn't be turned away from services at the time they are presenting, even if the service can't provide immediate care (Public Health England, 2017). This should also include assessment of current crisis and ensuring that someone is safe from harm, rather than just providing a referral. This is particularly important for young people who may be more likely to self-harm and to undertake more risk-taking behaviours (Casey & Jones, 2010). The ethos of the current guidance is reliant on staff having the required training to undertake suitable screening and referral and outlines the importance of the networks and referral pathways across mental health and alcohol services. Furthermore, qualitative research has highlighted the importance of the therapeutic relationship in building trust and reducing the distress experienced by those with co-occurring problems during the treatment process (Chilton et al., 2020).

## Barriers to Accessing Care in Young People

Given that co-occurring problems are the norm rather than the exception for people with alcohol use disorders, this is not reflected in practice. People with co-occurring problems can be turned away from services because they don't meet the eligibility criteria (Jackson et al., 2024), for example, if mental health services require someone to have reduced their alcohol use before they can be seen. A review of the barriers to treatment experienced by people with co-occurring problems found that these range from individual barriers, such as personal characteristics and beliefs around the value of attending a treatment service, fear and stigma of seeking support, to structural barriers (Priester et al., 2016). In young people, beliefs about stigma may go beyond the individual level, with parental and family beliefs having the potential to prevent someone from seeking support (Hawkins, 2009). Structural barriers include the availability of services (e.g., opening hours or accessibility of the location), under-identification of co-occurring problems, training of the provider to deal with co-occurring problems, and service provision in terms of someone's eligibility (Priester et al., 2016). These structural barriers are likely to be compounded during the transition from adolescence to adulthood, when young people may fall between children's and adult services, they may not want to disclose problems to their family and they may be more likely to experience prejudices around their behaviours and concerns may not be taken seriously.

Given that young people with co-occurring problems are more likely to experience poorer outcomes than those with a single problem (Erskine et al., 2015), including poorer treatment outcomes and involvement with the criminal justice system, it is important that appropriate treatment is provided early. This needs to be seen in the context that younger people may have less motivation to engage in treatment and often have less insight into their problems (Ramchand et al., 2015), so may be less likely to seek out treatment for both problems if this is not detected by services. Recent UK research has shown that young people may find it difficult to access formal mental health services due knowledge on where to go, that they delay talking to friends and family due to stigma and furthermore they may be told they are not eligible for treatment due to their age or use of substances and so have found it easier to self-medicate (Sumnall et al., In Preparation). These themes highlight the importance of implementing preventative approaches and screening and brief intervention, to identify problems earlier and before more intensive treatment is required.

## Conclusion

Despite alcohol use declining in young adults, there is clear evidence that particular groups of young adults are still at risk of alcohol-harms, such as those with a mental health problem. The findings outlined in this chapter support existing theories on the relationship between alcohol and mental health, whereby alcohol may be used by young adults to cope with poor mental health or that heavy drinking leads to a decline in mental health, but the directionality of this relationship is still unclear. This is further complicated given recent global changes, such as the rise in digital technology and the COVID-19 pandemic, both of which contribute to poor mental health and have changed the ways in which young adults socialise. The management and treatment of co-occurring alcohol and mental health problems are complex in any population yet are further complicated when treating young adults who may face additional barriers due to eligibility or fears of stigma. To ensure young adults with co-occurring problems receive co-ordinated care and to prevent adverse outcomes, future research and public health policies should focus on (1) widening conversations around alcohol as a coping response to raise awareness among carers and teachers, (2) developing preventative approaches to identify alcohol problems early, (3) bridging the gap between child and adult services for both mental health and alcohol problems, and (4) supporting the integration of mental health and alcohol services.

## References

Anda, R. F., Whitfield, C. L., Felitti, V. J., Chapman, D., Edwards, V. J., Dube, S. R., & Williamson, D. F. (2002). Adverse childhood experiences, alcoholic parents, and later risk of alcoholism and depression. *Psychiatric Services, 53*(8), 1001–1009.

Atkinson, A., Meadows, B., & Sumnall, H. R. (2024). 'You're in the alcohol Matrix, then you unplug from it, and you're like 'Wow': Exploring sober women's management, negotiation and countering of alcohol marketing in the UK. *Drugs: Education, Prevention and Policy, 31*(1), 54–69.

Bakhshaie, J., Storch, E. A., & Zvolensky, M. J. (2021). Obsessive-compulsive symptoms and problematic alcohol use: The explanatory role of drinking motives. *Addictive Behaviors, 115*, 106734.

Bandura, A., & Walters, R. H. (1977). *Social learning theory* (Vol. 1). Prentice Hall.

Bell, S., & Britton, A. (2014). An exploration of the dynamic longitudinal relationship between mental health and alcohol consumption: A prospective cohort study. *BMC Medicine, 12*(1), 1–13.

Berkowitz, A. D. (2003). Applications of social norms theory to other health and social justice issues. In *The social norms approach to preventing school and college age substance abuse: A handbook for educators, counselors, and clinicians, 1*. Jossey-Bass/Wiley.

Bhattacharya, A. (2016). *Youthful abandon: Why are young people drinking less.* https://www.ias.org.uk/uploads/pdf/IAS%20reports/rp22072016.pdf

Bhatti, S. N., Fan, L. M., Collins, A., & Li, J.-M. (2020). Exploration of alcohol consumption behaviours and health-related influencing factors of young adults in the UK. *International Journal of Environmental Research and Public Health, 17*(17), 6282.

Blumenthal, D., Gokhale, M., Campbell, E. G., & Weissman, J. S. (2001). Preparedness for clinical practice: Reports of graduating residents at academic health centers. *Jama, 286*(9), 1027–1034.

Boniface, S., Lewer, D., Hatch, S. L., & Goodwin, L. (2020). Associations between interrelated dimensions of socio-economic status, higher risk drinking and mental health in South East London: A cross-sectional study. *PloS One, 15*(2), e0229093.

Boson, K., Berglund, K., Wennberg, P., & Fahlke, C. (2016). Well-being, mental health problems, and alcohol experiences among young Swedish adolescents: A general population study. *Journal for Person-Oriented Research, 2*(3), 123–134.

Boys, A., Farrell, M., Taylor, C., Marsden, J., Goodman, R., Brugha, T., Bebbington, P., Jenkins, R., & Meltzer, H. (2003). Psychiatric morbidity and substance use in young people aged 13–15 years: Results from the Child and Adolescent Survey of Mental Health. *The British Journal of Psychiatry, 182*(6), 509–517.

Caldwell, T. M., Rodgers, B., Jorm, A. F., Christensen, H., Jacomb, P. A., Korten, A. E., & Lynskey, M. T. (2002). Patterns of association between alcohol consumption and symptoms of depression and anxiety in young adults. *Addiction, 97*(5), 583–594.

Caluzzi, G., Livingston, M., Holmes, J., MacLean, S., Lubman, D., Dietze, P., Vashishtha, R., Herring, R., & Pennay, A. (2022). Declining drinking among adolescents: Are we seeing a denormalisation of drinking and a normalisation of non-drinking? *Addiction, 117*(5), 1204–1212.

Caluzzi, G., Pennay, A., & MacLean, S. (2021). Reflexive habitus and the new obligation of choice: Understanding young people's light drinking and alcohol abstinence. *Journal of Youth Studies, 24*(7), 886–900.

Casey, B. J., & Jones, R. M. (2010). Neurobiology of the adolescent brain and behavior: Implications for substance use disorders. *Journal of the American Academy of Child & Adolescent Psychiatry, 49*(12), 1189–1201.

Castillo-Carniglia, A., Keyes, K. M., Hasin, D. S., & Cerdá, M. (2019). Psychiatric comorbidities in alcohol use disorder. *The Lancet Psychiatry, 6*(12), 1068–1080.

Chan, Y.-F., Dennis, M. L., & Funk, R. R. (2008). Prevalence and comorbidity of major internalizing and externalizing problems among adolescents and adults presenting to substance abuse treatment. *Journal of Substance Abuse Treatment, 34*(1), 14–24.

Chilton, J., Crone, D. M., & Tyson, P. J. (2020). 'The group was the only therapy which supported my needs, because it helped me feel normal and I was able to speak out with a voice': A qualitative study of an integrated group treatment for dual diagnosis service users within a community mental health setting. *International Journal of Mental Health Nursing, 29*(3), 406–413.

Coakley, K. E., Lardier, D. T., Holladay, K. R., Amorim, F. T., Mechler, H., & Zuhl, M. N. (2021). Mental health severity is associated with increases in alcohol consumption in young adult students during the COVID-19 pandemic. *Alcoholism Treatment Quarterly, 39*(3), 328–341.

Conroy, D., & de Visser, R. O. (2018). Benefits and drawbacks of social non-drinking identified by British university students. *Drug and Alcohol Review, 37,* S89–S97.

Conway, K. P., Swendsen, J., Husky, M. M., He, J. P., & Merikangas, K. R. (2016). Association of lifetime mental disorders and subsequent alcohol and illicit drug use: Results from the national comorbidity survey-adolescent supplement. *The Journal of the American Academy of Child & Adolescent Psychiatry, 55*(4), 280–288. https://doi.org/10.1016/j.jaac.2016.01.006

Cooper, M. L. (1994). Motivations for alcohol use among adolescents: Development and validation of a four-factor model. *Psychological Assessment, 6*(2), 117. https://doi.org/10.1037/1040-3590.6.2.117

Cooper, M. L., Frone, M. R., Russell, M., & Mudar, P. (1995). Drinking to regulate positive and negative emotions: A motivational model of alcohol use. *Journal of Personality and Social Psychology, 69*(5), 990. https://psycnet.apa.org/doi/10.1037/0022-3514.69.5.990

Corre, T., Barrense-Dias, Y., & Suris, J.-C. (2023). The growing trend of young people abstaining from drinking alcohol: A literature review. *Substance Use & Misuse, 58*(1), 77–84.

Coulter, R. W., Blosnich, J. R., Bukowski, L. A., Herrick, A., Siconolfi, D. E., & Stall, R. D. (2015). Differences in alcohol use and alcohol-related problems between transgender-and nontransgender-identified young adults. *Drug and Alcohol Dependence, 154*, 251–259.

Cox, W. M., & Klinger, E. (1988). A motivational model of alcohol use. *Journal of Abnormal Psychology, 97*(2), 168. https://psycnet.apa.org/doi/10.1037/0021-843X.97.2.168

Creswell, K. G., Hisler, G. C., Lyons, G., Carrillo-Álvarez, F. A., Fairbairn, C. E., & Wright, A. G. (2024). Changes in alcohol consumption and alcohol problems before and after the COVID-19 pandemic: A prospective study in heavy drinking young adults. *Nature Mental Health,* 2, 728–739. https://doi.org/10.1038/s44220-024-00247-9

de Visser, R. O., Hart, A., Abraham, C., Graber, R., Scanlon, T., & Memon, A. (2014). How alike are young non-drinkers, former-drinkers, low-risk drinkers, and hazardous drinkers? *Addictive Behaviors, 39*(8), 1258–1264.

El-Guebaly, N. (2007). Investigating the association between moderate drinking and mental health. *Annals of Epidemiology, 17*(5), S55–S62.

Erskine, H., Moffitt, T. E., Copeland, W., Costello, E., Ferrari, A., Patton, G., Degenhardt, L., Vos, T., Whiteford, H., & Scott, J. (2015). A heavy burden on young minds: The global burden of mental and substance use disorders in children and youth. *Psychological Medicine, 45*(7), 1551–1563.

Evans, S., Alkan, E., Bhangoo, J. K., Tenenbaum, H., & Ng-Knight, T. (2021). Effects of the COVID-19 lockdown on mental health, wellbeing, sleep, and alcohol use in a UK student sample. *Psychiatry Research, 298*, 113819.

Fat, L. N., Cable, N., Marmot, M., & Shelton, N. (2014). Persistent long-standing illness and non-drinking over time, implications for the use of lifetime abstainers as a control group. *Journal of Epidemiology and Community Health, 68*(1), 71–77.

Geisner, I. M., Varvil-Weld, L., Mittmann, A. J., Mallett, K., & Turrisi, R. (2015). Brief web-based intervention for college students with comorbid risky alcohol use and depressed mood: Does it work and for whom? *Addictive Behaviors, 42*, 36–43.

Goldman, E., & Najman, J. M. (1984). Lifetime abstainers, current abstainers and imbibers: A methodological note. *British Journal of Addiction, 79*(3), 309–314.

Goodwin, L., Norton, S., Fear, N., Jones, M., Hull, L., Wessely, S., & Rona, R. (2017). Trajectories of alcohol use in the UK military and associations with mental health. *Addictive Behaviors, 75*, 130–137.

Gore, F. M., Bloem, P. J., Patton, G. C., Ferguson, J., Joseph, V., Coffey, C., Sawyer, S. M., & Mathers, C. D. (2011). Global burden of disease in young people aged 10–24 years: A systematic analysis. *The Lancet, 377*(9783), 2093–2102.

Griffiths, R., & Casswell, S. (2010). Intoxigenic digital spaces? Youth, social networking sites and alcohol marketing. *Drug and Alcohol Review, 29*(5), 525–530.

Gudjonsson, G. H., Sigurdsson, J. F., Sigfusdottir, I. D., & Young, S. (2012). An epidemiological study of ADHD symptoms among young persons and the relationship with cigarette smoking, alcohol consumption and illicit drug use. *Journal of Child Psychology and Psychiatry, 53*(3), 304–312.

Hawkins, E. H. (2009). A tale of two systems: Co-occurring mental health and substance abuse disorders treatment for adolescents. *Annual Review of Psychology, 60*, 197–227.

Hobden, B., Bryant, J., Carey, M., Baker, A. L., Farrell, M., Oldmeadow, C., Mattick, R. P., Shakeshaft, A., & Sanson-Fisher, R. (2018). Finding the optimal treatment model: A systematic review of treatment for co-occurring alcohol misuse and depression. *Australian & New Zealand Journal of Psychiatry, 52*(8), 737–750.

Hoel, S., Magne Eriksen, B., Breidablik, H.-J., & Meland, E. (2004). Adolescent alcohol use, psychological health, and social integration. *Scandinavian Journal of Public Health, 32*(5), 361–367.

Holmes, J., Fairbrother, H., Livingston, M., Meier, P. S., Oldham, M., Pennay, A., & Whitaker, V. (2022). Youth drinking in decline: What are the implications for public health, public policy and public debate? *International Journal of Drug Policy, 102*, 103606.

Hoy, A. R. (2017). Which young people in England are most at risk of an alcohol-related revolving-door readmission career? *BMC Public Health, 17*, 1–16.

Hughes, K., Bellis, M. A., Hardcastle, K. A., Sethi, D., Butchart, A., Mikton, C., Jones, L., & Dunne, M. P. (2017). The effect of multiple adverse childhood experiences on health: A systematic review and meta-analysis. *The Lancet Public Health, 2*(8), e356–e366.

Jackson, K., Kaner, E., Hanratty, B., Gilvarry, E., Yardley, L., & O'Donnell, A. (2024). Understanding people's experiences of the formal health and social care system for co-occurring heavy alcohol use and depression through the lens of relational autonomy: A qualitative study. *Addiction, 119*(2), 268–280.

Jacob, L., Smith, L., Armstrong, N. C., Yakkundi, A., Barnett, Y., Butler, L., McDermott, D. T., Koyanagi, A., Shin, J. I., & Meyer, J. (2021). Alcohol use and mental health during COVID-19 lockdown: A cross-sectional study in a sample of UK adults. *Drug & Alcohol Dependence, 219*, 108488. https://doi.org/10.1016/j.drugalcdep.2020.108488

Jones, E. A., Mitra, A. K., & Bhuiyan, A. R. (2021). Impact of COVID-19 on mental health in adolescents: A systematic review. *International Journal of Environmental Research and Public Health, 18*(5), 2470.

Jordan, C. J., & Andersen, S. L. (2017). Sensitive periods of substance abuse: Early risk for the transition to dependence. *Developmental Cognitive Neuroscience, 25*, 29–44.

Kauhanen, L., Wan Mohd Yunus, W. M. A., Lempinen, L., Peltonen, K., Gyllenberg, D., Mishina, K., Gilbert, S., Bastola, K., Brown, J. S., & Sourander, A. (2023). A systematic review of the mental health changes of children and young people before and during the COVID-19 pandemic. *European Child & Adolescent Psychiatry, 32*(6), 995–1013.

Khantzian, E. J. (1987). The self-medication hypothesis of addictive disorders: Focus on heroin and cocaine dependence. In *The cocaine crisis* (pp. 65–74). Springer.

Khantzian, E. J. (1997). The self-medication hypothesis of substance use disorders: A reconsideration and recent applications. *Harvard Review of Psychiatry, 4*(5), 231–244.

Khokhar, J. Y., Dwiel, L. L., Henricks, A. M., Doucette, W. T., & Green, A. I. (2018). The link between schizophrenia and substance use disorder: A unifying hypothesis. *Schizophrenia Research, 194*, 78–85.

Kraus, L., Room, R., Livingston, M., Pennay, A., Holmes, J., & Törrönen, J. (2020). Long waves of consumption or a unique social generation? Exploring recent declines in youth drinking. *Addiction Research & Theory, 28*(3), 183–193.

Kuppens, S., Moore, S. C., Gross, V., Lowthian, E., & Siddaway, A. P. (2020). The enduring effects of parental alcohol, tobacco, and drug use on child well-being: A multilevel meta-analysis. *Development and Psychopathology, 32*(2), 765–778.

Kushner, M. G., Sher, K. J., & Beitman, B. D. (1990). The relation between alcohol problems and the anxiety disorders. *The American Journal of Psychiatry, 147*(6), 685–695.

Lai, H. M. X., Cleary, M., Sitharthan, T., & Hunt, G. E. (2015). Prevalence of comorbid substance use, anxiety and mood disorders in epidemiological surveys, 1990–2014: A systematic review and meta-analysis. *Drug & Alcohol Dependence, 154*, 1–13. https://doi.org/10.1016/j.drugalcdep.2015.05.031

Larm, P., Åslund, C., Raninen, J., & Nilsson, K. W. (2018). Adolescent non-drinkers: Who are they? Social relations, school performance, lifestyle factors and health behaviours. *Drug and Alcohol Review, 37*, S67–S75.

Laukkanen, E. R., Shemeikka, S. L., Viinamäki, H. T., Pölkki, P. L., & Lehtonen, J. O. (2001). Heavy drinking is associated with more severe psychosocial dysfunction among girls than boys in Finland. *Journal of Adolescent Health, 28*(4), 270–277.

Levy, S. J., Williams, J. F., & Committee on substance use and prevention (2016). Substance Use Screening, Brief Intervention, and Referral to Treatment. *Pediatrics, 138*(1), e20161211. https://doi.org/10.1542/peds.2016-1211

Lima, F., Sims, S., & O'Donnell, M. (2020). Harmful drinking is associated with mental health conditions and other risk behaviours in Australian young people. *Australian and New Zealand Journal of Public Health, 44*(3), 201–207.

Marel, C., Siedlecka, E., Fisher, A., Gournay, K., Deady, M., Baker, A., Kay-Lambkin, F., Teesson, M., Baillie, A., & Mills, K. L. (2022). *Guidelines on the management of co-occurring alcohol and other drug and mental health conditions in alcohol and other drug treatment settings* (3rd ed.). The Matilda Centre for Research in Mental Health and Substance Use.

McCarthy, E., & Petrakis, I. (2010). Epidemiology and management of alcohol dependence in individuals with post-traumatic stress disorder. *CNS Drugs, 24*(12), 997–1007.

Mehta, K., Hoadley, A., Ray, L. A., Kiluk, B. D., Carroll, K. M., & Magill, M. (2021). Cognitive-behavioral interventions targeting alcohol or other drug use and co-occurring mental health disorders: A meta-analysis. *Alcohol and Alcoholism, 56*(5), 535–544.

Merikangas, K. R., He, J.-P., Burstein, M., Swanson, S. A., Avenevoli, S., Cui, L., Benjet, C., Georgiades, K., & Swendsen, J. (2010). Lifetime prevalence of mental disorders in US adolescents: Results from the National Comorbidity Survey Replication–Adolescent Supplement (NCS-A). *Journal of the American Academy of Child & Adolescent Psychiatry, 49*(10), 980–989.

Molina, B. S., Pelham, W. E., Gnagy, E. M., Thompson, A. L., & Marshal, M. P. (2007). Attention-deficit/hyperactivity disorder risk for heavy drinking and alcohol use disorder is age specific. *Alcoholism: Clinical and Experimental Research, 31*(4), 643–654.

Newcomb, M. E., Hill, R., Buehler, K., Ryan, D. T., Whitton, S. W., & Mustanski, B. (2020). High burden of mental health problems, substance use, violence, and related psychosocial factors in transgender, non-binary, and gender diverse youth and young adults. *Archives of sexual behavior, 49*, 645–659.

Ng Fat, L., & Shelton, N. (2012). Associations between self-reported illness and non-drinking in young adults. *Addiction, 107*(9), 1612–1620.

Ng Fat, L., Shelton, N., & Cable, N. (2018). Investigating the growing trend of non-drinking among young people; Analysis of repeated cross-sectional surveys in England 2005–2015. *BMC Public Health, 18*(1), 1090.

Niedzwiedz, C. L., Green, M. J., Benzeval, M., Campbell, D., Craig, P., Demou, E., Leyland, A., Pearce, A., Thomson, R., Whitley, E., & Katikireddi, S. V. (2021). Mental health and health behaviours before and during the initial phase of the COVID-19 lockdown: Longitudinal analyses of the UK Household Longitudinal Study. *The Journal of Epidemiology and Community Health, 75*(3), 224–231. https://doi.org/10.1136/jech-2020-215060

O'Hare, T., & Sherrer, M. (2011). Drinking motives as mediators between PTSD symptom severity and alcohol consumption in persons with severe mental illnesses. *Addictive Behaviors, 36*(5), 465–469.

Office for Health Improvement & Disparities. (2023). *UK clinical guidelines for alcohol treatment: Specific settings and populations*. https://www.gov.uk/government/consultations/uk-clinical-guidelines-for-alcohol-treatment/uk-clinical-guidelines-for-alcohol-treatment-specific-settings-and-populations#people-with-co-occurring-mental-health-conditions

Otasowie, J. (2021). Co-occurring mental disorder and substance use disorder in young people: Aetiology, assessment and treatment. *BJPsych Advances, 27*(4), 272–281.

Parker, H., Aldridge, J., Measham, F., & Haynes, P. (1999). *Illegal leisure: The normalisation of adolescent recreational drug use*. Oxford University Press.

Patalay, P., & Gage, S. H. (2019). Changes in millennial adolescent mental health and health-related behaviours over 10 years: A population cohort comparison study. *International Journal of Epidemiology, 48*(5), 1650–1664.

Patel, V., Flisher, A. J., Hetrick, S., & McGorry, P. (2007). Mental health of young people: A global public-health challenge. *The Lancet, 369*(9569), 1302–1313.

Patrick, M. E., Terry-McElrath, Y. M., Miech, R. A., Keyes, K. M., Jager, J., & Schulenberg, J. E. (2022). Alcohol use and the COVID-19 pandemic: Historical trends in drinking, contexts, and reasons for use among US adults. *Social Science & Medicine, 301*, 114887.

Pedrelli, P., Borsari, B., Merrill, J. E., Fisher, L. B., Nyer, M., Shapero, B. G., Farabaugh, A., Hayden, E. R., Levine, M. T., & Fava, M. (2020). Evaluating the combination of a Brief Motivational Intervention plus Cognitive Behavioral Therapy for Depression and heavy episodic drinking in college students. *Psychology of Addictive Behaviors, 34*(2), 308.

Pijnenburg, L. J., Kaplun, A., de Haan, L., Janecka, M., Smith, L., Reichenberg, A., Banaschewski, T., Bokde, A. L., Quinlan, E. B., & Desrivières, S. (2023). Autistic traits and alcohol use in adolescents within the general population. *European Child & Adolescent Psychiatry, 32*(9), 1633–1642.

Pitchforth, J., Fahy, K., Ford, T., Wolpert, M., Viner, R. M., & Hargreaves, D. S. (2019). Mental health and well-being trends among children and young people in the UK, 1995–2014: Analysis of repeated cross-sectional national health surveys. *Psychological Medicine, 49*(8), 1275–1285.

Preston, P., & Goodfellow, M. (2006). Cohort comparisons: Social learning explanations for alcohol use among adolescents and older adults. *Addictive Behaviors, 31*(12), 2268–2283.

Priester, M. A., Browne, T., Iachini, A., Clone, S., DeHart, D., & Seay, K. D. (2016). Treatment access barriers and disparities among individuals with co-occurring mental health and substance use disorders: An integrative literature review. *Journal of Substance Abuse Treatment, 61*, 47–59.

Public Health England. (2017). *Better care for people with co-occurring mental health, and alcohol and drug use conditions*. GOV.UK: Public Health England Retrieved from https://www.gov.uk/government/publications/people-with-co-occurring-conditions-commission-and-provide-services

Puddephatt, J.-A., Booth, M., Onwumere, J., Das-Munshi, J., Coomber, R., & Goodwin, L. (2024). Exploring experiences with alcohol and how drinking has changed over time among minority ethnic groups with a diagnosed mental health problem. *Social Science & Medicine, 348*, 116803.

Puddephatt, J.-A., Jones, A., Gage, S. H., Fear, N. T., Field, M., McManus, S., McBride, O., & Goodwin, L. (2021). Associations of alcohol use, mental health and socioeconomic status in England: Findings from a representative population survey. *Drug & Alcohol Dependence, 219*, 108463.

Puddephatt, J.-A., Makin, H., Gage, S. H., Jones, A., & Goodwin, L. (2023). Understanding alcohol use and changes in drinking habits among people with a severe mental illness: A qualitative framework analysis study. *Frontiers in Psychology, 14*, 1282086.

Puddephatt, J.-A., Onwumere, J., Gage, S. H., Coomber, R., Das-Munshi, J., & Goodwin, L. (Preprint). How does the prevalence of alcohol use and associations with psychological distress differ across ethnic groups in England: A cross-sectional analysis of eight national surveys. 19 April 2024, PREPRINT (Version 1) available at Research Square [https://doi.org/10.21203/rs.3.rs-4251689/v1]

Puddephatt, J. A., Irizar, P., Jones, A., Gage, S. H., & Goodwin, L. (2022). Associations of common mental disorder with alcohol use in the adult general population: A systematic review and meta-analysis. *Addiction, 117*(6), 1543–1572. https://doi.org/10.1111/add.15735

Ramchand, R., Griffin, B. A., Hunter, S. B., Booth, M. S., & McCaffrey, D. F. (2015). Provision of mental health services as a quality indicator for adolescent substance abuse treatment facilities. *Psychiatric Services, 66*(1), 41–48.

Raninen, J., Larm, P., Svensson, J., Livingston, M., Sjödin, L., & Karlsson, P. (2021). Normalization of non-drinking? Health, school situation and social relations among Swedish ninth graders that drink and do not drink alcohol. *International Journal of Environmental Research and Public Health, 18*(21), 11201.

Roberts, N. P., Lotzin, A., & Schäfer, I. (2022). A systematic review and meta-analysis of psychological interventions for comorbid post-traumatic stress disorder and substance use disorder. *European Journal of Psychotraumatology, 13*(1), 2041831.

Salom, C. L., Betts, K. S., Williams, G. M., Najman, J. M., Scott, J. G., & Alati, R. (2014). Do young people with comorbid mental and alcohol disorders experience worse behavioural problems? *Psychiatry Research, 219*(2), 372–379.

Sawyer, S. M., Afifi, R. A., Bearinger, L. H., Blakemore, S.-J., Dick, B., Ezeh, A. C., & Patton, G. C. (2012). Adolescence: A foundation for future health. *The Lancet, 379*(9826), 1630–1640.

Sinclair, J. M., Aslan, B., Agabio, R., Anilkumar, A., Brosnan, M., Day, E., Dowling, N. A., Flood, C., Grant, J. E., & Halliday, R. (2023). Identifying the most important research, policy and practice questions for substance use, problematic alcohol use and behavioural addictions in autism (SABA-A): A priority setting partnership. *Comprehensive Psychiatry, 124*, 152393.

Skogen, J. C., Sivertsen, B., Lundervold, A. J., Stormark, K. M., Jakobsen, R., & Hysing, M. (2014). Alcohol and drug use among adolescents: And the co-occurrence of mental health problems. Ung@ hordaland, a population-based study. *BMJ Open, 4*(9), e005357.

Strandheim, A., Holmen, T. L., Coombes, L., & Bentzen, N. (2009). Alcohol intoxication and mental health among adolescents—A population review of 8983 young people, 13–19 years in North-Trøndelag, Norway: the Young-HUNT Study. *Child and Adolescent Psychiatry and Mental Health, 3*, 1–7.

Sumnall, H., Bloomfield, H., Langella, R., Knowles, H., Atkinson, A., Goodwin, L., Hope, V., Jones, L., Measham, F., & Stevens, A. (In Preparation). AMOUNT: A mixed methods investigation of the individual, sociocultural, and societal factors that underlie the recent increase in substance use among young people to inform policy.

Teesson, M., Newton, N. C., Slade, T., Chapman, C., Birrell, L., Mewton, L., Mather, M., Hides, L., McBride, N., & Allsop, S. (2020). Combined prevention for substance use, depression, and anxiety in adolescence: A cluster-randomised controlled trial of a digital online intervention. *The Lancet Digital Health, 2*(2), e74–e84.

Tembo, C., Burns, S., & Kalembo, F. (2017). The association between levels of alcohol consumption and mental health problems and academic performance among young university students. *PloS One, 12*(6), e0178142.

Thompson, K., Holley, M., Sturgess, C., & Leadbeater, B. (2021). Co-use of alcohol and cannabis: Longitudinal associations with mental health outcomes in young adulthood. *International Journal of Environmental Research and Public Health, 18*(7), 3652.

Tomáš, J., & Lenka, Š. (2023). Prevalence of dual diagnoses among children and adolescents with mental health conditions. *Children, 10*(2), 293.

Toner, P., Böhnke, J. R., Andersen, P., & McCambridge, J. (2019). Alcohol screening and assessment measures for young people: A systematic review and meta-analysis of validation studies. *Drug and Alcohol Dependence, 202*, 39–49.

Treur, J. L., Munafò, M. R., Logtenberg, E., Wiers, R. W., & Verweij, K. J. (2021). Using Mendelian randomization analysis to better understand the relationship between mental health and substance use: A systematic review. *Psychological Medicine, 51*(10), 1593–1624.

Vashishtha, R., Livingston, M., Pennay, A., Dietze, P., MacLean, S., Holmes, J., Herring, R., Caluzzi, G., & Lubman, D. I. (2020). Why is adolescent drinking declining? A systematic review and narrative synthesis. *Addiction Research & Theory, 28*(4), 275–288.

Weitzman, E. R. (2004). Poor mental health, depression, and associations with alcohol consumption, harm, and abuse in a national sample of young adults in college. *The Journal of Nervous And Mental Disease, 192*(4), 269–277.

Whitaker, V., Curtis, P., Fairbrother, H., Oldham, M., & Holmes, J. (2023). Young people's explanations for the decline in youth drinking in England. *BMC Public Health, 23*(1), 402.

Yule, A. M., & Kelly, J. F. (2019). Integrating treatment for co-occurring mental health conditions. *Alcohol research: current reviews, 40*(1), arcr.v40.1.07. https://doi.org/10.35946/arcr.v40.1.07

# 18

# Conclusion and Reflections on Future Directions

Dom Conroy and Fiona Measham

A recurrent theme throughout the production of both editions of this book has been a sense of the emergence of new discourses, methodologies and terminologies which expand our understanding of young adult drinking practices. A starting point in the inception and development of this collection—carried through to communication and discussion with collaborators—was the need to bring together disparate strands of research from different disciplines and different methodological traditions which each were grappling with a sense of change. What we had not anticipated upon complete of the first edition was quite how much the world, the hospitality and events industries and alcohol consumption itself would change in just a few months' time. We hope that this second

D. Conroy (✉)
Faculty of Arts and Social Science, The Open University, London, UK
e-mail: d.conroy@open.ac.uk

F. Measham
Department of Sociology, Social Policy and Criminology,
University of Liverpool, Liverpool, UK
e-mail: f.measham@liverpool.ac.uk



D. Conroy, F. Measham (eds.), *Young Adult Drinking Styles*, Sustainable Development Goals Series, https://doi.org/10.1007/978-3-031-98528-7_18

edition of the book helps contribute towards reflecting on how drinking practices changed in pandemic and post-pandemic times and steering the trajectory of future research but clearly there is much work still to be done.

The compilation of this new collection continues its mission to capture researchers' ruminations on the relevance of dualisms to our understanding of young adult drinking practices. By dualisms we mean the well-established conceptual polarisation of the attitudes and behaviours surrounding young adult drinking practices which can produce coarse, and therefore potentially unhelpful, ways of making sense of these phenomena.

One example of these dualisms concerns drinking practices as rigid/enduring on the one hand, and fluid/inconsistent on the other. This dualism is apparent in the context of Martina Martinic's chapter on 'Life Transitions, High-risk Drinking, and 'Maturing Out' which demonstrated how particular life events and life changes may be linked to drinking modes and practices specific to that time and place in the life course. This dualism was also apparent in the second half of Dom's chapter with Emma Banister and Maria Piacentini where the conceptual and real-world limitations of employing 'drinking categories' (e.g. 'non-drinker', 'light drinker', 'binge drinker') to understanding young adult drinking practices were exposed and explored.

Another dualism can be understood in debates around whether and how young adults' drinking practices can be cast in terms of being 'safe versus unsafe' or 'responsible versus irresponsible'. For example, does the fall in alcohol consumption amongst many young people discussed throughout this collection provide evidence of a growing commitment to 'safer' consumption levels and a growing level of 'responsibility' among young adults? We might suggest that merely posing the question exposes the political assumptions and potential biases that are tightly embedded in the terminology surrounding notions of safety and responsibility in the context of alcohol, and indeed drug consumption of any kind. Notions of 'safe health behaviour' have been critically explored in other areas—notably by Paul Flowers in his studies of 'safe sex' (Flowers et al., 1997) and have revealed the difficulties and dangers involved in restricted definitions of risk and safety regarding particular health behaviours.

A third dualism also appears to be important and this has been touched on in several of the chapters—a dualism concerning the 'pleasurable versus problematic' in young adult drinking and drink-related behaviours. There is a recognition in the alcohol field of the importance of understanding the pleasures of drinking alcohol and even of drunkenness, if one is to paint a comprehensive picture of the motivations for consumption. Drinking to drunkenness may happen on an occasional basis and may be related to the environment within which such consumption occurs, but as Tim Turner and Fiona Measham remind us in their chapter, such drinking practices can occur amongst occasional as well as regular drinkers and therefore we must be wary of overgeneralising about 'typical' young adult behaviours. The English Festival Survey found that the average female as well as male UK festival-goer is likely to have consumed binge drinking levels of alcohol by late afternoon, together with friends, at festivals. Whilst such environments might be characterised as higher risk, however, Turner and Measham also note that leisure venues provide opportunities to provide welfare and harm reduction services, to engage with young adults 'where they are at', providing advice and information to drinkers who are otherwise not in touch with medical professionals or alcohol counsellors.

Clearly, these dualisms offer just one way of making sense of emerging themes in research concerning contemporary young adult drinking practices. Pinning down overarching themes designed to capture a body of work from such a diverse, heterogenous and multi-disciplinary group of international researchers and authors may be unhelpful. In reviewing the contributions to this collection and from our own experience as writers and researchers we simply appeal to colleagues whose field work concerns young adult drinking practices to sustain high levels of criticality, openness and willingness to engage in bold and sophisticated research designs; novel methods for analysing research findings; creative and participatory approaches to dissemination; and effective, evidence-based and politically nuanced policy recommendations. In this sense, finding a way to locate research on young adult drinking practices that acknowledges but does not succumb to dualisms feels important in developing a research agenda which is progressive and compassionate to its subject matter.

There are numerous strands present in this collection that alcohol researchers may wish to pursue in future research. Literature on young adult drinking behaviour in the transition from adolescence to adulthood, highlighted in Martinic's chapter, is one area which may warrant further research attention. For example, in-depth contemporary studies of initiation into alcohol consumption among young people and how this initial period of drinking (and perhaps non-drinking) practice may blur into later phases of a relationship with alcohol, feels valuable. In an area like life transitions, there is clearly scope for more research which adopts longitudinal designs and obviously significant funding commitments are called for here. Such research would be well-positioned to explore how drinking beliefs and practices at one stage of life (e.g. middle adolescence aged 14–17 years) might give way to different modes of drinking in young adulthood (e.g. 18–30 year olds) when circumstances around education, employment, living status, partner status, peer group norms and complexion may all be prone to radical change.

There is also an emerging and changing policy context relevant to drinking practices among young adults which needs ongoing monitoring and evaluation. The growing evidence base on the impact on alcohol consumption and alcohol-related problems from minimum unit pricing, restrictions on retail and promotional practices and licensing legislation in several national contexts indicate the extent of policy impact on young adult drinking practices (Angus et al., 2016; Stockwell et al., 2012), with an appreciation of the unintended as well as intended consequences of policy change (Holmes, 2023; So et al., 2021; Wyper et al., 2023). Ensuring the impact of policy change on young adult drinking styles in qualitative, quantitative and mixed methods studies will be an important ongoing concern of future research programmes.

The first section of this book included chapters concerning the latest data and discussion concerning changing trends in alcohol consumption and some evidence of decline in consumption levels among young adults. Ongoing research needs to not only chart these changing trends but also draw us towards a deeper understanding of the range of socio-economic, political and cultural factors at play. Conversely, drinking frequency and quantity of consumption both remain high among older adults; for example, in the UK, 85% of 55–74-year-olds consumed alcohol during the last 12 months compared with 62% of 16–24 year olds, and 18% of adults aged 55–64 years, compared with 9% adults aged 25–34 years, were classifiable as increasing risk drinkers (i.e., consumed between 14 and 35 UK alcohol units per week) (NHS England, 2022). We suggest here that the fall in young adult drinking warrants greater scrutiny in this context, not just as a phenomenon in and of itself, but in relation to the question "what can we learn from young adults changed (and changing) drinking practices and how might this be applied to health promotion and risk communications amongst older adults?"

There is also the interesting possibility of how the current phenomenon of 'drinking less' amongst youth and young adults around the world might also involve comparative consideration of other potentially 'addictive', dependency-inducing or compulsive practices and behaviours. Specifically, alcohol consumption may have been outcompeted by the attractions presented by smartphone and computer gaming technologies which give young adults opportunities for accessible immersion on platforms that offer hybrids of social media communication, video gaming on devices that offer private and immediate sources of entertainment and the emergent possibilities of virtual reality. These declines in young adult consumption have also occurred during a period of emergence and rapid rise in New Psychoactive Substances (NPS), chemicals whose availability was facilitated by advances in both the dark and clear web leading to new psychoactive landscapes for future generations (Mounteney et al., 2016). The lines between legal and illegal drugs, licit and illicit markets, and industry and organised crime are all increasingly blurred (Measham, 2020).

Whilst there might be displacement between legal and illegal drug *markets*, the chapter by Turner and Measham also reminds us to pay close attention to the relationship between legal and illegal drug *use*, including their combined use in situations of atypical or 'extreme' intoxication in contexts such as music festivals and nightlife resorts. There is a long-standing coupling of alcohol (a depressant) with a range of legal and illegal stimulants, from *Buckfast* (a nineteenth-century wine infused with caffeine made by English monks), *Vin Mariani* (a nineteenth century French wine infused with cocaine endorsed by the Pope) through to vodka *Red Bull* (a vodka and caffeine energy drink mixer popular with millenials). A further area for future research is to explore atypical, poly-drug using and displaced consumption, cultures and contexts. Holidays may buck the broader young adult trend towards reduced consumption, with unusually large amounts of alcohol consumed in combination with unusually large amounts of illegal drugs, making polydrug use a distinction of young adult holidays and adding a layer of additional risk at a time of relaxation and potential lowering of usual safeguards. This may be increasingly significant from a health perspective as the contrast between moderation and excess becomes more pronounced within individual lives.

A further key strand of emerging research concerns online drinking identities and social media use involving exposure to alcohol-related content among young adults. This emerging work is well-illustrated in this collection where, in Chap. 12 for example, Ian Goodwin and Antonia Lyons discussed how the range of social media platforms and opportunities for social media activities exert influences over the real-time dynamics of drinking choices and leisure time activities among young adults. The expansion of the Internet, smartphones and apps as technologies which offer instantaneous immersion in online social networks is something which alcohol researchers must strive to keep abreast of if only to understand and assess the ways in which these networks are targeted and utilised by alcohol industry, health promotion and harm reduction organisations. Exploring drinking practices in the context of social media engagement presents, again, significant methodological challenges to produce an account of the dynamic and sometimes reciprocal interplay between 'online' and 'real world' activities and also how alcohol-related beliefs and narratives are rhetorically employed in these circumstances. Work drawing on the innovative qualitative methods is employed by Antonia Lyons and colleagues which have involved integration of data from focus groups, individual interviews alongside online material in work designed to understand the complex dynamics involved in young adults' social networking and drinking practices (see Lyons et al., 2015 for more details). Thus changing drinking preferences and practices must be contextualised within broader changes in online as well as real-world leisure.

As part of the process of producing the first and second editions of these collections, we have been excited to learn about the work being conducted by our contributors and field colleagues. Through these dialogues, we have learnt about the range of topic areas, relevant theory and methodological approaches employed in the study of changing young adult drinking practices in a variety of different national and local settings. The risk of stereotyping and reaching premature assumptions about 'typical drinking behaviour' among young adults was raised as a concern in the introduction and throughout this book. Clearly, we cannot refer to the variety of topic areas covered in this book to make general claims about styles of young adult drinking practices in the first quarter of the twenty-first century. That said, there is evidence that young adult drinking is at an exciting juncture: the growing normative acceptability of not drinking during social occasions explored in the first edition is bedding in with this cohort; alongside a recognition of a responsive relationship between policy, industry and young adults, warranting this continued focus on young adults as a discrete group for research attention. Indeed, as hinted at earlier in this concluding chapter, there might be grounds to believe that lessons might be learnt from young adults and applied to middle-aged and older drinking cohorts in terms of developing more nuanced approaches to alcohol-related health and well-being.

We hope that you have enjoyed reading this second edition and the range of contributions included in the book. We hope also that the work included in this collection inspires colleagues to foster new collaborations designed to deliver new research projects which offer critical and considered accounts of the varied styles of young adult drinking practices present in contemporary cultures.

## References

Angus, C., Holmes, J., Pryce, R., Meier, P., & Brennan, A. (2016). *Model-based appraisal of the comparative impact of Minimum Unit Pricing and taxation policies in Scotland.* ScHARR, University of Sheffield.

Flowers, P., Smith, J. A., Sheeran, P., & Beail, N. (1997). Health and romance: Understanding unprotected sex in relationships between gay men. *British Journal of Health Psychology, 2*(1), 73–86.

Holmes, J. (2023). Is minimum unit pricing for alcohol having the intended effects on alcohol consumption in Scotland? *Addiction, 118*(9), 1609–1616.

Lyons, A. C., Goodwin, I., McCreanor, T., & Griffin, C. (2015). Social networking and young adults' drinking practices: Innovative qualitative methods for health behavior research. *Health Psychology, 34*(4), 293.

Measham, F. (2020). The NPS imposters, merging and emerging drug markets and the contribution of drug checking. In D. Bewley-Taylor & K. Tinasti (Eds.), *Research handbook on international drug policy* (pp. 341–354). Edward Elgar.

Mounteney, J., Griffiths, P., Sedefov, R., Noor, A., Vicente, J., & Simon, R. (2016). The drug situation in Europe: An overview of data available on illicit drugs and new psychoactive substances from European monitoring in 2015. *Addiction, 111*(1), 34–48.

NHS England. (2022). Health Survey for England, 2021 part 1. https://digital.nhs.uk/data-and-information/publications/statistical/health-survey-for-england/2021/part-3-drinking-alcohol#trends-in-maximum-alcohol-consumption-on-any-day-in-the-last-week-by-survey-year-age-and-sex

So, V., Millard, A., Katikireddi, S., Forsyth, R., Allstaff, S., Deluca, P., Drummond, C., Ford, A., Eadie, D., Fitzgerald, N., & Graham, L. (2021). Intended and unintended consequences of the implementation of minimum unit pricing of alcohol in Scotland: A natural experiment. *Public Health Research, 9*(11), 34699154.

Stockwell, T., Auld, M. C., Zhao, J., & Martin, G. (2012). Does minimum pricing reduce alcohol consumption? The experience of a Canadian province. *Addiction, 107*(5), 912–920.

Wyper, G., Mackay, D., Fraser, C., Lewsey, J., Robinson, M., Beeston, C., & Giles, L. (2023). Evaluating the impact of alcohol minimum unit pricing on deaths and hospitalisations in Scotland: A controlled interrupted time series study. *The Lancet, 401*(10385), 1361–1370.

# Index[1]



[1] Note: Page numbers followed by 'n' refer to notes.



D. Conroy, F. Measham (eds.), *Young Adult Drinking Styles*, Sustainable Development Goals Series, https://doi.org/10.1007/978-3-031-98528-7